PERIMENOPAUSE

Changes in
Women's Health
After 35

James E. Huston, M.D.
L. Darlene Lanka, M.D.

New Harbinger Publications, Inc.

Distributed in the U.S.A. by Publishers Group West; in Canada by Raincoast Books; in Great Britain by Airlift Book Company, Ltd.; in South Africa by Real Books, Ltd.; in Australia by Boobook; and in New Zealand by Tandem Press.

Copyright © 1997 James E. Huston and Darlene Lanka
New Harbinger Publications, Inc.
5674 Shattuck Avenue
Oakland, CA 94609

Cover design by SHELBY DESIGNS AND ILLUSTRATES.
Edited by Dusty Bernard.
Text design by Michele Waters.
Index by Carol Burbo.

Library of Congress Catalog Card Number: 97-66079
ISBN 1-57224-085-7 Paperback

Printed in Canada on recycled paper.

New Harbinger Publication's Website address: www.newharbinger.com

00   99   98

10   9   8   7   6   5   4   3

Table of Contents

Foreword

"Oh, no! Not another book on menopause. Hey, wait a minute, Lois, do not be so quick to dismiss this book. Take another look and you will see it is exactly what the doctor ordered!" These words were the exact conversation I had with myself when I was asked to write a Foreword for this book. Writing the Foreword did not seem to be the chore, but reading another book on menopause was not what I really wanted to do for a weekend. Wow, once I settled into the first few sentences I was glued for the entire piece. Rather than writing a Foreword to another "me, too" book for others to read, I was asked to write the Foreword to a wonderful, gentle introduction to the next phase of my life. Although, I have actually written two books on the menopause, perhaps I, too, was struggling with the notion that one day I would experience all the ups and downs of menopause. So I wrote the books as though I was writing about a different species and that all that was in store really did not apply to me. In fact, when I was asked to market the books, I politely declined. I did not want to be known as "Miss Menopause." The power of my denial is not at all uncommon, as I learned from the beginning of this book. I am among over thirty-one million women who are part of the "mighty baby boomer generation" and thus are facing the perimenopausal years. Rather that preparing and correcting my deviations from healthy attitudes, I just chocked up my mood swings, weight gain, hair, skin, and nail changes to "stress." If an endocrinologist, trained in the care of postmenopausal women could deny the perimenopausal changes so obviously happening, then how could a general doctor, let alone the general women on the street, properly prepare for the rest of her life? This book stuck a harmonious chord in my musical shift to a minor key. Now discordant sounds can be placed in a rhythmic pattern to produce a beautiful, melodious result. Thank you Drs. Lanka and Huston!

From the first chapter on what changes to expect I almost skipped past important information, but the good doctors knew that I might be cheating and caught me page turning. I laughed out loud when they told me not to cut this chapter. How did they know? They seem to know a lot of other very personal things about me, too. Such as the subtle changes in my menstrual cycle, my irritability and my concern about the few extra pounds which seemed to come out of the air. How could I be so dumb? Perhaps it was because I never really thought about the perimenopausal state as being part of life and a part of my life which I had control over. After the astute introduction which had me "hooked," I passionately read every word, searching for "truth and justice." Each and every chapter then taught me a thing or two which definitely will make me a better physician for my female patients. Such things as changes in fertility, premenstrual syndrome in these transition years, prevention strategies to minimize the complications of cardiovascular disease and osteoporosis, a new look at thyroid disease as "a masquerader" of menopause (a notion which I really had not thought of before, and if I haven't thought of it, imagine how many other physicians have also been amiss . . .).

Thank goodness the good Drs. Lanka and Huston offer ways to change the odds. Rather than merely pointing out to the reader the changes of the perimenopause, and what's in store for the future, this book provides concrete, bonafide therapies to make a difference for the rest of our lives. Yes, I did know most of the literature on hormonal replacement therapy, after all I am an endocrinologist. However, the stuff on alternative medical disciplines was an eye opener for me. I guarantee you, even the best medical school in the Bronx (I am an Einstein alum) did not teach me one wit about Chinese medicine, herbs, acupuncture, homeopathic remedies, and mind/body exercises. My savvy patients ask me about these alternatives all the time. Previously, I just dismissed the conversation, hiding behind my ignorance, now I am prepared to advise, guide, and succeed in helping to incorporate these alternatives into a plan to change the odds.

Although I have a good background in nutrition, I did not know of a good reference for my patients to read. Thus, I would find myself trying to provide a makeshift educational piece on this very important area of care. This book is now mandatory for all my female patients. After all, we are what we eat, but more importantly, we will be what we eat! Because this book has the expertise of a great gynecological surgeon, the section on gyne-cological surgery and cosmetic surgery is a wonderful reference for any or all of my patients who are faced with the news that they need a hysterectomy. This section is informative and written with a comforting, loving perspective of "you needed that hysterectomy and you don't miss your uterus—so why are you so sad?"

As a grand finale, the authors leave us taking charge of our destiny. What started as a drudgery and a tremendous resistance to accepting that I too am aging and needing a bit of guidance through this phase of my life, ended in an invigorated response to work on my lack of attention to impor-tant things in my life. Better than a New Year's resolution, this book has given me the rationale and thus empowered me to stick to a healthier diet, to increase my exercise program, and to try techniques to minimize the stresses and episodes of depression. Yes, this book has made me wiser, and one weekend older, but it also has made me a better physician and given me the strategies to be a better me, despite the perimenopause!

Lois Jovanovic, M.D.
Sansum Medical Research Foundation
Santa Barbara, California

Preface

Jim's Note

My interest in women's health care came to the forefront when I was just a young pup in family medical practice. It stimulated me to leave practice for residency training in obstetrics and gynecology. That was a good decision because I have enjoyed my career in women's health care immensely. I was fortunate enough to establish a warm rapport with the women I served, so we both benefited. In 1994, I had a mild stroke. Recovery was complete; but I retired from active practice. I felt obligated to withdraw since a recurrence can come without notice. Much of what an Ob/Gyn does is without an assistant and I was not willing to risk injury to a patient or her baby.

With time on my hands, I began to reflect on my career and the women I have known as patients. I must confess that I do not miss the enormous stress to which obstetricians are subjected from time to time. But I do miss the women I knew so well, and the to and fro exchange of information that was so free between us. Bringing a newborn baby into the world was an enormous "high" for me right up to the very last one I delivered. If it was in the middle of the night, I usually couldn't get to sleep when I got home because I was so keyed up by the exhilaration of having been a participant in one of life's paramount experiences. There were thousands of those highs for me. The sustaining and enduring satisfaction of my career in women's health care however, was in the one-on-one educational efforts I was able to accomplish for the women who entrusted me to teach them. That was a fulfilling accomplishment, and that was what made it a good career for me.

Since physicians are basically health educators who also possess various skills to improve the health status of their patients, my thoughts after retirement turned to the education component of my career. The hands-on aspect of medical service is behind me, true enough. But then I realized that I am not cut off from the teaching aspect of health care; and writing became my focus. My thoughts isolated on women's midlife health. This was the area where I always spent the most time in educational efforts—an area of great concern to women and yet an area of clouded understanding. I was also directed to this area by experiences in my personal life. My wife Victoria is just completing her perimenopausal transition, and I have lived these years with her. I have seen her mood swings, lived through her PMS and felt her insecurities as she perceived that she was in unfamiliar territory. We weathered her changes together and successfully. I don't have the faintest notion of how it could have happened so quickly; but I have two daughters from a previous marriage who are in their perimenopausal transition. I hope Janet and Jeni will benefit from this book.

Perimenopause is generally regarded as those few years before menopause when menstrual periods become irregular. Actually it begins in your mid-thirties when your female hormone production begins to diminish ever so slightly. A lot happens in the next fifteen years, and that is the subject of this book. I was at first reticent to write on a medical topic because my medical background does not include the university medical center teaching credentials that most physician writers possess. When I considered however that private medical practice has put me closer to the women for whom I would be writing, I realized that I might be as well qualified, and in some ways perhaps better qualified than the folks in academia.

Another daunting thought occurred: I am the wrong gender! Most of the writers on women's health are not only academics and/or professional writers, they're also women. That's when Dr. Darlene Lanka came center stage in my thoughts. Dr. Lanka and I have been acquainted for most of three decades. We became friends during our residency training in obstetrics and gynecology, and have remained so since then. Her career led to an Ob/Gyn practice with a large medical group, and mine to a solo practice. Both of us worked in the San Francisco Bay Area. That we would one day collaborate in writing a book about perimenopause never crossed our minds as we pursued our careers, raised families, and enjoyed sailing and skiing together with our spouses. When I approached her about writing a book about perimenopause, her enthusiasm for the project was unbridled. Darlene is that kind of lady. She is a midlife woman who is at the peak of her career, and on the forefront of medical advances in this area of healthcare. So, with our backgrounds in women's health care, and our personal experiences with perimenopause, we felt we could be a good writing team.

Darlene and I both realize that one-on-one teaching of our patients is valuable; but we also realize it doesn't reach nearly enough women. We feel a book would be a better way. Very little has been written that focuses on the perimenopausal transition, and yet a very large number of women are in this era now. As a matter of fact, there are 38,000,000 women of your baby boomer generation out there who are approaching or in their peri-menopausal transition. Based on our personal experiences with you, a great deal more needs to be known about this time than has been provided for you. We hope our book will improve your fund of knowledge about peri-menopause, and empower you to smooth your way through a watershed era of change in your life after 35.

Darlene's Note

I've lived this book. I was a first year medical student at UC San Francisco the year I got married. My husband was a graduate student at Berkeley. Because my class schedule was so overwhelming, Alan would meet me every evening in the student cafeteria where we would buy a "fast-food meal." I was too overworked and too stressed out to cook. We ate dinner every night with the only other woman in my class who was married. Her husband was also a Berkeley grad student.

Like many of you today, I thought that doctors were men. I never considered becoming one until in my junior year of college. I realized I was getting the "A's" and the pre-med men were getting the "C's". So I went to medical school. I was one of eight women in a class of 105. The harassment was unbelievable; but all of it, to the credit of my classmates, was offered in the spirit of fun. I was never subjected to "sex for grades" as I understand has happened to more than one graduate student. My professors and class-mates kidded me mercilessly—so I kidded them right back and survived.

I became a doctor and went on to an Ob/Gyn residency. There were very few women in Ob/Gyn residencies at that time. It was a man's field. When I interviewed for the position as a first year resident, I had to promise the chief to take birth controls pills throughout my residency. . . . Let someone try to get away with that today. We've come a long way, baby!

One or another of my fellow residents would periodically ask me if I had "taken my pill?" I never once asked any of them if they had remembered to use their condoms, though that would have been a good come back, now that I think of it. Jim and I met when he was a first year resident, and I was his chief resident. I walked him through his first hysterectomy, and he did a wonderful job of it too. That year we both celebrated big birthdays. He turned forty and I turned thirty. For each of us, those were milestone years.

After finishing my training, I got a job. I thought my biological clock was running out, so I went off my birth control pills, and guess what? I didn't get pregnant. I was hypothyroid. Happy ending. . . . I had my children even though I was in the "high risk age group." I turned out to be very fertile, so I had to figure out the best and safest birth control methods to use as a thirty-something woman to limit my family.

My practice has been interesting and absorbing. I quickly found that I had to budget my time between being wife, doctor, mom, and daughter. While all of this was going on, my own mom was shrinking in front of my eyes. She went on to break just about every bone in her little body. She had osteoporosis because she hadn't taken estrogen. She just exercised and took calcium. When my husband hit his male menopause, or andropause, as Jim likes to call it, he bought a sailboat. I was thrilled that maybe this would be the extent of his "midlife crisis." He went on to change jobs and buy a sports car; but I think I got off easy.

He didn't fair as well with me though during my perimenopause. The wicked witch of the west used to arrive at our house once a month in my place. There were many PMS evenings when I would take off on a drive by myself because Alan or one of the kids had done something "monumental" to start me off. All three would just look at me in wonder, but not dare to say a word. Fortunately, they were saved when I went back on birth control pills because of heavy bleeding. The pills stopped my heavy bleeding and my terrible PMS symptoms.

Throughout the years, I have struggled with my patients through everything discussed in this book. Over the past thirty years there has been little research into women's health issues. Now because of the equal rights initiative and affirmative action, lots of women are going into every field of science. What do these women study? . . . you guessed it, women's issues, and it's about time. There is more and more out there about our health, and what we can do to help ourselves reach a happy healthy maturity.

When Jim called me to say he was planning to write a book about perimenopause, and asked if I would like to co-author the book with him, I immediately said yes. There are very few good self-help books out there for perimenopausal women. Almost everything written has been about menopause, or about trendy treatments of one kind or another which don't seem to help.

Both Jim and I feel perimenopause is an important transitional stage in a woman's life. We both hope that our endeavor to educate you will help you reach your maturity healthier and more mentally strong and confident. So enjoy the book. We wrote this book like we talk to our patients. Everything we wrote is researched and as accurate as we could make it.

Section I:

The Changes

1

What Changes? An Overview

We can almost hear what you're thinking: "Changes? You mean I'm already changing, and I'm only thirty-seven?" Yes, it's true. "Is this the *Change of Life?*" No, it's not menopause. "What's causing it?" Your female hormones are declining. "I can stop it though, right?" Not a chance. "What should I do?" Read this book from cover to cover.

Change is what life is about. Whether for good or for ill, all of us continually change as time passes. As for hormonal change, there is a gender difference. Males change in a steady, slow fashion. Females are rhythmic. The difference is mediated by hormones. Every month your uterus builds a new lining and then, if a pregnancy is not begun, sheds it. Every month your breasts change in concert with this rhythm. Think of the other patterns of change you experience on a rhythmic basis: in appetite, skin, mood, sexual desire, and energy, among many others.

Then there are the macro-hormone changes of puberty, pregnancy, and menopause. The engine of the rhythmic pattern of change is female hormone production. It follows, then, that a change in hormone output will alter your rhythms. In this book you will learn about the changes that occur in your body and in your life as a result of decreasing hormone levels. A transition is gradually taking place that you can prepare for and influence in a positive fashion. This book is a guide to maintaining good health during these transition years. It will teach you how to prepare for the best half of your life.

Let's Talk Hormones

Estrogen and progesterone are the female hormones that regulate many of the changes we've mentioned. Of the two, estrogen is the most influential in causing the changes we will be discussing in this book. The life peak of estrogen production is reached at age twenty-seven to twenty-eight. Then a faintly declining plateau is maintained until about thirty-five. Although there is a slight decline in the plateau years, there is always sufficient estrogen to fully support your body. After age thirty-five, though, the average amount of estrogen production per cycle begins to decline sufficiently to produce subtle changes in your body. This marks the earliest beginning of perimenopause. Figure 1-1 demonstrates your estrogen level at various ages. Dr. Bernard Eskin reported in 1995 that the decline is in the amount of estrogen you produce in the second half of your cycle after ovulation. Estrogen output in the first half of your cycle remains sufficient to cause ovulation for many more years. Most people, including many health care professionals, don't know this. The decline is not a landslide. You will not suddenly (nor need you ever) become the stereotypic "little old lady." In your forties the decline accelerates, and by age fifty-one to fifty-two, female hormone output is minimal. This book is about those fifteen years from age thirty-five to fifty, and a few years beyond.

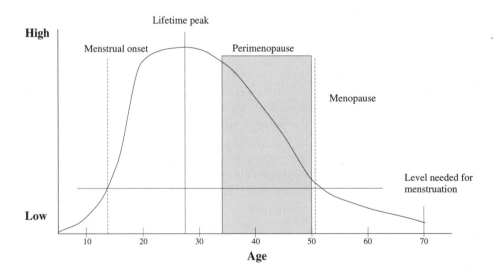

Figure 1.1.   Estrogen Levels By Age

The Boomers Are Coming

You are not alone in this period of life. Seventy-six million babies were born in the United States during those years, thirty-eight million of you are women, and about 31 million of you are perimenopausal. You are part of the mighty "baby boomer" generation born after World War II, between 1946 and 1964. According to a widely reported 1995 study by the National Council on the Aging (Graham 1995), the first "boomer" turned fifty on January 1, 1996. The youngest of your generation will turn thirty-five in 1999. Your boomer cohorts are entering and completing their transitional years at the rate of about two million women per year. Yours is the largest group of American women ever to pass through this stage of life. Your group is also the most inquisitive, the most energetic, and the most vocal.

Your generation is not content to accept things as they are simply because that's the way they have always been. For example, you changed birthing methods in the U.S. by advocating natural childbirth with fathers in attendance, making it a family event. Our culture has come to understand that you will demand and expect to receive accurate information about whatever interests you or confronts you. For this reason, the expectation is that you will more likely *change* your transitional years than be changed *by* them. As always, you first need up-to-date, accurate information about your potential changes; then you can unleash your collective imagination and energy to deal with these changes in innovative ways. If this book furthers that ability, it will have been wildly successful.

An Overview of Change

This chapter provides you with a general description of what happens during these years, how it happens, and the role of hormone diminution in causing changes. This is a normal process in every woman—no exceptions. There is plenty you can do, however, to control these changes. The medical term for these transitional years is perimenopause, which means the period of time leading up to, and the period of time just after, menopause. Menopause itself refers to the point in time right after your last menstrual period has happened. Postmenopause refers to the years of life following menopause.

In the past two decades, perimenopause has been regarded as those four to six years after the mid-forties when the symptoms and effects of hormone decrease begin to become quite noticeable. The changes include irregular menstrual cycles, menstrual flow variability, hot flashes, fragmented sleep, mood swings, short-term memory loss, unexplained fatigue, diminished sexual desire, and others (see Chapter 2). The reality is that these changes begin a decade earlier than the mid-forties, but they are not signaled by dramatic symptoms—they don't suddenly grab you one morning as you step out of the shower. If you are attuned to your body rhythms, you may be able to detect the subtle changes that are taking place.

What is the significance of these changed body rhythms and feelings, and what should you do about them? Your initial response might be to ignore them or to deny the possibility that they are a result of hormone decline. If you do seek advice, you may find that your doctor knows little more than you about these changes and, if you are still having menstrual periods, may not recognize that your hot flashes, fatigue, and sleep disruptions might be from hormone depletion. You might hear statements like, "You're just tense; you need to relax" or "You're too young for hormonal decline." In this case, it might be time to change doctors; and the more you educate yourself about the transitional years and the biological markers you may experience, the easier it will be to find a health-care advisor who can help you during this phase of your life. Then, you and your doctor can work together to smooth the way for your own transitional years.

Biological Markers

Let's take a look at the changes in body function and behavior, as well as the cognitive changes, that may arise for you in the transitional years. There is enormous variation among women in terms of which of these symptoms they experience, and to what degree. Some of them may seem unpleasant, and some of them can even be threatening to your health. Throughout this book, you'll find ways of managing the troublesome changes.

- **Ovarian slowdown:** At birth, a female infant has all the eggs (ova) she will ever have. (This is in contrast to males, who manufacture new sperm throughout life. Each egg in the ovary is contained in a structure called a *follicle.* Female sex hormones, *estrogen* and *progesterone,* are produced by the cells of the follicle walls. As egg release (ovulation) takes place on a monthly basis, your follicles gradually diminish in number. This reduction begins to be noticeable after age thirty-five in a measurable decrease in average monthly hormone production (Eskin 1995). The reduction proceeds over about fifteen years to an eventual point at which not enough hormones are produced to cause menstrual periods; they cease entirely (menopause). Menopause doesn't just pop up at age fifty-one or fifty-two. It is a process that has its beginnings in the mid-thirties as the result of the natural aging of the reproductive system. The reduced estrogen availability has an enormous influence on your body and the way it functions. For example, a woman forty years old may have difficulty becoming pregnant because the eggs her ovaries supply are also forty years old and may have lost some of their reproductive efficiency.

- **Menstrual cycle and menstrual period changes:** Changes in your menstrual cycle and menstrual period can vary tremendously. Cycles may become longer or shorter or fall into a "no-pattern" pattern. Menstrual bleeding may be heavier or lighter, more prolonged or shorter, or entirely absent. Variable and declining hormone production is the cause.

- **Hot flashes:** Decreased estrogen availability changes the heat release and conservation mechanisms in your body. This results in flushing of the upper body, head, and neck. Hot flashes most commonly begin in the mid-forties, but they can also affect women in their thirties.

- **Reduced stamina:** It is most commonly women who are not fit to begin with who experience reduced stamina in the transitional years. A decrease in muscle tone and strength bears a direct relationship to a woman's diet and how much she exercises.

- **Changes in the skin, vagina, and hair:** The most common time for changes in the skin, vagina, and hair is after the mid-forties. With lessened estrogen, natural secretions diminish, and tissues become thinner and drier than they had been. *Atrophy* is the medical term for these changes; it refers to the loss of tissue in any part of the body as a result of diminished tissue nutrition. In the transitional years, the tissues most likely to show atrophic change are the skin and mucous membranes, including the face, neck, chest, hair, vagina, and bladder. Diminished natural secretions result in thinning and drying of these tissues, resulting in wrinkles, loss of luster in hair, lessened vaginal lubrication, and urinary tract infections. Skin damage and wrinkling can be accelerated by ultraviolet sunlight exposure and by smoking.

- **Premenstrual Syndrome (PMS) may worsen:** If PMS symptoms worsen, it is usually in the late thirties and early forties. PMS usually diminishes after the mid-forties and disappears about the time of menopause. Chapter 4 presents a full discussion of perimenopausal PMS.

- **Cognitive changes:** Brain cells have what are known as estrogen receptors. If these receptors don't get their regular supply of estrogen. they can cause wide swings in emotional responses, including transitory episodes of moodiness, short-term memory loss, unexplained sadness, decreased sexual desire, and lessened ability to concentrate.

- **Osteoporosis:** Loss of bone mass, and therefore bone strength, is a well-proven result of estrogen loss. Other factors, such as a poor diet, lack of exercise, and smoking, also contribute to a deteriorating skeleton, but the fundamental causative agent and the cornerstone for prevention is estrogen. Osteoporosis tends to be a late event in the perimenopausal-menopausal transition. Nonetheless, be aware that a major deterrent to this crippling and potentially life-threatening problem is to develop a sturdy skeleton *before* you reach mid-life.

- **Cardiovascular disease (CVD):** It is important to point out that heart disease is the number one cause of death for women between the ages of fifty to seventy-five (in other words, after menopause). It may surprise you to learn that heart attack deaths are five times more common than breast cancer deaths (Henderson 1986). A major goal for you in the transitional years of life is to find out how to maintain cardiovascular fitness.

- **Thyroid problems:** The thyroid requires estrogen to function normally. A lack of estrogen can lead to underactive thyroid hormone production (hypothyroidism). This condition can leave you feeling weak and lethargic, depressed and moody. If your thyroid is found to be sluggish and you are transitional, your estrogen production may be at the root of it.

- **Decreased sexual desire:** Decreased sexual desire can (but not necessarily does) occur during the transitional years. This is a complex issue, and when it does occur, the symptom may have its roots in a number of areas, including relationship problems, lifestyle excesses, and self-esteem issues, as well as hormone loss.

The Ovary Connection

To help you better understand the topics covered in this book, let's take a look at some anatomy and a little physiology. (Wait! Don't slam the book shut. It will be in plain language, and it won't take long.)

The Anatomy

By the time a female fetus is twenty weeks old, her ovaries contain about 7,000,000 egg follicles (Speroff 1989). Over the remainder of intrauterine life, the growing ovaries gradually push the surface follicles out of the ovaries into the abdominal cavity, and they disintegrate. At birth, a baby girl has about 2,000,000 follicles left. This number continues to diminish so that at puberty, about 400,000 remain. Does it worry you that this may not be enough? Turns out that it's plenty. The rate of loss slows from an average of 250,000 follicles per week during fetal life to about 2,500 per week in childhood, and after puberty it is less than 1,000 per month. A woman ovulates only 400 to 500 times during the childbearing years, so the numbers work out okay.

Each month several hundred follicles are readied for release of an egg. Usually only one is released at ovulation, and the rest of the follicles shrink away. Occasionally, of course, multiple ovulations take place, producing a multiple pregnancy. Humans are not well designed for litters, however, and single egg release is the usual result. By the mid-thirties and beyond, the number of follicles will have diminished sufficiently to result in a decreased blood level of estrogen and progesterone, the female sex hormones. As this process continues, perimenopausal changes begin and the ability to achieve a successful pregnancy declines.

Menopause is ultimately reached by about age fifty-one, at which time the childbearing years of life are concluded. Clearly, it is not a sudden process. In fact, in light of the inexorable decrease of ovarian follicles culminating in menopause, one might make the case that the process of menopause begins in fetal life!

The Physiology

Alphabet Soup	
GnRH	Gonadotropin releasing hormone
FSH	Follicle stimulating hormone
LH	Leuteinizing hormone (LH)

To understand the changes of perimenopause, it is important to know how the ovarian cycle, or menstrual cycle, works. Then it becomes easier to understand what happens when it doesn't work.

The cycle is really sort of a daisy chain, as you can see in Figure 1-2. (Don't worry—we'll explain the fine print in a moment.) The chain involves three hormone-producing glands:

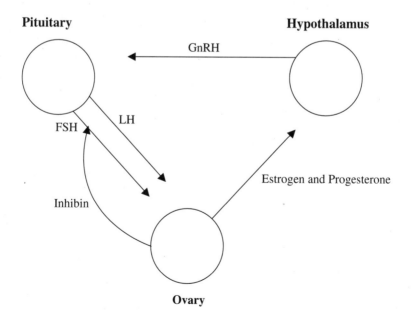

Figure 1.2.   Ovarian Cycle

- The *hypothalamus,* in the brain
- The *pituitary,* in the brain
- The *ovaries,* in the pelvis

These glands work in concert with each other. Each produces hormones that are recognized by the other two, acting as chemical messengers that are carried to their targets by your bloodstream. Some of these hormones influence the ovarian cycle.

We need to start our discussion somewhere in the cycle, so let's enter it at the end of a menstrual period, after the uterine lining has been shed. At this point, your ovaries are producing low levels of estrogen and progesterone, as the chart shown in Figure 1-3 demonstrates. The hypothalamus detects this and sends a hormone called *gonadotropin releasing hormone* (GnRH) to the pituitary. In response, the pituitary releases two hormones that target the ovaries: *follicle stimulating hormone* (FSH) and *leuteinizing hormone* (LH). FSH stimulates the ovaries to do two things: start producing more estrogen (which, among other things, rebuilds the lining of the uterus) and get a follicle ready for ovulation. At mid-cycle, estrogen reaches a critical level, which triggers a sudden surge of LH from the pituitary; this causes ovulation.

After the follicle has released its egg, it turns into a structure called the corpus luteum, which manufactures progesterone and a glycoprotein called *inhibin.* Progesterone increases the blood supply in the uterine lining and fills the glands of the lining with *glycogen* (a sugar). This prepares the lining of the uterus for receiving and nourishing a fertilized egg. Inhibin, another substance produced by the corpus luteum, may instruct the pituitary gland to inhibit production of FSH when the ovaries no longer need it. (Note: Recent studies are questioning whether this in fact is true.)

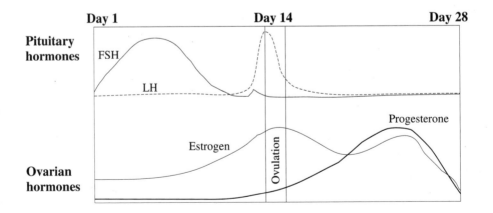

Figure 1.3.   Hormone Levels in Menstrual Cycle

At this point the bloodstream contains high levels of estrogen, progesterone, and inhibin. In response, the hypothalamus reduces the GnRH level, signaling the pituitary to cut back on FSH and LH. This in turn causes the ovaries to decrease estrogen and progesterone production. The net result is that, once again, the bloodstream contains a low level of female hormones. The lining of the uterus is no longer supported by hormones, and it is shed—in other words, a menstrual period occurs. Then the cycle, which usually takes about four weeks, begins again.

Diagnosis of Perimenopause

As we mentioned earlier in this chapter, if you are still having menstrual periods, you may find it hard to believe that hormone depletion may be causing the symptoms you've been having—and equally hard to have this confirmed by a doctor. There are steps you can take, though, to ensure proper diagnosis and treatment of the symptoms you experience during the transitional years.

Get Smart: Educate Yourself

Health care in the U.S. today is less personalized than it used to be, and it has become increasingly important for people to become more personally involved in maintaining their own wellness. The responsibility for initiating certain procedures, such as screening exams, falls more and more into the individual's own hands.

Diagnosing perimenopause (or any other altered body state, for that matter) is a process that you can actually initiate by becoming aware that a change has taken place in your body. We're not talking about an occasional change in menstrual flow or timing or occasionally tender breasts, excess fluid retention, or an increase in skin blemishes; variations of this type are normal. What we *are* talking about is an awareness of a *persistent* and *recurring* change—you can look back over recent cycles and realize that they are different from those in prior years. The more you know about your body, the better able you are to observe these changes.

An important aspect of educating yourself is becoming aware of your personal risk factors for particular health problems. How you live your life, what foods you eat, how well you exercise, the toxins to which you are exposed, preexisting conditions, and in some cases, inheritance, can play major roles in your current and future health. For example, if you are a smoker, then cancer, heart disease, and osteoporosis may all be part of your future. Also, try to find out as much as you can about your family's health history, which can provide further clues to your own risk factors. The risk factors you identify for yourself can help decide the kinds of screening tests you might need, and their frequency. The goal, of course, is to avoid illness or to treat it early. (Specific risk factors for heart disease, osteoporosis, and cancer are covered in Chapters 5 and 7.)

Once you have chosen a doctor (see the next section), you can arrange for a complete physical exam, which is also important to your understanding of your body. The exam should include your height, weight, blood pressure, head (including eyes, mouth, throat, ears), neck (including thyroid, lymph glands, blood vessels), chest, breasts, armpits with lymph glands, heart, abdomen, pelvic with rectal, extremities, pulses, skin, and neurological. A complete exam is a must for your first visit to the doctor you choose; but if you are in good health in your transitional years, it isn't necessary to have a complete exam every year.

Choosing Your Health Care Advisor

You need a competent and compassionate professional to work with you in maintaining good health during your transitional years. Unfortunately, many talented physicians and alternative medical professionals are not yet well informed about the health concerns of women in transition or the hormonal changes that can occur, so be sure the person you choose is familiar with these issues. Good candidates are gynecologists, internists, family practitioners, and endocrinologists (hormone specialists). In addition, many clinics specialize in women's health care, and others limit their services to menopause and perimenopause. Be alert to whether your consultant is truly listening to you; skillful health professionals know that taking a careful medical history can help pinpoint a problem.

Testing Hormone Levels

Until recently, doctors often tested women for follicle stimulating hormone (FSH) to determine whether their ovaries were producing enough estrogen. The FSH testing was based on the knowledge that in menopausal women, the FSH level is high because of low production of estrogen. The pituitary gland is sending out high levels of FSH in an effort to get the failing ovaries to produce more estrogen. The problem with FSH testing in perimenopausal women, however, is that estrogen production may wax and wane from one month to the next, so consistent results are not possible. For this reason, most doctors no longer rely on FSH blood levels to diagnose perimenopause. What other options are there?

One option, advocated by leading experts in the field, is to do a clinical test: give you a trial dose of a hormone supplement. If your perimenopausal symptoms are improved, you are on the right track. (If not, you and your doctor need to look elsewhere for a cause of the changes you are experiencing such as thyroid abnormalities, ovarian disease, or perhaps stressful events in your life. Some women are now opting to use low-dose birth control pills during their entire perimenopause. They can control perimenopausal symptoms, help prevent long-term problems such as heart disease and osteoporosis, and prevent pregnancy.

CAUTION! If you have abnormal uterine bleeding, it must not be treated with hormones unless it is clearly established that you do not have uterine disease. (Chapter 15 covers this topic in detail.)

Your Hormones Are Down a Little— Should You Worry?

You may be wondering why generations of women before yours didn't worry about perimenopausal symptoms. One reason was that relatively little was known about menopause, and the term *perimenopause* was not even used until the late 1970s or early 1980s. Menopause was neither a topic of conversation nor a subject of research.

Another reason is that prior to the twentieth century, women often did not live many years after the childbearing years. In the last hundred years or so, though, women have been living longer, thanks to improvements in areas like nutrition, sanitation, medical care, housing, clothing, work savers, and accident prevention. The current life expectancy for American women is just over eighty years.

What hasn't changed, however, is the age at which female hormones decline. It has been happening in a woman's forties for many centuries, and it still is. For American women, the average age of menopause is fifty-one. (The age differs in other cultures.) The simple arithmetic is that women now live more than one third of their lives after their childbearing role is completed. For many, this is a forty-year span. Staying healthy during these years takes some advance planning and preparation.

Planning and Preparation

During the transitional years of perimenopause, you have a good shot at keeping the balance of your life healthy and enjoyable. If you don't have to have hot flashes, moodiness, and short-term memory loss, why put up with them? Granted, these symptoms are not life threats, and they will subside in a few years even if you do nothing. Still, controlling or eliminating these symptoms can improve your quality of life. In addition, you now have an opportunity to prevent or modify your risk for a few more ominous problems that can plague significant portions of the last half of your life.

With the help of your health consultant, you can follow a proactive program of prevention ranging from hormone replacement, to lifestyle changes, to use of alternative medical remedies, to more aggressive preventive care, including screening techniques and a fitness program. Life is a journey, so why not enjoy the trip?

Table 1.1. Symptoms and Signs of Estrogen Loss	
Irregular periods	Hot flashes
Mood swings	Fragmented sleep
Short-term memory loss	Difficulty concentrating
Irritability	Anxiety
Minor depression	Skin dryness
Wrinkling	Reduced sexual lubrication
Vaginal dryness	Decreased sexual desire
Reduced muscle tone	Reduced stamina
Constipation	Recurrent urinary tract infection
Breast sag	Eye dryness
Underactive thyroid	Osteoporosis
Rise in cholesterol	Beginning risk of heart disease

Hormone Replacement—The Easy Part

If the primary cause of perimenopausal change is decreased estrogen production, *hormone replacement therapy* (HRT) is a logical option for dealing with it. There has been much debate in recent years on the appropriateness of this form of management. Certainly, there are risks in using HRT, but there are also risks in failing to do so. Take a look at Table 1-1, which lists the changes caused by estrogen loss through the transitional years and beyond. This a daunting list of potential problems, but you may experience few or none of them. The point of Table 1-1 is to demonstrate that estrogen is widely utilized throughout your body, and that HRT is not recommended solely for the relief of relatively minor symptoms. Estrogen levels affect your entire body; and reduction of this hormone changes the way your body looks and operates.

Be aware that a variety of not as yet mainstream alternative treatment modalities other than HRT are available for perimenopausal changes. Some, like Chinese herbal medicine, predate Western medicine by many centuries. Many perimenopausal changes are considerably helped by these alternative remedies, but unfortunately, there is a scarcity of information from the medical community as to their safety and effectiveness. Homeopathy, Chinese herbal medicine, acupuncture, holistic medicine, and mind/body medicine are discussed in Chapter 9.

Lifestyle Changes—The Hard Part

You might think at this point that all you need is to load up on hormone replacement and go merrily on with your life. Alas, there is much more to maintaining good health and vitality than HRT. These are the major issues:

- **Fitness:** has been embraced by boomers as by no other generation of Americans. In Chapter 10 you will learn about diet and exercise, the two major components of fitness—be sure not to skip that chapter!

- **Stress management:** In our culture of busy, striving-to-keep-afloat individuals and two-income families, stress management is of signal importance to us all. Stress may be magnified during your perimenopausal transition, so it is helpful for you to know how to deal with it. When poorly controlled, stress takes a serious toll on relationships important to you—those with your partner, children, co-workers, relatives, and friends—and it takes its toll on your body as well. Chapter 12 provides a discussion on a variety of ways to manage stress.

- **Alcohol, tobacco, and other deleterious drugs:** Lifestyle choices that include use of harmful drugs may contribute to many of the adverse perimenopausal changes. Chapter 11 takes a look at why these substances can harm you.

Summary

Consider carefully the forty or so years ahead of you. How well you prepare for the second half of life may be the most important quality-of-life consideration you will ever make. The balance of this book is devoted to showing you how to do just that.

O O O

2

Changes You Can See and Feel: Symptoms and Signs of Perimenopause

Estrogen and progesterone are "behind the scenes" support players, some-what akin to the stage hands in a play. They aren't visible to the audience or actors during the performance, but the show functions smoothly only as long as the stage hands are doing their job. If they don't show up for work or forget the correct placement of a prop, chaos may erupt on stage. Estrogen is like that unheralded stage hand: You don't appreciate all that it does for you until it stops doing it. Then a host of new feelings and changes begin to show up. In this chapter you will learn what to expect in terms of menstrual changes, hot flashes, cognitive changes, wrinkles, vaginal dryness, decreased sexual desire, and urinary incontinence.

Each of these changes usually makes its own individual appearance, without relation to the others. Figure 2-1 shows the approximate timeline for the appearance of various perimenopausal symptoms. Ultimately, there may be more than one such change taking place simultaneously. For the most part they are individually manageable; but for some women (perhaps 20 percent), the sum of the changes can make coping with them very difficult. Their symptoms are severe enough to disrupt their everyday functioning in important spheres such as marriage, occupation, and relationships with children, parents, co-workers, and friends.

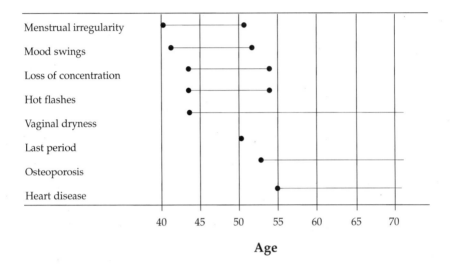

Adapted from: Nancy Lee Teaff and Kim Wright. 1996. *Perimenopause: Preparing for the Change*. Rocklin, Calif.: Prima Publishing

Figure 2.1. Approximate Timeline for Perimenopausal Symptoms

As mentioned in Chapter 1, the realization that a given change you experience may be related to hormonal decline is often delayed by your lack of awareness of this possibility or by your doctor's low index of suspicion. The hot flash is a high-profile event and one of the defining symptoms of perimenopause, so you'd be unlikely to miss its significance. On the other hand, if the first thing that shows up is short-term memory loss, you and your doctor may write that off to your busy life and the myriad distractions you face in organizing life around your family and your occupation. If you start your perimenopausal symptoms with sleep disruption and all the secondary effects of chronic fatigue, including irritability and minor depression, without recognizing them as hormonal changes, you may find yourself filling prescriptions for sleeping pills or spending needless time with a therapist.

The point is that perimenopause produces a constellation of changes, which you can identify if you know what to look for. Taken individually, your symptoms can suggest a confusing array of problems, or even no problem at all. However, if you and your doctor can step back and view these symptoms together, a clear picture will arise. The following sections describe what you should be looking for and offer some suggestions for minimizing your symptoms.

Menstrual Irregularity

Menstrual irregularity is one of the early changes you can expect. This can start in your thirties, but the changes are usually so subtle that you will not notice. By your forties, however, there will be differences that you won't miss. The most common pattern begins with a shortening of your cycle by a few days; you have a normal flow; but it starts sooner than expected. Later, your cycle lengthens to more than its usual twenty-eight days; later still, you miss an occasional period; and ultimately, your periods stop altogether. You can expect up-and-down changes in the amount of flow once menstrual irregularity begins because of up-and-down levels of hormone production. The variations can be considerable; but they usually fall into some combination of the following categories:

- **Too often:** The number of days in your cycle has decreased by a few days from your accustomed average of twenty-eight. This happens because you have started producing less estrogen. The lining of the uterus, called the *endometrium,* loses its hormonal support earlier than usual, and you shed it sooner than expected. This can lead to some unwelcome surprises, but for the most part, if the difference is only a day or two, it is little more than an eyebrow raiser. On the other hand, if you find your cycle shortened to fewer than twenty days from the first day of one period to the first day of the next, talk to your doctor.

CAUTION! A menstrual pattern in which the cycle is shortened to fewer than twenty days from the first day of one period to the first day of the next is abnormal and may signal a disease in your endometrium. In this situation, an endometrial biopsy should be done—an office procedure in which a thin, flexible canula (hollow tube) is inserted into the uterus to remove a sample of tissue for microscopic examination.

- **Not often enough:** The cycle lengthens when ovulation does not occur. This results when not enough progesterone is produced to halt the thickening of the lining of your uterus and prepare it for shedding at the usual time. This tends to provoke cries like "Holy mackerel! I'm overdue." A home pregnancy test will probably be at the top of your agenda on that occasion. Skipping two and three periods at a time is referred to as *oligomenorrhea.* A consultation with your doctor may be in order when this first happens, to make sure the absence of menstrual periods has not resulted from more ominous causes, such as an ovarian tumor or other hormonal disturbance.

- **Too much:** The medical term for heavy flow is *hypermenorrhea* but flooding, is what we are referring to, and all the embarrassments associated with it. It is caused by the absence of ovulation, which results in low progesterone levels. In this instance, estrogen levels are adequate; but with- out progesterone to check its growth, the endometrium becomes too thick. Shedding a thickened endometrium takes longer and bleeding is heavier.

- **Too little:** A scanty menstrual period is called *hypomenorrhea*. This symptom is rarely a source of concern. It results from low levels of both estrogen and progesterone. The endometrium is thin and does not require much shedding.

- **None:** Absence of menstrual bleeding for more than three months is called *amenorrhea*. Neither estrogen nor progesterone is being supplied in sufficient quantities to build up the endometrium, and there is nothing to shed.

TIP! Keeping a menstrual calendar is a great help in determining what may be happening to your cycles. Just mark each day you have bleeding with an *L*, *N*, or *H* for light, normal, heavy, and *S* for spotting.

Menstrual irregularity is rarely a serious problem. Anemia can result from prolonged heavy periods, but no one dies from it. You may come to regard this symptom as a frustrating inconvenience, in which case you have a lot of company. If you prefer to have more control of your menstrual cycles, hormone supplements may be the answer.

Low-dose birth control pills serve this purpose quite well for most perimenopausal women. The low-dose pill has been approved by the FDA for use in women up to age fifty who are in good health and nonsmokers. The low-dose pill, not only controls your cycles, it can improve many other perimenopausal symptoms, including mood swings, sleep disruption, hot flashes, and others. You can use the low-dose pill right up to menopause, and a few years after, if you wish. Then you can stop the low-dose pill and, if you choose, switch to hormone replacement therapy (HRT). The time to switch will be signaled by symptoms during the week off hormones. Hot flashes, insomnia, and just not feeling well are common if menopause has occurred. The estrogen dose with HRT is about 75 percent less than the low-dose pill. The lowered dose will still control estrogen deficiency symptoms and is adequate for osteoporosis and cardiovascular protection.

CAUTION! If your bleeding pattern changes, do not ignore it. Talk to your health advisor. Abnormal uterine bleeding can result from a number of serious conditions, so a diagnosis must be established before treatment is undertaken. (See Chapter 15 for a thorough discussion of the various causes of abnormal uterine bleeding and their management.)

Hot Flashes, Hot Flushes, and Vasomotor Instability

Alphabet Soup	
ANS	Autonomic nervous system
HRT	Hormone replacement therapy
SPF	Sun-protecting factor
UV	Ultraviolet

Doctors call it a flush and professors call it vasomotor instability; but women with this symptom call it like it is: *a hot flash!* You may hear yourself making comments like these: "My makeup felt like it was raised about an inch off my face." "The first course was cold gazpacho soup, and yet there I sat sweating like I had jogged to the dinner party." Yes, they're hot flashes, and hot flash is the term we use in this book.

Dr. Fredi Kronenberg (1990) reported that about 85 percent of American women experience hot flashes in the perimenopausal-postmenopausal years. They can start as early as the late thirties for some, but they are more common after the mid-forties. Following menopause, hot flashes recede in three to four years to infrequent occurrences, although the duration in years of hot flashes varies widely. Table 2-1 shows the results of Kronenberg's 1990 study of hot flashes.

What Is a Hot Flash, Anyway?

Hot flashes occur when the blood vessels in your skin dilate and bring large amounts of blood to the surface. This is what makes your skin red when you are having a hot flash. Your body normally has a heat release and conservation mechanism. (For example, in cold weather, when you are in a heat conservation mode, these surface vessels constrict to keep blood deeper inside your body, and your skin looks pale; in hot weather, your vessels dilate to help get rid of the heat.) A hot flash occurs when this conservation/release system gets off kilter and the vessels dilate even though it isn't necessary to get rid of any heat. Everyone else around you may be quite comfortable, but you are inappropriately sweating buckets.

A typical hot flash lasts three to five minutes, but on rare occasions, it may persist for thirty to sixty minutes. It is preceded by an *aura* of about a minute—you may experience a sense of anxiety or dread, plus a stepped-up heart rate and a feeling of weakness. This phase is caused by a release of adrenaline. The aura is soon followed by sudden dilation of your skin's surface vessels over your upper body, head, and neck. The increased blood flow may raise skin temperature (not body temperature) by up to 7 degrees. This is when the skin becomes reddened. Then comes profuse sweating, which can melt your hairstyle, run your eyeliner, and ruin your new shear blouse. Air movement across your skin (such as fanning yourself with the menu or rolling down the window when it's 15 degrees outside) starts evaporation of the abundant skin moisture. Evaporation itself is a cooling process, and *now* you may actually get a chill. Complete recovery can take up to half an hour.

Table 2.1. Duration of Hot Flashes	
1–2 years	Up to 75%
5 years	20–50%
Indefinitely	10%

What Causes Hot Flashes?

Remember the hypothalamus from the discussion in Chapter 1? It does more than help regulate your ovarian cycle; among its numerous other regulatory functions, it is your body's thermostat. The hypothalamus is aided and abetted by the *autonomic nervous system* (ANS), which controls blood vessel dilation and constriction. Estrogen receptors exist in the hypothalamus, and keeping the receptor sites occupied with estrogen is necessary to its proper functioning. It is thought that a lack of estrogen is the culprit that disturbs the usual smooth coordination between the hypothalamus and the ANS, the two temperature regulators. In the absence of adequate estrogen, the hypothalamus changes its set point; and this signals the ANS to throw open those surface blood vessels and release some heat. It may not be the right time for you to be a heat exchanger, but the hypothalamus did not receive its estrogen "fix," and that made it get crazy. Well, there you are. It's estrogen again.

How Bad or Frequent are Hot Flashes?

The experience of most women is that hot flashes are, at worst, unpleasant and inconvenient. For some, they are an expected event in the transitional years, easily tolerated. However, as Kronenberg reported in 1993, 10 to 15 percent of women find hot flashes to be a debilitating influence on their lives. These women are devastated by the intensity and frequency of hot flashes.

Hot flashes can range in frequency from one to four per day, or night. As a matter of fact, hot flashes most commonly occur at night. This seems to be related to the fact that the hypothalamus is involved in fewer regulatory functions during sleep. With less estrogen available and some free time, it seems to start fiddling with the thermostat, permitting the ANS to cause a hot flash. Guess what that does to your sleep? You may wake up with your hair wet, your pillow soaked, the covers thrown back, and your partner wondering what the devil all the thrashing around is about. Chronic sleep deprivation from nighttime hot flashes is widely regarded as the primary cause of irritability, moodiness, fatigue, short-term memory loss, and other common perimenopausal changes.

TIP! If you are on HRT, try taking your estrogen at bedtime. Many women find that the improved estrogen level during sleep prevents or substantially diminishes their hot flashes. You can call this a "hot tip."

What Can You Do About Hot Flashes?

Many things can help you control hot flashes, including:

• Replacing the estrogen

• Exercise

• Alternative medical remedies

• Avoiding trigger situations

The simplest and quickest solution is to go after the basic cause: replace the estrogen you lack. If you're concerned about that not being a natural remedy, you can use 17 beta *estradiol,* the natural, native estrogen your ovaries produce. It is available both as a tablet and as a skin patch. Estrogen replacement reliably relieves hot flashes in one to four weeks. The low-dose birth control pill works the same wonders for hot flashes, in addition to controlling or preventing several other transitional changes (not to mention pregnancy). (See Chapter 8 for a full discussion of the various estrogen preparations and their routes of administration.)

Exercise does a good job in controlling hot flashes. A brisk walk can be helpful during a hot flash. This isn't a particularly convenient means to deal with it if it's 3:00 a.m. when your hot flash engulfs you, so regular aerobic exercise for thirty to forty-five minutes, three to four times weekly, is a more sensible routine. (See Chapter 10 for a discussion of effective exercise techniques.)

Many women are reporting favorable results from alternative medical remedies. These include homeopathic remedies, herbs, acupuncture, mind/ body techniques, and holistic approaches. (See Chapter 10 for the details.)

Avoiding situations that trigger hot flashes can be helpful. A big meal is a common source because digestion brings large amounts of blood into the abdomen. This raises your core body temperature, and your hypothalamus reacts accordingly. Other situations to consider are the weather, overheated rooms, overdressing, too many blankets, hot tubs, hot drinks, alcohol, and stress. If you are underweight, you may have more hot flashes. (This is because a weak form of estrogen, called *estrone,* is made from body fat. If you're slender, a few more pounds might decrease hot flash symptoms.)

Brain Changes

Estrogen receptors exist throughout the brain. A receptor site is much like a lock-and-key arrangement. An estrogen molecule (the key) fits only into a receptor site (lock) that is specifically designed for it. When an estrogen molecule is plugged into a cell receptor site, it directs the cell to perform certain metabolic functions that benefit you. When the available estrogen is inadequate, the cell does not function normally. If this occurs in brain cells that happen to control such things as emotions, moods, thinking, heat regulation, or sexual circuits, the cells don't send their usual signals, and some unusual symptoms can result. To understand how these symptoms occur, let's take a look at how the brain works.

Neurotransmitters

Brain cells are called *neurons.* Each neuron is capable of receiving messages from millions upon millions of other cells The messages, or electrical impulses, travel along the nerve fiber of a neuron to its end point, or *synapse.* A synapse is the connecting point with other nerves. It's like a junction. For the message to cross the synapse to an adjacent neuron and continue along its way, neurotransmitter chemicals are necessary. There are many neurotransmitters, but the main three are *norepinephrine, dopamine,* and *serotonin.* Each of them is produced in the neuron and is stored inside the neuron near the synapse. When your brain is sending a message (such as "Take your finger off that hot stove"), a nerve cell generates the impulse and releases a neurotransmitter to transport the impulse across the synapse. On the other side of the synapse, the neurotransmitter molecule plugs into a receptor on the next nerve cell and passes the impulse along. This process continues from nerve cell to nerve cell until the message gets to its destination (in this example, your hand, and you move that toasty finger). Every cell has multiple receptors, so one cell can receive and transmit multiple impulses. After the message has been sent, the neurotransmitter is returned to the brain cell to await the next transmission job.

By their presence or absence, certain chemicals, including hormones like estrogen, can influence the ability of the receiving cell to pick up the message being sent. It can get garbled if estrogen receptors on the cell are not well supplied. In the brain, estrogen receptors are especially concentrated in the cerebral cortex and the limbic system. The *cerebral cortex* is the center for thinking and integrating thoughts. The *limbic system* is a collection of structures deep in the middle of the brain; it is the major center for regulating sleep, memory, mood, sex drive, pain, and appetite. Multiple connections exist between the limbic system and other parts of the brain, including the spinal cord. The cord is the pathway for messages being sent from your brain to all other parts of your body and back again. Do you see where this is leading? If the limbic system doesn't get its normal allotment of estrogen, it's going to be out of sorts and start sending some strange messages, or maybe no messages at all. This changes brain function, and especially mood.

Changes in Memory

In her landmark book *The Silent Passage,* Gail Sheehy (1991) put it well when she said, "At forty you can't read the numbers in the phone book. At fifty you can't remember them." Short-term memory loss isn't a disaster. You won't need to start wearing a wristband with your address on it so someone can take you home. It's little things that get away from you, like forgetting your point halfway through a scintillating conversation. Vocabulary selection becomes labored as you struggle to bring just the right word to your narrative. Thinking gets slower, logic gets fuzzy, and if it isn't on your list of things to do, it doesn't get done.

Disturbed sleep resulting from nighttime hot flashes may be a major contributor to short-term memory loss. Memory and sleep are controlled by the limbic system, and the adequacy of both is related to how well those limbic system receptor sites are occupied by estradiol. Campbell and White-head reported in an elegant study (1977) that hot flashes caused sleep dis-ruption; and sleep deprivation triggered short-term memory loss, fatigue, irritability, diminished sexual desire, and mood swings. When estrogen was supplemented, the hot flashes disappeared, sleep improved, and a domino effect took over, with improvement in all the other parameters of change. Campbell and Whitehead found that taking estrogen at night was most bene-ficial in controlling hot flashes.

There are other steps you can take to enhance your memory:

- Eat a balanced diet in smaller meals and at regular intervals. This keeps a steadier flow of nutrients to your brain.

- Do aerobic exercise four to five times per week. Several studies have demonstrated that exercise improves memory and learning ability in all age groups. This is especially true if the activity involves complex movement, such as aerobic dancing as opposed to aerobic walking, but both work.

- Stop smoking. Brain oxygenation will be improved. (Smoking can also cause an earlier menopause and therefore an earlier perimenopause.)

- Eliminate or reduce alcohol. Ever had so much you couldn't remember how much you had?

- Get enough sleep, and don't use sleeping pills. (You may need to wean yourself from a sleeping pill habit.)
- Challenge your brain by learning a new skill or examining new ideas. Brain exercise with new learning has been shown to increase the actual number of connections between nerves cells.

Moods

During perimenopause, you may feel helpless to control your mood swings. It's as though someone else is inside you pulling the levers and you can do nothing but watch yourself respond in out-of-character ways. Perhaps you burst into tears when the paper deliverer throws the newspaper into the birdbath again, or you cancel an entire appointment because it's going to start ten minutes late. These changes from your usual demeanor can be frustrating and embarrassing. Fortunately, changes like these are not a constant, everyday thing; they come and go. For many, the fluctuations are not severe at all. Perhaps you simply feel on edge and have a sense that you are not coping as well as you used to. Don't worry—none of these are signs of mental illness. But what causes them, and what can you do about them?

It is tempting to point a finger at estrogen deficiency as the source of mood swings and leave it at that. Hormone levels are certainly a factor (and hormone replacement has been reliably shown to even out your unreliable production of estradiol and to relieve mood swings), but the real stress behind mood swings may come from other areas of your life. You may have responsibilities and conflicts in a relationship, or in terms of your children or your occupation; you may have social and community obligations; and perhaps you are looking at the prospect of your parents becoming dependent on you and how that will change your lifestyle. You are used to orchestrating the ebb and flow of these important aspects of your life. Then, either suddenly or gradually, keeping all the balls in the air is not as simple as it used to be. It's important to understand that a changed equilibrium in your hormone balance has come into play; you are not being beset by mental illness. Your moods, and the frequency of their changes, are not entirely in your control.

TIP! Talk to your family and others close to you about your mood swings. You can ask them not to confront you with divisive issues when one of these moods is upon you, but to wait until your equanimity has returned. Then a productive discussion is possible.

Depression may be part of the mood-swing scenario. In most cases, it is *minor depression*, characterized by its brief episodes—a day, or a few days, at a time. It is not a serious mental illness. Depression that hangs on for weeks could be a major depression, a more serious condition. Women who have been teetering on the brink of major depression may be nudged into it by perimenopausal changes such as mood swings; but there is little like-lihood that a major depression will result from hormone decline alone (Avis 1997). (See Chapter 12 for more information on depression.)

Decreased Sexual Desire

The good news is that you may not experience any loss of sexual desire The bad news is that you might. Sexuality has diverse origins and influences. Changes in any of them are capable of altering your sexual response. The most important sex organ is your brain, which is why sexuality is included in this section about perimenopausal brain changes. Your intellectual percep-tion of sex has a powerful influence on how pleasurable it is. Cultural ex-pectations, prior experiences, partner sensitivity, and a huge array of other background input are all factors in your current attitude about your sexuality. Your brain is also influenced by whether or not its female sex hormone re-ceptors are being adequately supplied. Not only that, your small but im-mensely important production of male hormone has a profound impact on your sexual desire and sexual fantasies.

Sexuality is also influenced by the responsiveness of your genital anat-omy. Inadequate sexual lubrication, a chronically dry vagina, and diminished clitoral sensitivity all have a dampening effect on sex. These changes are a direct result of inadequate estrogen and respond well to estrogen replacement. Vaginal dryness with painful sex and clitoral insensitivity typically make their appearance late in the transitional years; often they are not a problem until the early postmenopausal years. On the other hand, you may notice dimin-ished sexual lubrication in your early forties. (See Chapter 13 for a full dis-cussion of sexual issues during the transitional years.)

Wrinkles

Our culture is obsessed with looking young. For some women, the de-velopment of wrinkles is a distressing event. Perpetually young skin isn't a realistic expectation, of course, because skin wrinkling occurs as the body ages, and no one has figured out how to avoid aging. There are several reasons for skin wrinkling and dryness:

- **Ultraviolet light:** Dermatologists worldwide advise that ultraviolet (UV) light from sun exposure is *the* major cause of aging skin. (This is called *photoaging.*) After the age of forty, the skin contains less mela-nin, a pigment that protects the skin from UV damage. With less mela-nin, the skin absorbs more UV light and burns more easily. This leads to damage of *collagen* (a type of connective tissue in the skin) and a dry, mottled appearance. The only solution is to avoid excessive sun exposure. You can do so by wearing protective clothing and using a sun-blocking cream (sunscreen) with a sun-protecting factor (SPF) of 15 or more. Apply it fifteen to thirty minutes beforehand to allow it to bond to your skin. Perimenopausal suntans are not cool. (See Chapter 14 for a more thorough discussion of skin care.)

- **Diminished estrogen:** A reduction in estrogen adversely affects production of collagen and *elastin* (also a connective tissue of the skin). These two tissues give skin its thickness, pliability, and elastic qualities. With adequate collagen and elastin, skin is able to shape itself smoothly over the various body contours. With loss of collagen and elastin, skin becomes thinner, and it becomes drier from decreased secretion of skin oils. Skin aging and wrinkling result from decreased production of these connective tissues or as a result of their deterioration or damage. Estrogen loss plays a key role in the lessening of these essential skin elements. Estradiol receptors are known to exist in skin, especially on the face and neck. By age sixty, women who have been on HRT through their perimenopausal-postmenopausal years have skin thickness up to twice that of nonusers (Nachtigall 1995). When HRT is begun, collagen production improves and skin plumps up ... up to a point. Once you have wrinkles, you can choose from a variety of nonsurgical and surgical cosmetic remedies (see Chapter 14).

- **Smoking:** Smoking causes skin wrinkling at an earlier-than-expected age. The theory, according to many dermatologists, is that it damages small blood vessels and diminishes cell nutrition. Smokers are well known to have an earlier menopause, and therefore an earlier perimenopause. The cause seems to be a toxic effect on the ovaries. In addition, women in their forties who smoke sometimes have wrinkles as prominent as women in their sixties. Typical smokers' wrinkles are deep smile lines about the eyes and radial wrinkles around the mouth.

- **Genes:** Genes play a role in terms of skin wrinkling. Dark-skinned people have thicker skin and more skin oils than fair-complexioned people, so their wrinkles come later in life. In addition, all the cells in the body are programmed genetically to age at a predetermined rate. This is an inherited determinant that influences wrinkling. More on this in Chapter 14.

Urinary Incontinence

Involuntary loss of urine is a common problem during the transition. Somebody tells a devastatingly funny joke, and there you are laughing like the others, but with wet pants. You urge your partner to stop the car at the very next available restroom because you really "gotta go," but you can feel urine leaking out as you scurry across the parking lot. How frustrating. You have just emptied your bladder; but upon returning to your guests and sitting down on the couch, some more urine squirts out! Doctors call these three conditions *stress incontinence, urge incontinence,* and *overflow incontinence.* Each has its own root cause, but a contributing factor they all have in common is loss of estrogen.

It is estimated that American women spend $10 billion annually on products marketed to cope with incontinence—not to treat it, but just to put up with it. If the cost of treatment is included, the annual bill is $16 billion (Brown 1996). The products include pads, panty liners, vaginal support devices, and training classes. This reflects a mindset that involuntary urine loss is just a part of aging, and you must learn to live with it. The good news is that you can do plenty to cure or reduce incontinence. (For a full discussion of this topic, see Chapter 15.)

Summary

Hormonal decline is an inevitable event in the transitional years of life. The particular combination of symptoms and physical changes, and their severity, vary widely among women. There is no way to predict exactly what will happen to you as an individual. If you know what can happen, you can be prepared for whatever does happen. This chapter has shown you that gradual, fluctuating estrogen decline is behind the plethora of changes you may experience. This hormone is of nearly universal use throughout the body, so it is no surprise that loss of estrogen affects so many bodily tissues. In the rest of this book, you will discover the many things you can do to minimize these changes, including, in Chapter 8, the benefits and risks of hormone replacement therapy.

○ ○ ○

3

Changes in Fertility: Pregnancy, Infertility, and Contraception

Alphabet Soup	
CVS	Chorionic villus sampling
FAS	Fetal alcohol syndrome
HBV	Hepatitis B virus
NTD	Neural tube defect
STD	Sexually transmitted disease

This chapter is about pregnancy. It's for those of you who will, those of you who won't, and those of you who can't have children during the transitional years. First we take a look at the special risks of having a baby when you are over thirty-five and what you can do to eliminate or minimize these risks. Then we talk about why you may not be able to get pregnant; as you approach the end of your reproductive life, you may experience some confounding problems while trying to conceive. This chapter examines the causes of difficulty in conceiving, the methods for diagnosing those causes, and the variety of fertility aids available when you can't get pregnant. The final part of the chapter is for women who don't want to have babies during the transitional years. As you reach perimenopause, your contraceptive needs change somewhat. Preventing pregnancy is actually easier during perimenopause, but sometimes you can really get tripped up. This chapter discusses each of the contraceptive methods now available, as well as the pros and cons of choosing each method.

Figure 3-1 illustrates a woman's normal pelvic anatomy. You might find it helpful to refer to this **diagram while reading th**is chapter.

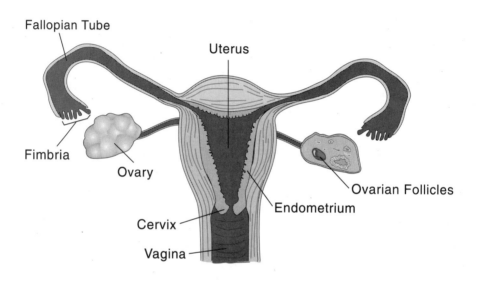

Figure 3.1.　**Normal Pelvic Anatomy**

Pregnancy

Twenty years ago, if a woman thirty-five years old had a child, her doctor would probably assume that she didn't want any more children and might even offer to tie her tubes, especially if the delivery was a cesarean. Today, attitudes have changed, and many women over thirty-five are choosing to have children. Many women delay marriage and then choose to establish their careers before considering a family. Many women don't finish their families until they are in their early forties. What has happened that makes being pregnant at thirty-seven okay today, when it was not okay twenty years ago?

The major difference today is the safety and reliability of fetal diagnosis (Rose et al. 1994). The chances of your having an abnormal child today are the same as they were fifty years ago (Cuckle et al. 1987). The difference is that now doctors can diagnose most of these abnormalities during pregnancy, and you can make a decision about whether to carry the child to term. These choices give women freedom that wasn't possible in their parents' day.

CAUTION! In addition to the specific risk factors discussed in this section, the usual list of risk factors applies: the use of cigarettes, drugs, and alcohol have all been implicated in abnormalities in fetal development.

Abnormal Pregnancies

Every year you age increases the risk of an abnormal pregnancy. For example, if you are over forty, the chance of miscarriage increases to almost 50 percent (Gindoff and Jewelewicz 1986, Asch and Marrs 1993). The risk of bearing a child with trisomy (Down syndrome, which we explain in a moment) also increases. These abnormalities are usually caused by an abnormal egg. Every cell in your body except your eggs contain forty-six chromosomes (the components of the cell nucleus that contain genes). Genes determine your various body characteristics, such as eye and hair color. Your forty-six chromosomes are pairs, with twenty-three from your father's sperm cell and twenty-three from your mother's egg. The chromosomes from your father and mother are separate until ovulation occurs. Then the chromosomes from your father and mother intertwine, exchanging genetic material before splitting apart. An egg cell begins with forty-six chromosomes, but at ovulation, it discards twenty-three of them. The twenty-three remaining chromosomes contain genes from both your mother and your father. Your egg is now ready to receive the sperm, which has gone through a similar process of discarding twenty-three of its chromosomes. As you age, though, variations can occur, resulting in an egg with an extra chromosome (twenty-four instead of twenty-three), and the fertilized egg develops into an embryo with forty-seven chromosomes. This condition is called trisomy. (Trisomy is always due to an extra chromosome from the egg. Sperm containing more than twenty-three chromosomes can't swim, and if they can't swim, they can't penetrate an egg.)

Most trisomies are incompatible with life. An exception, and the best known of these conditions, is trisomy 21, or *Down syndrome*. In younger mothers, Down syndrome results from the attachment of extra genes from chromosome 21 to another chromosome. In older women, two number 21 chromosomes in the egg combine with one 21 chromosome in the sperm cell. The child born with this syndrome has mental retardation, a sweet personality, and a distinctive facial structure, as well as heart and bowel problems. As you get older, your risk of bearing a child with Down syndrome increases, as you can see in Table 3-1 (Cuckle et al. 1987, Polamaki et al. 1995). Eighty percent of Down syndrome babies are born to women under age thirty-five (American College of Obstetricians and Gynecologists 1991), and women over

Table 3.1
Risk of Down Syndrome by Age

Age	Risk	Age	Risk
20	1:1353	41	1:75
25	1:1196	42	1:57
30	1:802	43	1:44
33	1:508	44	1:33
34	1:419	45	1:25
35	1:340	46	1:18
36	1:272	47	1:13
37	1:214	48	1:9
38	1:167	49	1:7
39	1:129	50	1:5
40	1:99		

Adapted from: Cuckle et al. Palomali et al.

thirty-five account for fewer than 10 percent of all pregnancies. However, they account for 20 percent of all cases of Down syndrome.

Single Gene Abnormalities

Unlike trisomies, most single gene abnormalities, such as hemophilia, cannot be detected before birth. While certain single gene abnormalities are discovered through fetal chemical changes, which a doctor may look for because of prior family history, the majority are not detected. Trisomy has been linked to older mothers, but single gene abnormalities have been linked to older fathers. (Finally, there is something they can't blame on women!)

Abnormal Pregnancies Not Related to Age

Abnormal pregnancies in women of all ages can also result from neural tube defects (NTDs), viral infections, and other conditions. Starting prenatal vitamins containing 0.4 to 0.8 mg of folic acid before you get pregnant markedly reduces your risk of having a baby with a neural tube defect (MRC Vitamin Study Research Group 1991, Werler et al. 1993, ACOG 1993 (editorial), Lancet 1991). The risk of these abnormalities does not appear to increase in perimenopause.

Testing for Abnormal Pregnancies

Let's take a look at some tests your doctor can perform to diagnose an abnormal pregnancy.

Amniocentesis and Chorionic Villus Sampling (CVS)

One way your doctor can diagnose trisomies is by using a procedure called *amniocentesis,* which involves testing the *amniotic fluid,* the liquid that surrounds the growing fetus. Another procedure for testing trisomies is called *chorionic villus sampling* (CVS); it involves taking tissue from the *placenta* (the so-called "after birth") instead of the amniotic fluid. CVS is more dangerous for the fetus, but it can be done earlier in pregnancy, which makes the results available at an earlier stage in fetal life (California Department of Health Services 1995). Amniocentesis is offered to women who, when they give birth, will be thirty-five or older.

To perform an amniocentesis, the doctor places a thin needle through the abdominal wall, into the uterus, and into the amniotic sac containing the fetus, using ultrasound for guidance. An *ultrasound* machine sends sound waves through the tissues. Because different body tissues are of different densities, they reflect the sound waves differently. The echoes are evaluated electronically, and the picture this creates can be seen on a monitor. The amniocentesis needle also shows up on the ultrasound screen. The doctor then removes a small amount of amniotic fluid and sends it to a laboratory, where a laboratory technician cultures the fetal cells for Down syndrome, other chromosomal abnormalities, and NDT. These abnormalities can almost always be detected by an amniocentesis.

Although the risk of Down syndrome gradually increases every year, an amniocentesis is not recommended until after age thirty-five, when the risk for giving birth to a baby with Down syndrome exceeds the risk of the test. Most health centers today will do an amniocentesis on younger women when they ask for it and understand the risk to the fetus. An amniocentesis costs between $1,000 and $1,500, but most insurance policies pay for the test (California Department of Health Services 1995).

In *chorionic villus sampling (CVS)*, the doctor takes cells from the developing placenta) rather than from the amniotic fluid. CVS is done between the tenth and twelfth weeks of pregnancy, and the cells can be obtained in one of two ways. Using ultrasound as a guide to locate the placenta, the doctor can pass a thin needle through the lower abdomen to extract some cells. Alternatively, depending on the location of the placenta, the doctor can obtain the cells by passing a thin tube through the cervix. The placental cells, which have the same chromosomal makeup as the fetus, are then grown and examined for abnormalities. With CVS, Down syndrome can be detected 98 percent of the time, but CVS can not detect neural tube defects. Women who choose a CVS first have an AFP blood test (see the next section) to screen for neural tube defects between the fifteenth and eighteenth weeks of pregnancy. The advantage of a CVS over an amniocentesis is an earlier diagnosis and an earlier choice for women who would choose to not carry an abnormal fetus. The disadvantage is a higher miscarriage rate of about 3 per 100. The cost of a CVS is between $1,200 and $1,800. Not all insurance companies pay for this test.

Triple Marker

A combination of three blood tests, called the *triple marker*, can screen for neural tube defects and for the risk of Down syndrome, as well as other abnormalities. The advantage of these tests is that they are maternal blood tests, so they avoid invasion of the pregnancy itself.

A laboratory technician tests the mother's blood for three substances: alpha-fetoprotein (AFP), human chorionic gonadotropin (hCG), and unconjugated estriol (UE). The test can be done between fifteen and twenty weeks of pregnancy; but the most accurate results are between the sixteenth and seventeenth weeks. The triple marker doesn't make a diagnosis, but it gives the percentage of risk for the abnormalities it tests for. If this risk is low, nothing more needs to be done. If it is high, further testing may be done, including an ultrasound and possibly an amniocentesis.

Handling the Test Results

The purpose of all these tests is to see whether the baby you are carrying is normal. If your decision will be to carry the baby to term, regardless of any abnormality that may show up in tests, there may no point in having the tests performed—especially in the case of amniocentesis, which puts the fetus at risk. On the other hand, you may want to know, before birth, whether your child will have Down syndrome. This way you can prepare yourself and your family emotionally and find out about the resources available to help your child, including support groups that can help you understand and cope with raising a child with Down syndrome. Schooling starts very early for Down babies and seems to help them become healthier and more productive adults. People with Down syndrome live well into middle age. Today, their nutrition is better, the abnormalities common to these children are repaired, and they are not institutionalized. Early intervention, within the first six months to a year, has helped them join mainstream society (Rudolph 1989).

Other Factors to Consider

This section examines some other factors you should consider before becoming pregnant that can help decrease the chance of fetal abnormalities.

"High-Risk" Pregnancies Over Age 35

Traditionally, pregnant women over thirty-five have been regarded as being "high risk" in terms of their own health. There is some doubt as to whether that point of view is accurate. Drs. Edge and Laros (1983) studied over 800 women having their first pregnancy at age thirty-five or older. They found no increased incidence of chronic diseases—specifically, heart disease, high blood pressure, diabetes, and lupus. They did find an increase in *preeclampsia* (pregnancy-induced high blood pressure and fluid retention), *fibroids* (noncancerous tumors of the uterus), pregnancy-induced diabetes, fetal distress in labor, and abnormal labor patterns, and, as a result of these symptoms, a higher incidence of cesarean section than younger mothers. Their babies, though, were just as big and healthy as babies of younger mothers.

Extra Care for Chronic Diseases

Some women have medical conditions that require special care before, during, and sometimes after pregnancy. A pregnancy puts increased demands on the body. A health problem that was well controlled, before pregnancy might be more troublesome once pregnancy occurs. For example, if you have high blood pressure, your antihypertensive medication may need to be changed, prior to conception, to a drug that is safe for a developing baby. If you are diabetic, it's important to have your blood sugars at target level before conception to ensure a normal baby. If you have thyroid disease, be sure your thyroid levels are monitored. (There is a high incidence of thyroid problems occurring for the first time in the initial three months after your baby is born. See Chapter 6 for a more detailed discussion of this subject.)

Known Familial Diseases

If your family has a history of a particular disease or diseases, be sure to discuss this issue with your doctor before conception. That way, you can make informed decisions as to the best way to have a healthy pregnancy.

Stopping Birth Control Pills

Birth control pills regulate your menstrual periods. When you decide to get pregnant and quit taking them, your menstrual periods may become irregular for a while. If you become pregnant before your periods are regular again, it makes establishing the duration of your pregnancy more difficult. Your endometrium (uterine lining) will have been thinned during your years of taking birth control pills. It needs time to develop into the lush, sugar-filled glandular tissue needed to support an embryo. Therefore, it is a good idea to stop taking the pills several months before getting pregnant. However, using birth control pills before you become pregnant does *not* cause birth defects, regardless of how close to pregnancy you stop taking them.

Cigarettes, Alcohol, and Drugs

Tobacco, alcohol, and social drugs have adverse effects on a developing baby. This is true both during the time the organs are forming and throughout fetal life. Let's take a look at what can happen.

Smoking is associated with low-birth-weight babies, an increase in fetal death, and an increase in crib death called Sudden Infant Death syndrome (SIDS). Children raised in a house of smokers have a 50 percent increase in their lifetime chance of developing cancer (Stjernfeldt et al. 1986, John et al. 1991). Quitting smoking helps you *and* your baby.

Fetal alcohol syndrome (FAS) occurs when a woman drinks heavily during her pregnancy. This syndrome results in abnormal facial features and mental retardation. The amount of alcohol needed to cause FAS varies from person to person. As few as two drinks a day can cause a child to be born with this syndrome, although most children with FAS are born to women who drink considerably more. It doesn't matter whether you drink wine, beer, or hard liquor; they all cause the fetal alcohol syndrome (Dorris 1990). If you are trying to get pregnant, it is a good idea to abstain from drinking. In the event of an unplanned pregnancy, stop drinking immediately. If you think you might have a problem with alcohol abuse, get help before you try to get pregnant.

In case you haven't heard, using cocaine, crack cocaine, or heroin while pregnant will seriously damage—if not kill—a fetus. "Crack babies" have short attention spans, are irritable and hyperactive, and have trouble learning. More information will no doubt be forthcoming on the continuing negative effects of maternal drug use during pregnancy as these children grow up, and the picture won't be a pretty one.

It takes time to quit a habit. According to research in human learning, it takes six weeks to six months for nerves to shrivel and new neural pathways to form in their place (Soares 1996). Don't be embarrassed if you have a habit that is difficult to quit. Ask your health provider for support and medical advice. The decision to quit may be one of the most difficult things you've ever done, but one of the most worthwhile.

Viral Infections

Infections with measles, mumps, chicken pox and rubella (German measles) during your pregnancy can cause serious birth defects or illness in your baby. Vaccination against these viral infections can prevent them. Find out if you are immune to these diseases prior to pregnancy. If not, get vaccinated and then pregnant, but in that order.

Hepatitis B (HBV), a viral infection, is the most common cause of hepatitis in the United States (U.S. Dept. Health, Education and Welfare 1977, Teufel et al. 1992). It results in 300,000 new cases of acute hepatitis yearly. If you are a carrier of this virus, you can give it to your infant during birth or immediately afterwards. Over 16,000 babies are at risk each year. A baby that becomes infected may become a chronic carrier. Twenty-five percent of chronic carriers eventually develop cancer or cirrhosis of the liver. As a result, when you first become pregnant, your doctor will test to see whether you are an HBV carrier. If you aren't but are in a high-risk group, you should be immunized to prevent the disease. If you are in a high-risk group, you should be tested before you get pregnant and then immunized as soon as possible. Your risk for being an HBV carrier is increased if you are

- Originally from the Orient or from Oceania, or a Native American Eskimo
- Use illicit drugs
- Have acute or chronic liver disease
- Have had a blood transfusion
- Are a health care worker
- Have multiple sex partners
- Have had any sexually transmitted diseases

If you are identified as a carrier, your baby will be given HBV prophylaxis immediately after birth to prevent this disease. It is common practice to immunize babies after birth, but if you are diagnosed early, your baby gets an extra boost toward preventing infection.

Sexually Transmitted Diseases (STDs)

Sexually transmitted diseases (STDs) are diseases you get through sexual contact. These include gonorrhea, chlamydia, genital herpes, syphilis, warts (human papilloma virus), and AIDS. Not only can they adversely affect your ability to get pregnant, they can infect and harm your baby. Certain contraceptive methods, such as condoms, spermicides (contraceptive foams or creams), and even birth control pills (by thickening your cervical mucus) lower your risk of contracting an STD. Once you are trying to get pregnant, however, you obviously stop using these methods. This places you at a higher risk level for contracting an STD, especially if you or your partner is non-monogamous. If you think you or your partner has a sexually transmitted disease, see your health provider right away and get treatment. Then abstain from sex until both of you have completed treatment and been rechecked.

Infertility

Perhaps you have delayed your first pregnancy until your career is set, and you may have bought your first home. You have started prenatal vitamins, you've seen your health provider, and you're healthy. You may have even stopped your birth control pills three months ago. You are ready to get pregnant, but nothing happens. You find this pregnancy business isn't going the way you had planned. Well, you are not alone. You have probably heard stories of women who tried to get pregnant for years but became pregnant only after they had stopped trying. Actually, that sort of pregnancy doesn't happen very often. Most of the time, if you are having trouble getting pregnant on your own, you need help from your health provider.

There are numerous possible factors responsible for a couple's lack of conception. This section takes a look at those most likely to be responsible for failure to conceive during the perimenopausal years.

(Note: It is estimated that 40 percent of all infertility is caused by the male factor [Jaffe and Jewelewicz 1991]. If you are having infertility problems, make sure your partner is not causing over-warming of the scrotum [warm sperm are sluggish] by wearing tight underwear, jeans, or padded bicycle shorts or taking hot showers, and ask him to be tested for sperm count.)

- **Ovulation:** After the age of thirty-five, your ovaries have fewer eggs and gradually produce less and less estrogen and progesterone. (See the next section for a full discussion of ovarian issues.) This is coincident with the inevitable reduction in the number of eggs left to be ovulated, as we discussed in Chapter 2. These coinciding factors reduce your chances of conception. Figure 3-2 illustrates the relationship between pregnancies and age. If progesterone levels fall too much, the endometrium does not produce enough sugar (glycogen) to support a little embryo. As a result, even when you conceive normally, you have an increased miscarriage risk.

- **Tubal disease:** Twenty percent of all infertility is due to tubal or uterine disease. Several factors contribute to this high rate. Contemporary women are delaying their childbearing. The net result is that not only are they running out of good eggs; they are allowing more time and more chances to be exposed to sexually transmitted diseases (STDs), such as gonorrhea and chlamydia. These STDs have increasingly damaging effects on fallopian tubes and fertility with each occurrence of the infection.

- **Thyroid disease:** Thyroid hormone, either too much or too little, can cause infertility. Chapter 6 is devoted to this issue.

- **Frequency of sex:** Couples have sex less often as they age for a variety of reasons. Once you are in your late thirties, you will have intercourse half as often as you did when you were younger (Menken et al. 1986).

- **Age of partner:** As you age, so does your partner; as his interest in having sex decreases, so does the pregnancy rate.

- **Postponement of childbearing:** If you choose a career outside of the home, you probably graduated from college, went on to graduate school, found a job, got established, and then decided to have children. All of this takes time and each year you wait, the fewer fresh grade AA eggs you have left to be fertilized.

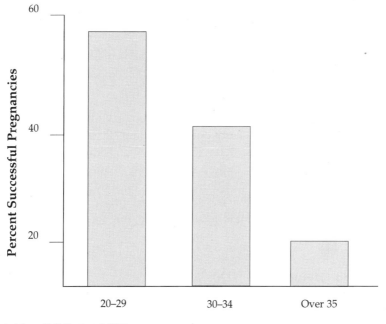

Adapted from: R. T. Scott et al. 1995.

Figure 3.2. Percent of Pregnancies vs. Age

Ovarian Problems and Infertility

You know that you have to ovulate to get pregnant and have healthy fallopian tubes to transport your embryo. Your partner has to have an above-target sperm count and motility to impregnate you, and your pituitary gland needs to be functioning for all of this to happen. If you've made sure you have no problems in those areas and you still haven't been able to conceive, your ovaries may be the culprit.

As you reach perimenopause, you're getting older, and so are your eggs. Your estrogen and your progesterone levels just "ain't what they used to be." Even if you are lucky enough to ovulate a grade AA egg, the follicle from which the egg emerged may not make enough progesterone in the *luteal phase* (the two weeks after ovulation) to sustain an embryo.

Production of progesterone must be constant during the luteal phase to prepare the endometrium for pregnancy. If your progesterone level begins to fall, the embryo can't implant in your uterus, and a miscarriage results. This is called a *luteal phase defect*.

Your doctor can diagnose a short luteal phase by "dating" your endometrium. The procedure involves taking a sample of the endometrial lining, using a small hollow tube that is placed into the uterus. Suction is then applied to extract a small amount of tissue. The endometrial biopsy is usually performed two or three days before your next period is due. A pathologist looks at the endometrial lining and accurately "dates"—that is, determines, from the size and character of your endometrial lining when your next period is due. If your endometrial lining is out of phase by two days or more (that is, you don't have your period within the time predicted by the pathologist), you have a luteal phase defect. You are not making enough progesterone to support a pregnancy. (Note: Your doctor can also order a simple progesterone blood level drawn on day twenty-one to tell you whether you are making enough progesterone (Jaffe and Jewelewicz 1991). Although a blood test is certainly less painful than an endometrial biopsy, your doctor cannot as accurately diagnose a luteal phase deficiency by a blood test.)

The usual treatment for a shortened luteal phase is progesterone suppositories. Progesterone shots are also available, but they don't work as well as suppositories.

Assisted Reproductive Technologies

Pregnancy rates decrease with age. There are many reasons for this decline but one of the main reasons is fewer normal eggs. Remember, you only produce one egg per month. If there is a defect in your egg, it is less likely to be fertilized. The incidence of these defects increases with age (Palomski et al. 1995, Cuckle et al. 1987, Asch and Marrs 1993). To increase your chance of pregnancy, your doctor may recommend a fertility-enhancing drug (clomiphine citrate, human menopausal gonadotropins, human chorionic gonadotropins) to help you produce more than one egg per month. (Believe it or not, gonadotropins at present are made by purifying urine collected from menopausal Italian nuns!) Multiple eggs increase the likelihood that one or more of them will be successfully fertilized and you will be on your way to motherhood.

Fertility-enhancing drugs don't always work. When they don't, a number of assisted reproductive technologies (ARTs) are available for women trying to conceive. These include *in vitro fertilization (IVF),* or fertilization in a laboratory dish or test tube, as illustrated in Figure 3-3, and *GIFT,* a procedure that places the sperm and egg in the fallopian tube to allow fertilization, shown in Figure 3-4. Two others are *assisted hatching,* an enhancement of IVF in which the cells around the fertilized egg are removed to help the fertilized egg implant in the uterus, and *intracytoplasmic sperm injection (ICSI),* which is the placement of a single sperm into a single egg. Several other techniques are used less frequently. If you are under forty, your success rate with IVF any given month compares favorably with the natural pregnancy rate of the general fertile population (33.6 percent per cycle) (Society for Assisted Reproductive Technology 1996). If you are over forty, your chance of having a successful pregnancy with IVF is only about 8 percent (Asch and Marrs 1993). The addition of ICSI and assisted hatching increases that rate to 17 percent (Society for Assisted Reproductive Technology 1996).

When fertility enhancing drugs and assisted reproductive technologies don't work, then the use of an egg donor should be considered. This may seem very radical, but remember that donor sperm have been used for twenty-five or thirty years with wonderful success rates. With a donor-egg pregnancy, the sperm comes from your partner, the egg comes from a younger woman, and you carry the pregnancy. The advantage of this over surrogate pregnancy, where another woman carries the baby to term, is that you are in control of the food, drugs, and alcohol to which your baby is exposed. You carry the baby to term, and your maternal gene (recently discovered in humans as well as mice), is turned on (Brown et al. 1996).

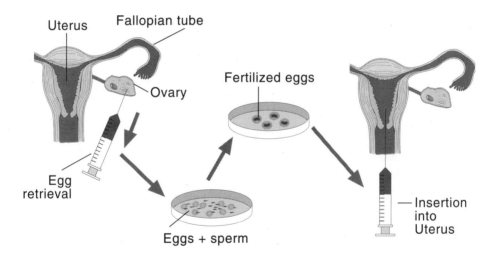

Figure 3.3. In Vitro Fertilization

Contraception—If You Would Rather Be 40 Than Pregnant

When you arrive at perimenopause, your cycles often lose their regularity. You may have used the rhythm method for years, but be careful: It no longer works, because your cycles are no longer rhythmic!

Some women nearing the end of reproductive life spot a little blood when they ovulate. This can last for several days. If this happens to you, don't be fooled into assuming this is the beginning of your menstrual period (especially if it is overdue). Continue using contraception to be sure of avoiding pregnancy.

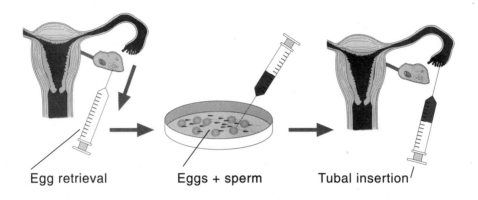

Egg retrieval   Eggs + sperm   Tubal insertion

Figure 3.4.   Gamete Intrafallopian Transfer (GIFT)

Contraception in Perimenopause

A variety of contraceptive methods are available for use by women. (This discussion doesn't include the topic of vasectomy, a surgical procedure performed on men.) Let's take a look at what's available and what makes sense for you during perimenopause.

Barrier Methods—Foam, Condoms, and Diaphragms Work Well

Once you are perimenopausal, barrier methods work better than ever before . . . as long as they are not left in the dresser drawer. Why better than before? Because you are less fertile. You aren't infertile, though, so use your diaphragm, cervical cap, condom, contraceptive foam, or cream all the time. Even if you think you are having your menstrual period, don't take chances. If used, the barrier methods are nearly foolproof at this age. Barrier methods include

- **Condoms:** This is an effective method; but not if you use a torn condom. Your vagina lubricates more slowly than it used to, and a lack of adequate lubrication makes a condom more likely to tear. For this reason, use a contraceptive jelly or foam as an adjunct to the condom.

- **Diaphragm:** The incidence of bladder infection is two and a half times higher in women who use the diaphragm as their birth control method compared to other forms of birth control. This increased rate is due to the spermicidal jelly used with the diaphragm. The jelly kills normal bacteria in the vagina, but allows infection-causing bacteria to survive and get into the bladder. If you have a history of recurrent bladder infections, you shouldn't use a diaphragm.

- **Spermicides:** Grimes noted in 1997 that spermicides are a very safe method of birth control because using them does not present a risk of birth defects if a woman becomes pregnant while using them.

- **Cervical cap:** This is a variation on the diaphragm that fits over the mouth of the womb (cervix) and can be worn for several days at a time. This allows a greater element of spontaneity in lovemaking. Like the diaphragm, there is a potential risk of increased bladder infections.

- **Contraceptive sponge:** This method has been taken off the market. It was an effective method for women who had never had a child, but much less so for women with children.

- **Female condom:** This is the first totally woman-controlled method intended to protect against pregnancy and sexually transmitted diseases. However, Grimes noted that the pregnancy rate for women using the female condom is 12 percent over six months. This unacceptably high pregnancy rate means that this method isn't used.

The Intrauterine Device (IUD)—Safe and Effective, but with a Bad Reputation

The *intrauterine device* (IUD) is a great method of birth control. Unfortunately, because of the serious problems that occurred in women using the Dalkon Shield a few years ago, the IUD has been blamed for infertility. It has been estimated that, during the 1980s, over 300,000 women worldwide were injured by infections caused by the Dalkon Shield (Grimes 1997). Other safe IUDs were "guilty by association" and were taken off the market. American women lost a valuable method of birth control.

Gradually, the truth about infection and IUDs became known: The number of sex partners a woman has, not the IUD, is responsible for pelvic infection and subsequent sterility (Darney 1996, Grimes 1997). The risk of significant infection occurs only in the first month after insertion and, for the most part, can be prevented by giving prophylactic antibiotics, which prevent chlamydia, to all women at the time of insertion. Doxycycline, given to you at the time your doctor inserts your IUD, does not prevent infection unless you take it for ten days. A single dose of azithromycin will prevent an infection, however (Grimes 1997).

There are two types of IUDs on the American market. The first is the Copper "T." It is quite small, easy to insert, and good for ten years. The copper acts as a spermicide so pregnancy doesn't occur either in the uterus or in the tube. The second type is also a "T," but it has progesterone instead of copper as the active ingredient. The progesterone "T" is also small, easy to insert, and decreases your menstrual flow and cramps, but it must be replaced each year. The progesterone reduces your uterine lining, which acts as a barrier to sperm migration. The World Health Organization has concluded that "today's copper and hormone-bearing devices are among the safest and most effective reversible methods of contraception in the world" (Grimes 1997).

Several new IUDs are on the horizon. A new progesterone IUD containing levonorgestrel, a more potent progestin (a synthetic progesterone; more on that subject in a moment), is in use in Finland and is in FDA-mandated clinical trials in the United States; these IUDs last seven years. Brill noted in 1995 that this new IUD decreases menstrual flow by over 80 percent—good news if you have heavy periods. In addition, it decreases menstrual cramps.

CAUTION! This IUD is not advisable if you have had an ectopic pregnancy in the past because it carries an increased risk of tubal pregnancy

The latest IUD in clinical trials is a bodiless copper IUD. It has a monofilament string and six copper bands; but there is no body onto which the copper is mounted. (The body in other IUDs is what causes cramping.) Another prototype being considered has very pliable arms that point downward to prevent its expulsion. No one knows which will get the FDA nod; but it is encouraging to see advances being made in the important area of contraception (Grimes 1997).

Birth Control Pills—Now?

Birth control pills are an excellent option for you during perimenopause. Doctors prescribe them for perimenopausal women who experience heavy or irregular bleeding, including women who have had their tubes tied. For many women, taking the pill during perimenopause is multipurpose: It serves as a method of birth control, bleeding control, and perimenopausal symptom control.

There is, unfortunately, a large group of women who can not use the Pill safely after age thirty-five. They include women with the following health issues:

- **Smoking:** If you smoke, your risk of having a heart attack on the Pill is seventy-seven times higher than for women not taking the Pill. This statistic is for all women. It only becomes a significant risk to you, though, once you are over 35, when the risk of heart disease begins to rise for all women (Darney 1996).

- **Diabetes:** Older forms of birth control pills (Loestrin, Triphasil, Ovcon, and Ortho-Novum 777, to name a few) make management of diabetes more difficult. For insulin-dependent diabetics, fasting blood sugars are raised and insulin dose regulation gets tricky. If you take oral antidiabetic pills or use diet to control your diabetes, the older varieties of birth control pills may also make management of your blood sugar a bit of a problem. Newer birth control pills on the market (such as

Desogen and Ortho Tri-Cyclen) have not proven to be superior to the older types of birth control pills except for women with diabetes or acne. If you have diabetes, the new pills will not affect your blood sugar at all. The insulin dose regulation that you normally require from time to time is easy when you are on the new pill (Burkman et al. 1992, Becker 1990, Huber 1991).

CAUTION! Troglitazone, a new oral agent for treating diabetes, negates the contraceptive affects of the birth control pill! Don't count on any birth control pill, new or old, to protect you if you start this medication (Norton 1997).

- **Hypertension:** Women with high blood pressure are cautioned not to take the Pill. Birth control pills raise blood pressure in susceptible people (Physician's Desk Reference 1997). Uncontrolled hypertension can lead to stroke and kidney failure. It is a silent illness, diagnosed only by blood pressure tests.

- **Fibroid tumors:** Fibroids are muscle tumors of the uterus. They tend to start growing in a woman's early forties. They can cause severe bleeding, as well as bladder and back problems. The engine for fibroid growth is estrogen, and birth control pills raise estrogen levels. If you have fibroids, these higher levels of estrogen may make the fibroids grow, causing more problems than you had to begin with.

- **Antitubercular and anticonvulsive drugs:** Rifampin (rifater), phenobarbitol, Dilantin (phenytoin sodium), and other anticonvulsive drugs activate liver enzymes that destroy the hormones in birth control pills, as well as the hormones in Norplant (described in the next section). The only safe birth control methods for you are Depo-Provera (also described in the next section) and barrier methods (Darney 1996, Grimes 1997).

- **Classic migraine headache:** Birth control pills may aggravate the symptoms of a migraine, or they may improve them. In any case, according to the Group for Study of Stroke in Young Women (1975), there is no increased risk of stroke in women using birth control pills that contain 35 micrograms or less of ethinyl estradiol or less (University of Minnesota 1997). If your migraines become more frequent after beginning birth control pills, or they occur for the first time after you begin birth control pills, however, you should consider a different form of birth control (Silberstein 1992).

If you are not affected by any of the factors described above, the birth control pill may be ideal for you. It regulates your periods, may decrease your PMS, protects you from getting pregnant, and delays your risk of osteoporosis. Many women continue to take birth control pills into the first five years or so of menopause itself, as their drug of choice for hormone replacement therapy. The Pill has little or no effect on cholesterol at all. In 1996, Darney quoted a study from Finland that showed a six-fold (600 percent) decrease in the risk of heart attack and stroke in Pill users over nonpill users. This dramatic difference continued for fifteen years after the women had discontinued using the Pill.

In terms of cancer risks, women who take the birth control pill for ten or more years have an 85 percent decrease in the risk of ovarian cancer, a 50 percent decrease in the risk of uterine cancer, and maybe a 35 percent decrease in the risk of breast cancer. There is disagreement among the various studies on the effect of birth control pills and breast cancer. Some studies have suggested a slightly increased risk of breast cancer on the Pill, but most find it to be safe and to lower the risk of breast cancer (Darney 1996, Grimes 1997).

One disagreeable side effect for perimenopausal women on the Pill is that up to 30 percent experience diminished sexual desire (Leventhal 1997). Taking the Pill reduces the available testosterone in your body, and testosterone is the source of sexual desire and sexual fantasies. One solution to this problem is the addition of a small dose of testosterone in tablet form; it is not necessary to go off the Pill. (Chapter 8 provides a full discussion of testosterone.)

Injectable Progestins: Norplant and Depo-Provera

Progestins are synthetic progesterones that can be taken in pill form. Natural progesterone, the hormone you make the second half of your menstrual cycle, can only be taken by injection or absorbed through your skin. Both Norplant and Depo-Provera contain long-acting progestins, which have three mechanisms for preventing pregnancy:

- **Hostile cervical mucus:** These contraceptive methods change the character of the cervical mucus so that sperm cannot penetrate it; in other words, it acts as a barrier.

- **Endometrial change:** The character of the endometrium is altered to make it hostile to sperm.

- **Halts ovulation:** There is no egg to fertilize.

Norplant (levonorgesterol implants) delivers levonorgesterol in six small permeable capsules These are placed under the skin of the inner side of your upper arm so they don't show. They are effective for five years and are almost as effective at the end of that time as they were at the beginning. After five years they need to be removed and replaced if contraception is still desired. The insertion and removal are done in the doctor's office under local anesthetic. Your arm may be black and blue for about a week after the procedure, but discomfort is not a major problem during either insertion or removal. A new version of Norplant is being studied that uses only two pellets, which are larger and easier to remove (Darney 1996, Nelson 1996, Grimes 1997).

Depo-Provera (depo-medroxyprogesterone acetate, or DMPA) is an injection given every three months (Physician's Desk Reference 1997). It has been the mainstay of contraception in the Third World for the last twenty-five years. DMPA is now used increasingly in the U.S. (Kaunitz 1996, Fraser and Dennerstein 1994). You may have irregular bleeding with DMPA, and some women feel mildly depressed, as with other progestins. In contrast to birth control pills, there is no contraindication to Depo-Provera use in women who smoke, have high blood pressure, or are on medication to prevent blood clotting. Dr. Nelson (1996) advises the use of Depo-Provera as contraception for women with mild estrogen depletion but who are not yet menopausal. She states that estrogen replacement therapy can be added for those women who need it. The addition of estrogen can control perimenopausal symptoms and prevent osteoporosis. In addition, Depo-Provera prevents pregnancy while decreasing the risk of uterine and ovarian cancer.

When the Norplant is removed, the hormone effects are gone immediately. Depo-Provera continues to have some effects for up to nine months after it is discontinued. Most women do not have periods while using either of these methods. The majority of women using Norplant or Depo-Provera are very satisfied with this method of contraception (Fraser and Dennerstein 1994, Kaunitz 1996), although side effects can include weight gain, irregular bleeding, headaches, acne, mild depression, and increased PMS. Women using Norplant may also have painful functional ovarian cysts; women using Depo-Provera do not. Fewer than 15 percent of women experience the side effects. Unlike birth control pills, Depo-Provera and Norplant are not affected by antibiotic usage. (Note: Norplant and birth control pills don't work for you if you are on anticonvulsive medications, but anticonvulsants have no adverse effect on Depo-Provera [Grimes 1996].)

Emergency Contraception— The Morning-After Pill

If you have had unprotected sex about the time you should be ovulating, emergency contraception using the so-called morning-after pill can be effective. It must be started within 72 hours of the time sex occurred. Several methods of emergency contraception are in use, but the one most frequently utilized is the called the Yuzpe method. This involves taking two doses of two oral contraceptive pills twelve hours apart for a total of four tablets. (Grimes 1997)

Other emergency contraception methods include the use of synthetic estrogens, conjugated estrogens (such as Premarin), insertion of an IUD, and anti-progesterones such as RU-486, the "French abortion pill." RU-486 is not yet available for use in the United States.

TIP! If you think you have some undesired sperm hanging around, you can call the following toll-free number to find out the correct medication to take for emergency contraception: 800-584-9911. If you can't remember that number and can't find this book, ask the 800 operator for the emergency contraception phone number.

What's New

Contraceptive research in the U.S. has slowed to a glacial pace since about the 1970s. Political posturing, liability concerns, and bureaucratic regulation have all played roles in the domestic slowing of research in the U.S. Other industrialized countries and even Third World countries have benefited much more from new contraceptive devices and techniques than we have (Reichman 1996, Grimes 1997). In spite of this, several new methods are on the horizon:

- Injectables that last six to eight months are being investigated, as compared to Depo-Provera, which lasts three months.

- Spermicides are being developed that are stronger and will inhibit HIV, chlamydia, trichomonas, and other infectious agents from multiplying in the vagina or from adhering to vaginal walls. They are being tested in new disposable diaphragms.

- Progestin gel may be available to rub into your skin.

- Biodegradable implants using only two capsules are on the horizon (Grimes 1997).

- Biodegradable pellets containing progestin are being developed. They are about the size of a rice kernel, can be injected under the skin, and dissolve after two years. A similar method using a biodegradable micro capsule containing a time-release hormone will be injected and is intended to provide contraception for one to six months.

- Research is under way on a vaccine to immunize against the pregnancy hormone hCG, which is necessary to maintain an early pregnancy. Vaccines may also be developed to attack sperm or to oppose a fertilized egg (Reichman 1996).

Permanent Sterilization

If you are interested in methods of permanent sterilization, you have several options.

Tubal Ligation

A *tubal ligation* is a permanent solution to birth control, right? Well, not exactly! The latest statistics show the failure rate to be 1.8 percent, not 0.1 as was thought in the past (Grimes 1997). The failure rates of the IUD and birth control pills are lower than that! The purpose of this surgical procedure is to obstruct the fallopian tubes, preventing the egg from traveling downstream and the sperm from traveling upstream. Several techniques may be employed to do this. The most common is to cut the tube, remove a segment of it, and tie off the cut ends. Other methods involve cauterizing the tube at one or more sites to obstruct it with scar tissue or pulling a loop of tube into a plastic ring, which then constricts and obstructs the tube. In some, but not all, cases, tubal ligation can be reversed.

Hysterectomy

If you have small fibroids, heavy periods, menstrual cramps, prolapse (sagging uterus), or stress incontinence, you will benefit from a vaginal *hysterectomy*. A hysterectomy is another form of permanent sterilization. A vaginal hysterectomy (removing the uterus through the vagina) has a shorter recovery period than an abdominal operation. Your ovaries can be left behind so you continue to produce hormones; but you won't bleed anymore, and you can't get pregnant. Also, with you uterus gone, when you reach menopause you can take estrogen alone instead of the combination therapy recommended for other women.

A lot has been made in recent years about the feeling that sex changes after a hysterectomy. Critics say that the cervix is necessary to normal sexual enjoyment and orgasmic competence. As a result, these assumptions and opinions have been carefully evaluated. Several investigators have studied the psychosexual impact of a hysterectomy and all found either no change or a better sex life after the operation. There was no difference in the incidence of orgasm whether the cervix was left behind or removed (Nathorst et al. 1993, Virtanen et al. 1993, Dwyer et al. 1993, Helstom et al. 1993). Masters and Johnson (1966) established that as a woman becomes sexually aroused, her vagina elongates, and the cervix and uterus are actually pulled out of the way during vaginal thrusting. After a hysterectomy, there is no change in either the length of the vagina or the sensations experienced.

Summary

Pregnancy during perimenopause may stir a variety of emotions, depending upon where you are in your life plan. You may be concerned that a pregnancy at this age will be fraught with health difficulties for you and risks for a fetus. You may fear that you cannot become pregnant, although you still want to try. You may feel you have completed your childbearing years and be concerned that you might become pregnant again. This chapter has addressed all these areas of uncertainty. As you have learned, all the answers aren't in yet, but you have a number of options for dealing with a midlife pregnancy.

O O O

4

PMS Can Change You: Premenstrual Syndrome in Your Transitional Years

Hippocrates (as in the Hippocratic Oath) wrote about menstrual disorders for the first time in recorded history. He coined the term *hysteria*, thought to be caused by the uterus "wandering" throughout the body, causing trouble wherever it went. Premenstrual tension was described in 1931 (Frank), but the term *premenstrual syndrome* was coined by Dr. Katharina Dalton in 1953. Who cares what it's called! It's real, and it can make you feel as though you aren't in control of your emotions. It's as though you are suddenly outside of yourself, watching in horror as you make really stupid mistakes and comments. The bad news here is that it gets worse during the perimenopausal years (Leventhal 1997, Revlin 1990). The good news is that it goes away once you reach menopause. This chapter will give you a clearer understanding of whether or not you have PMS, what causes it, and how you can treat it.

Diagnosis

Premenstrual syndrome (PMS) is defined as a variable collection of physical and psychological/emotional symptoms recurring on a regular basis in the week or two preceding a menstrual period. It includes symptoms such as mood disturbances, headache, bloating, and weight gain. PMS doesn't affect every woman, but some of the symptoms affect 85 to 90 percent of women (Parker 1994)—and maybe the other 10 to 15 percent just aren't paying attention! In diagnosing PMS, doctors look for the following general conditions:

- **Time of onset:** The symptoms must begin during the two weeks before your menstrual period is due—the luteal phase of your cycle.

- **Duration of symptoms:** The symptoms must resolve within one or two days after the start of your menstrual bleeding.

- **Symptom-free period:** There must be a symptom-free period during the first week after your menstrual period. The first two weeks of your cycle are called the *follicular phase.*

- **Persistence of symptoms:** Your symptoms must be present over several menstrual cycles, and they must not be accounted for by some other disorder.

- **Severity:** Your PMS symptoms *must* be severe enough to disrupt your normal lifestyle. Sound familiar? You are not alone. Ten percent of women experience symptoms severe enough to disrupt their lives (Parker 1995).

There are over 150 symptoms ascribed to PMS. The most common of these are insomnia, anger, depression, forgetfulness, sore breasts, weight gain, headaches (including menstrual migraines), tearfulness, acne, and recurrent cold sores. A more complete list can be found in Table 4-1. About 70 percent of PMS sufferers also report one or more *positive* symptoms, such as increased sex drive, greater creativity, and more energy. (At least there's a ray of light!)

Premenstrual syndrome is now recognized as a valid diagnosis by psychiatrists in the latest edition of the *Diagnostic and Statistical Manual of Mental Disorders.* There has been a move to change the name to premenstrual dysphoric disorder (PDD), although it's probably way too late to make a dent in the well-established public acceptance of the term *premenstrual syndrome.* To make the specific diagnosis of PDD, you must have one of the following four symptoms and four other symptoms, either from this list or from the Emotional or Behavioral list found in Table 4-1:

- Depressed mood

- Marked anxiety

- Sudden tearfulness, sadness, or increased sensitivity to rejection

- Persistent anger or interpersonal conflicts

Table 4.1.
Common Symptoms of PMS

Physical	Emotional or Behavioral
Breast swelling and tenderness	Anxiety
Fluid retention and weight gain	Depression
Headaches, migraines	Tearfulness
Bloating	Anger
Fatigue	Hostility
Acne, cold sores	Aggression
Heart palpitations	Mood fluctuations
Constipation	Irritability
Dizziness	Forgetfulness
Muscle aches	Poor concentration
Hot flashes	Insomnia
Sleepiness	Food cravings
	Sexual desire up or down
	Poor coping skills
	Panic attacks
	Suicidal attempts
	Feeling overwhelmed or out of control
	Lethargy

Adapted from: American Psychiatric Association. 1996. *Diagnostic and Statistical Manual of Mental Disorders.*

Causes of PMS

Whatever you call it, hormones from all over the body have been implicated in PMS. They include

- Ovarian hormones (estrogen and progesterone)
- Pituitary hormones (FSH, LH, and possibly prolactin)
- Endorphins (produced in the mid brain and hypothalamus) and adrenal hormones
- Neurotransmitters

Serotonin, a neurotransmitter in the brain thought to be responsible for chemical depression, is now felt to be the main player in PMS (Barnhart et al. 1995), but your symptoms probably come from a combination of factors.

Hormones

First of all, it really isn't just your raging hormones that are to blame. It is a combination of your ovarian hormones plus your cortisone, serotonin, endorphins, heredity, and life stresses. Premenstrual syndrome knows no boundaries. PMS does not correlate with race, culture, marital status, or education. It seems to be more prevalent in perimenopausal mothers who work outside the home (Ekholm and Backstrom 1994).

Heredity

You've probably heard this one: "PMS has been found to be hereditary—you get it from your kids!" Actually, it may indeed be hereditary. Studies of identical twins (Condon 1993; Kendler et al. 1992) show a 93 percent chance of their both having PMS. (There is a lesser correlation in fraternal twins.) If your mother had PMS, you are more likely to have it too (Wilson et al. 1991).

Diet

Certain dietary excesses are known to aggravate PMS, including the following:

- **Salt:** Most women experiencing PMS will have increased their salt and carbohydrate intake premenstrually and thereby unwittingly increased their PMS symptoms.
- **Sugar:** A high intake of sweets results in salt retention by your body. The increased presence of salt causes fluid retention and increases premenstrual bloating.
- **Caffeine:** Consumption of large amounts of caffeine, found in coffee, tea, colas, and chocolate, has been reported (Barnhart et al. 1995; Parker 1994) to worsen the symptoms of PMS. Caffeine can increase anxiety, tension, depression, and irritability and contribute to insomnia.

Nonhormonal Treatment of PMS

A wide variety of nonhormonal options are available to help you manage the symptoms of PMS.

Diet

In the last section, we pointed out several dietary factors that can contribute to PMS; changing what you eat and drink can make a difference. A diet rich in carbohydrates diminishes mood swings.

Sugars—including fructose and sucrose—are simple carbohydrates. Vegetables, fruits (but not fruit juice, which has no pulp), legumes, rice, pasta, and so on, are complex carbohydrates. Both vegetables and fruits have simple sugars within them. When cooked, some vegetables (potatoes and carrots, for example) release their simple sugars.

Serotonin building blocks are found in complex carbohydrates, so the "carbo-cravings" so common in PMS may indicate a natural need to increase serotonin levels. For years, the recommendation for PMS sufferers was to increase proteins and limit simple carbohydrates (donuts, cakes, sweets, and so on). More recently, however, there is increasing evidence that meals high in *complex* carbohydrates and low in protein improve mood symptoms of PMS sufferers, including depression, tension, anger, confusion, fatigue, and alertness (Barnhart et al. 1995).

Sweet attack! Sweet attack! You know that as you near your menstrual periods, you crave sweets. The fact is that hypoglycemia, or low blood sugar, does not occur premenstrually any more often than at any other time in your cycle (Barnhart et al. 1995). If you succumb to your sweet craving, the sugar you take aboard causes water retention and results in bloating. What to do about it? At times like this, change your *sweet attack* signal to a *complex carbohydrate attack.* You should try to limit sweets and emphasize grains, vegetables, pastas, and fruits. These are all complex carbohydrates that will help your symptoms. Watch out, though: One penalty for a sudden increase in complex carbohydrates, which dramatically increases your fiber intake, is that it can produce a lot of gas.

Fluid retention and bloating are common complaints during the premenstrual period. Many women gain more than five pounds each month. You might think that if you restricted your salt intake, water retention would be reduced. This sounds like it would work, but it doesn't. The solution to fluid retention and bloating, surprisingly enough, is to *increase* your water intake. Hard to believe it works, but it does. Increased water pulls salt from the tissues, and it is excreted in the urine. The more water you drink, the more salt-laden fluid your excrete.

Vitamins & Minerals

Let's take a look at the effects of several vitamins and minerals on decreasing or eliminating PMS symptoms.

Vitamin B6

In doses of 100 to 150 mg a day throughout the month, vitamin B6 may help symptoms of PMS. This vitamin is necessary in the synthesis of serotonin and prostaglandins, which play a role in PMS. *Prostaglandins* are chemicals manufactured throughout the body that exert a hormone-like effect and influence involuntary muscular contraction (including the uterus), circulation, and inflammation. B-6 supplements have been used in the treatment of PMS for years. Complaints of fatigue, irritability, and depression may respond to this vitamin.

CAUTION! More B6 is not always better. There have been many reports (Parker 1994, Dalton and Dalton 1987, London et al. 1991, Schaumburg et al. 1983, Parry et al. 1985) of permanent nerve damage with as little as 200 mg a day.

Vitamin E

Vitamin E offers some relief from sore breasts. The dosage needed is 600 to 800 units a day, not 400 units (Leventhal 1997, Severino and Moline 1995). Vitamin E is an antioxidant, and probably the only one that works as well in its synthetic form as in its natural food source. *Antioxidants* are the garbage collectors of the body. They neutralize toxins and clear them out of the body so they cannot link up and destroy normal body tissues. Vitamins A, C, and E are well-known antioxidants, but zinc, selenium, and beta-carotene are too.

TIP! While we're on the subject of antioxidants, the latest nutritional advice is to increase the intake of antioxidants by eating more foods that contain the various antioxidants, such as salmon and other cold water fish, broccoli, and other members of the cabbage family instead of ingesting beta-carotene supplements.

To date, no toxic effects have been noted with 400 to 800 units daily of vitamin E. This vitamin is also good for your heart and cholesterol, decreases breast tenderness, and decreases those little lumps in your breast called fibrocysts. In 1996, Dr. Jeanne Leventhal reported on vitamin E in a *double-blind study,* meaning that neither the woman nor the investigator knew who was on a placebo and who was on vitamin E. (A *placebo* is an inert compound that appears to be identical to a compound being tested in experimental research. In placebo studies, some participants take the substance being tested, and some take the placebo. Any benefit perceived by a participant taking the placebo is called the *placebo effect.*) Results: 85 percent of the women on vitamin E reported a significant reduction in breast symptoms. If breast tenderness is your major PMS complaint, vitamin E may help.

Calcium and Magnesium

Calcium and magnesium show modest success in reducing PMS symptoms. (Note: Single mineral therapy with other minerals, such as zinc and copper, have never been shown to diminish the symptoms of PMS.) Both are necessary for your nerves to transmit impulses. Several studies have shown both minerals to be of some benefit for PMS in the following doses: Calcium 1,000 mg a day (Thy-Jacobs et al. 1989); magnesium 1,080 mg, which is twice the dose recommended for ordinary use (Fachinetti et al. 1991). Both calcium and magnesium can help relieve mental as well as physical symptoms of PMS. Almost all over-the-counter PMS medications contain both magnesium and calcium.

CAUTION! In addition to causing loose stools, using twice the normal dose of magnesium can prevent adequate calcium absorption and increase your risk of osteoporosis in later years (see Chapter 5). For this reason, take the increased magnesium dose only premenstrually, and discontinue it as soon as your period starts.

L-Tryptophan

Taking an oral medication called L-tryptophan significantly reduces PMS symptoms, especially irritability (Steinberg 1991, Leventhal 1996). L-tryptophan converts to tryptophan in the body. Tryptophan is an *amino acid* (protein building block) that is in most common proteins, such as milk. Tryptophan helps PMS because it is a precursor for serotonin, a neurotransmitter that promotes relaxation. (That explains why mothers give babies warm milk before bedtime!) The usual dose of L-tryptophan is six grams per day.

The good news is that L-tryptophan is an over-the-counter medication that works. The bad news is that it is off the market because of a bad *batch* of the product in Japan, which caused several deaths. It was the filler in this batch, not L-tryptophan itself, that caused the problem, but it was removed from the market nonetheless.

Exercise

Muscle contractions of your lower legs force extra fluid out of your tissues and into your bloodstream. This is why walking, jogging, bicycle riding, and swimming all help get rid of those puffy feet. Aerobic exercise has been demonstrated to decrease the severity of the negative mood and some of the physical symptoms associated with PMS. Aerobic exercise (walking, jogging, swimming, biking) is superior to strength training (weight lifting) in reducing premenstrual symptoms (Moline 1993, Pearlstein et al. 1992). Research has shown that *frequency*, such as 30 minutes daily, rather than *intensity*, is the most important in ameliorating your symptoms and increasing your feeling of self-worth. There is, however, no evidence that increased *endorphins* (morphine-like chemicals made in the brain in response to exercise, pain, and stress) released in vigorous exercise have any effect on PMS. (For more information about exercise, see Chapter 10.)

Evening Primrose Oil

Evening primrose oil is extracted from the seeds of the evening primrose. The oil contains vitamin E, prostaglandins, linolenic acid, and several other active substances that are said to be responsible for its therapeutic effects on a number of conditions. There have been four trials comparing evening primrose oil with a placebo for the treatment of PMS (Kleijnenn 1994). These studies found some benefit in the treatment of premenstrual breast tenderness. In 1990, Khoo found no differences between evening primrose oil and a placebo in the treatment of other symptoms of PMS (Leventhal 1997).

Behavioral Modification for Mild PMS

Gaining control over your life and its stresses reduces the impact of PMS. Stress control, relaxation techniques, meditation, changes in your diet, and exercise programs have all been shown to help. Prayer is thought to be of benefit, possibly in the same way meditation has been shown to help. Unfortunately, for women with severe PMS, the symptoms themselves disrupt their lifestyle rather than the other way around—PMS turns out to be the stressor. Still, it's beneficial to have a handle on other stresses in your life. To improve your chances of successfully coping with PMS, the following are some stress management goals that can help:

- Try not to take everything personally.
- Learn to accept what you are not in a position to control.
- Avoid unnecessary complications; simplify your life.
- Do not procrastinate. (That's a big one!)
- Judge yourself by your own standards to bolster self-esteem.
- Avoid being judgmental of others.
- Exercise every day.

Do's and don'ts are easy to list; but they are frequently difficult to accomplish, especially when it comes to modifying your behavior. (For a more thorough discussion of stress management, be sure to read Chapter 12.)

Sleeping Aids

Insomnia and early awakening are very common complaints in peri-menopause. The cause of the insomnia is usually a hot flash during the night, or simply feeling warm. (You may not recognize it as a hot flash.) If you do sleep all night, you may still feel tired when you awaken. Regardless of your perception of what is wrong, it is almost always due to decreased estrogen. Estrogen supplements can make a big difference, especially if you take them at bedtime (Revlin et al. 1990, Leventhal 1997).

There are also several lifestyle changes you can make to help alleviate this disruptive occurrence. Sleeping pills do not work; after you have taken them for some time, your body adjusts to them, and you simply fall back to your old pattern of sleeplessness. Some further behavioral modification can help here:

- **Avoid caffeinated beverages after lunch:** If this doesn't help, stop them all together. As mentioned above, go off them gradually to avoid withdrawal symptoms.

- **Avoid alcohol within four hours of bedtime:** Although alcohol is a depressant, it has an excitatory phase following the sedative phase. If the four-hour restriction doesn't help, stopping altogether may.

- **Continue to exercise, but do so in the morning or afternoon:** If you exercise within three or four hours of going to bed, you may be too stimulated to get to sleep.

- **Do not eat a heavy meal just before retiring:** Take a light snack if you need food shortly before bedtime.

- **Do something relaxing for the hour or so before going to bed:** In other words, don't pay your bills, study for school, or work.

- **Stop worrying about getting to sleep:** This is the most important item! Just let it happen.

When PMS isn't helped by behavioral modification and diet changes, you may need to use medication.

TIP! You may be using melatonin to help you sleep. Melatonin has been reported to reduce serotonin levels, so you may find your PMS is becoming a lot worse. If so, it is best to avoid using melatonin during the second half of your menstrual cycle.

"Give Me Drugs!"

Many different medications have been used to decrease or eliminate PMS. Physical symptoms can usually be easily treated. None of them have proven to be a cure, but many are helpful. For example, diuretics reduce fluid retention, and a nonsteroidal anti-inflammatory drug (NSAID) like Naproxen or Ibuprofen will help headaches.

Prior to the advent of selective serotonin reuptake inhibitors (SSRIs), such as Prozac, Paxil, and Zoloff, the only effective medications for the psychological symptoms of PMS were those that worked by altering or halting ovarian activity. The problem with this approach is that your ovaries alone aren't responsible for PMS; however, ovarian function is necessary for PMS to flourish. Therefore, it isn't surprising that hormonal investigations were so extensive.

Let's take a closer look at some of these medications.

Diuretics

Most diuretics help reduce bloating, weight gain, fluid retention, and sore breasts. A type of diuretic called spironolactone has become the most popular for the treatment of PMS related fluid retention (Mortola 1994; Parker 1994; Barnhart et al. 1995). The dose is 25 mg twice a day, taken premenstrually. Although spironolactone is very effective for fluid excess, it has been disappointing in its effect on emotional symptoms. Potassium loss is a worry with spironalactone, as with all diuretics. Prolonged use of spironolactone also can cause cramping and diarrhea, drowsiness, headache, and (rarely) mental confusion. Other diuretics are generally reserved for patients who have no success with spironolactone therapy.

CAUTION! Diuretics sometimes become drugs of abuse, especially in women who are highly concerned about excess weight.

Nonsteroidal Anti-Inflammatory Drugs (NSAIDs)

Some women get menstrual cramps before their period begins. *Nonsteroidal anti-inflammatory drugs* (NSAIDs) helps both these cramps and cramps during the menstrual period. In 1980, Wood and Jakubowicz, in a double-blind study, found NSAIDs to show an improvement in PMS symptoms, including emotional disturbances. However, their patients included menstrual as well as premenstrual symptoms. NSAIDs help physical PMS symptoms and are the first choice for menstrual cramps, but don't help emotional symptoms as well as other medications (Mortola 1994).

The chemicals called prostaglandins are known to be responsible for menstrual cramps. Actually, they make the uterus contract during labor, too. Before they were discovered, menstrual cramps were thought to be psychological. The discovery that NSAIDs are anti-prostaglandins led to their use to temper the pain many women experienced. Ibuprofen and Naproxen have become the mainstays for treating menstrual cramps. In a 1980 double-blind study of NSAIDs, Wood and Jakubowitz reported an overall improvement in PMS symptoms, including emotional disturbances, headaches, dizziness, and weakness. The major usage of these drugs, however, is for the treatment of pelvic pain, backache, and menstrual cramps.

CAUTION! NSAIDs often cause stomach upset, can lead to ulcers, and, in the elderly and diabetic, may cause kidney problems if used over a prolonged period of time.

Selective Serotonin Reuptake Inhibitors (SSRIs)

The most commonly known *selective serotonin reuptake inhibitor* (SSRI) is Prozac. How do SSRIs work? As you know, serotonin is a neurotransmitter chemical. It is produced by the neurons (brain cells) and conducts electrical impulses across the synapse from one neuron to the next. Serotonin is stored inside the neuron, near the synapse. When a neuron sends an impulse, serotonin is released by that cell. The serotonin jumps the gap and attaches to a serotonin receptor site on the next neuron, from where it passes along the impulse. With us so far?

When serotonin is outside the neuron and attached to receptor sites, it has, among other influences, a calming effect on moods. Neurons can take the serotonin back inside, however, and when they do this in sufficient quantities, the calming effect is diminished or lost. An SSRI keeps the neurons from taking up serotonin. This is why SSRIs are so effective in the treatment of premenstrual symptoms (Stone et al. 1990). With more serotonin available, your sense of well-being is enhanced; serotonin lets you go a few extra miles.

Serotonin levels are decreased in the late luteal phase of women with PMS. This discovery has finally pinned down a chemical cause for severe symptoms of PMS and led the way to a treatment that works. In 1995, Steiner et al. reported on a PMS study involving seven university-affiliated clinics in Canada. They studied fluoxetine in patients with PMS severe enough to impair their daily lives. They were assigned randomly in a double-blind fashion to receive either fluoxetine (Prozac) or a placebo for six months. The results showed a 7 percent improvement in those patients using the placebo, but 44 to 52 percent improvement in the patients receiving fluoxetine. Twenty milligrams a day was the ideal dose for most patients. Four other earlier studies showed similar results using other SSRIs (Zoloft, Paxil, Effexor, and Serzone). These drugs become effective for PMS symptoms within three weeks of continuous use. One study even showed that a woman can take fluoxetine premenstrually only, as opposed to continuous use. It appears to improve mood, anxiety, concentration, and some physical symptoms, such as bloating.

CAUTION! Medications such as fluoxetine appear to be safe for everyone *except* people with a bipolar depression (what used to be called manic-depression). See Chapter 12 for a more complete discussion of this disorder.

The major problems with SSRIs are insomnia or disturbed sleep, sleepiness, shakiness, headache, and lack of orgasm. You can alleviate the sleep disturbance by changing the time you take the medication: If the medication makes you sleepy during the day, take it at night; if it keeps you awake, take it in the morning. Most people find the side effects decrease over time (Barnhart et al. 1995).

Tranquilizers such as Xanax (alprazolam), Ativan (lorazepam), Valium (diazepam), and Buspar (buspirone), which are not SSRIs, may help some mood changes. Some psychiatrists suggest taking these medications the week before a period is expected, to treat irritability. However, all of them except Buspar are addicting, and you may get withdrawal symptoms unless you decrease them gradually. By contrast, if you don't like the effects of an SSRI, you can just stop taking it, without fear of withdrawal symptoms.

There are some downside considerations. SSRIs work wonders for most people, but for about 5 to 30 percent of women and men, there may be problems with sexual desire or orgasm. Desire may be lessened and/or orgasms diminished or absent. (Some men experience the inability to ejaculate. It's the male version of anorgasmia.) If you consider that one of the only good things about PMS is your increased interest in sex, it may sound like you've thrown out the baby with the bath water. Luckily, this symptom is dose related and sometimes goes away on its own. If not, switching to a different SSRI may help. (Note: The older antidepressants, tricyclics [not SSRIs] like Tofranil and Elavil, have many more side effects than do SSRIs. The old-timers don't mess with your sex life, but they don't treat PMS either!)

There will soon be a new generation of SSRIs that will not have this annoying side effect. These SSRIs will be more site-specific than those currently available. In other words, the new SSRIs will be able to attach to only those receptors in your cells that influence your PMS or depressive symptoms. They will leave your sexuality alone (Leventhal 1997).

Hormone Treatment and PMS

Premenstrual syndrome is almost exclusively the result of normal menstrual cycles. Fluctuations in the hormones without ovulation have been associated with PMS-like symptoms, but those symptoms are rarely as severe as when ovulation takes place (Rubinow 1992). For thirty years, researchers and clinicians alike have thought that variations of estrogen and progesterone were in some way causative of the 150 PMS symptoms that plague so many perimenopausal women. Over the years, all sorts of hormonal manipulation has been tried, with varied success. With each subsequent generation, a new "cure-all" emerges. Each one claims to eliminate the plethora of annoying to life-altering symptoms we know as PMS. The latest of these brouhahas is the use of "natural" progesterone. Let's see whether progesterone in any form has any effect on the course or cure of PMS.

Progesterone Therapy—Does it Have An Effect of PMS?

In the early to mid-1980s it would have been hearsay to say that progesterone therapy had no effect on PMS! Let's look at the evidence that led investigators to conclude that progesterone was effective in treating PMS. Then we will discuss more recent research which demonstrates that progesterone is no more effective that a placebo in the treatment of PMS.

Investigators in the late seventies and early eighties concluded that progesterone was effective in treating most women with PMS. Here are the reasons. Mid-cycle, your progesterone levels rise, late in your cycle, your progesterone levels begin to drop and that's when PMS occurs. The drop in progesterone late in the cycle led researcher to believe that the addition of progesterone at that time might alleviate PMS symptoms, and it does: 60–80 percent of the time. Furthermore, seventy percent of women who take birth control pills no longer experience symptoms of PMS. Birth control pills contain *both* synthetic progesterone and estrogen and this provided further evidence that progesterone was effective in the alleviation of PMS symptoms.

Twenty to forty percent of women's symptoms were not helped by the addition of progesterone or birth control pills, so investigators continued to look for other ways to relieve PMS symptoms. Because women developed PMS when their *natural progesterone* levels fell, investigators reasoned that the addition of natural progesterone, as opposed to *synthetic* progesterone might help and it did—70 to 80 percent of the time.

We now know that natural progesterone is more gentle than synthetic progesterone without the same side effects, which account for the somewhat better results using natural instead of synthetic progesterones. The principal side effect of progesterone is the reduction of serotonin levels in the brain. Serotonin is a neurotransmitter that has a potent calming influence and helps modulate mood. Natural progesterone reduces serotonin levels less than does synthetic progesterone.

Natural progesterone suppositories were the main therapy for PMS during the eighties. At that time there was no way for natural progesterone to be absorbed if taken orally. The only way to get natural progesterone into the body was by injection or through the vagina with suppositories. The dosage of those suppositories ranged from 100 to 800 mg, and they were used twice daily. Natural progesterone therapy created quite a stir: specialty pharmacies that made the suppositories opened up, books were written, and advocates hit the lecture circuit. Up to 80 percent of the women using birth control pills or natural progesterone suppositories successfully treated their PMS. The remaining 20 percent were treated with diuretics and tranquilizers. Investigators were still hopeful that progesterone therapy would be the answer, so they continued their research.

Placebo double-blind studies were started to provide proof of benefit. To prove a medication helps PMS, it must show a higher efficacy than a placebo, and it must be possible for other investigators to duplicate the results. There is a high placebo effect when studying PMS—as high as 80 percent (Mortola 1992, Parker 1994) which compares to an 80 percent effective- ness of natural progesterone. In eight out of ten women, the placebo was just as effective as the progesterone. In the other 20 percent of women, neither the placebo nor the progesterone had any effects (Dennerstein et al. 1985, Magos and Studd 1985, Smith and Schiff 1993).

In 1990, Freeman, Rickels and Sondheimer studied placebos versus pro- gesterone suppositories of 400 to 800 mg and found *no difference* between the two groups in the reduction of PMS symptoms.

In 1991, Schmidt measured progesterone blood levels. He also measured progesterone precursors as well as progesterone breakdown products (meta- bolites). He found no differences between women suffering from PMS and those who did not.

Both of these studies concluded that PMS is not due to a progesterone state and that women are not benefited by the addition of progesterone, either natural or synthetic any more than from a placebo.

Phyto Hormones

Phyto hormones are found in a variety of plants. They are currently popu- lar for treating PMS because they occur naturally in plant life, and natural hormones are often perceived as safer or more effective than synthetic hor- mones. Phyto hormones are a form of natural progesterone. But think about this: Natural progesterone is the same hormone you make in the second half of your menstrual cycle, and the studies we described above have indicated that increased natural progesterone doesn't relieve PMS symptoms.

Progestins and PMS

Since natural progesterone cannot be absorbed if taken orally, the pro- gesterone molecule was chemically changed to make it absorbable. These synthetic hormones, called progestins, are one of the hormones in birth control pills and are used to control abnormal bleeding. Not only have progestins not helped in the treatment of PMS, they can make it worse; when given to postmenopausal women to help prevent abnormal bleeding and cancer, they can cause a PMS-like syndrome.

Micronized Natural Progesterone and Creams

Because of the problems with progestins, scientists have tried to find ways to adapt natural progesterone in the hopes of avoiding the side effects of the progestins yet retaining the benefits, which led to some interesting discoveries. Natural progesterone is extracted from wild Mexican yams and soy beans. It *can* be absorbed orally, but only when the progesterone has been pulverized into minute particles, a process called micronization. Micronized progesterone can be absorbed from the intestine. In this form, it can also be rubbed into the skin and absorbed. Several studies of the efficacy of progesterone cream for uses other than PMS are ongoing in Europe and are quite promising. There are, at last count, twenty-seven different progesterone creams on the market. These "natural progesterone creams" contain varying amounts of progesterone per ounce. Many of the phyto hormone creams add a number of other chemicals—chamomile extract, Chinese herbs (black cohosh, burdock root, and ginseng), aloe vera, and vitamin E—to the basic yam extract. They claim to help all sorts of female problems, but none have been reliably tested against a placebo.

The phyto progesterone creams, made from micronized natural progesterone, are rubbed into the skin. This allows them to be absorbed directly into the bloodstream without having to be processed by the liver. Women who use the creams hope to diminish their PMS symptoms. They start using the cream mid cycle, right after ovulation, and continue its use until their menstrual period begins. Although many of these women claim great relief from a myriad of PMS complaints, their reports have been anecdotal—reports of individual responses as opposed to formal scientific study. The double-blind placebo studies showed no difference between placebo and progesterone cream. Don't be fooled by the claims that these creams will help—they won't (Dennerstein et al. 1985, Magos and Studd 1985, Smith and Schiff 1993). European studies have shown that women get some relief from breast tenderness by rubbing small amounts of progestin or natural progesterone directly into the breast skin (Mauvais-Jarvis et al. 1978; Ayers and Jidwani 1983).

Estrogen May Help

Many pre-menopauseal women use the estrogen skin patch successfully to alleviate anxiety, migraine headaches and negative feeling associated with PMS. Drs. Jeanne Leventhal (1996) and William Bates (Revlin et al 1990) believe that estrogen is not a cure for most PMS but does *cure* the PMS that has its onset during the *premenopausal* years (the 5 years before the onset of menopause). Dr. Bates feels that premenopausal PMS is really due to a late luteal phase decline in estrogen levels. If you have never had significant PMS prior to age 45 to 50, extra estrogen (by either patch or pill) during the week to ten days before your period is due will usually relieve your symptoms. Unfortunately, your bloating, sore breasts or menstrual cramps will not be helped and your menstrual flow may get a little heavier.

How do you use the patch? Apply the patch once you begin to experience PMS symptoms. Place the patch away from your breasts and away from skin creases. The patch will begin to work within an hour.

CAUTION! Ten percent of women using the patch get a skin rash sufficient to discontinue its use.

If your PMS symptoms are very predictable, beginning like clockwork, you may get relief from taking oral estrogen, such as low dose Estrace. Estrace is taken every day beginning seven to ten days before the expected menstrual period.

Monocyclic birth control pills provide constant levels of estrogen and progesterone. This is in contrast to tricyclic birth control pills, in which both estrogen and progesterone doses vary throughout the month. Monocyclic pills produce significant relief from PMS for the majority of women (Cullberg 1972, Forrest 1979). This is thought to be due to the constant levels of estrogen and progesterone. Some women find their symptoms are worse on the pill, regardless of whether it is mono- or tricyclic; these women have an adverse sensitivity to progesterone (Leventhal 1996).

CAUTION! Migraine headaches may first appear with the use of birth control pills, in which case they must be discontinued.

Prevention of Ovarian Function

Prevention of ovarian function cures PMS, but the cure may be worse than the disease! It is known that ovarian function is necessary for PMS to occur, although many other factors come into play in production of the symptoms. This stimulated medical interest in determining whether inhibiting ovarian activity would be beneficial. The good news is that it does. The bad news is there are downside problems.

GnRH Agonists

GnRH agonists (Lupron-Depot, Synarel) relieve PMS but cause bone loss. Used to treat endometriosis, GnRH agonists prevent ovulation by shutting down the pituitary gland and, therefore, the ovary and its hormones. After the initial administration of a GnRH agonist, there is an outpouring of FSH and LH reserves from the pituitary gland, which increases estrogen and progesterone levels. PMS symptoms may get worse for a short period of time. Once the pituitary shuts down, though, PMS shuts down, too. Unfortunately, once a woman's estrogen level drops, she is thrown into a false menopause. With it come the accompanying risks for osteoporosis and heart disease, not to mention hot flashes, memory loss, and vaginal dryness. "Add-back" therapy, using low doses of estrogen with or without progesterone (discussed in Chapter 8), have been successful in the relief of these symptoms without worsening PMS in other ways. At about $400 a month, treatment with GnRH agonists is extremely expensive.

Danazol

Danazol is a testosterone derivative that also shuts down the pituitary and thereby suppresses ovarian hormones, so PMS symptoms are stopped. In double-blind studies (Watts 1987; Sarno 1987; Dalton 1987; Derzko 1990; Halbreich 1991), danazol is superior to placebos in reducing overall symptomatology, both physical and mental. However, danazol itself has side effects that can mimic those of PMS, including depression, weight gain, and bloating. Since the drug is derived from testosterone (see Chapter 8), it may also cause decreased breast size, acne, excess hair growth, and deepening of the voice. (If you use your voice professionally, be especially leery of taking this drug. Long-term danazol use may accelerate cardiovascular disease. If danazol is used only premenstrually, however, it markedly reduces breast tenderness, mood swings, and irritability without the long-term adverse effects. This is also an expensive medication, costing about $43 per cycle.

Ovarian Removal

All studies on the surgical treatment of PMS show that a hysterectomy *without* removal of the ovaries does nothing to improve PMS symptoms. Removal of the ovaries, however, does relieve the symptoms completely. If you are under forty and lose your ovaries, though, you will have great difficulty adjusting your estrogen replacement therapy (Riggs and Melton 1986). Inconsistent levels will result in an increase in the risk of osteoporosis and heart disease, even with replacement therapy. Therefore, ovarian removal should be considered only as an absolute last resort.

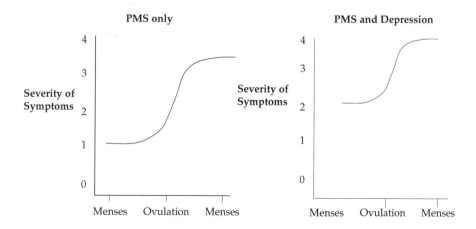

Figure 4.1. Premenstrual Syndrome with Depression

Depression and PMS

"I don't have any good days; my symptoms just get worse before my period." Does this sound like you? If it does, then you may have an underlying depression that is worsened by your PMS. Psychiatrists call this *premenstrual magnification*. Figure 4-1 illustrates the difference between PMS and depression worsened by PMS. As you can see from the graphs, severity of symptoms is the same in the second half of the cycle, after ovulation, but the symptoms increase in the first half. There are a number of depressive disorders ranging from major life-altering depression to disorders with only mild emotional effects, but they share similar symptoms. (See Chapter 12 for a fuller discussion of types of depression in relation to stress.

Menstrual Migraines

Menstrual migraines are severe headaches occurring a few days before your menstrual period is due to start, or the first few days of your bleeding. What is the difference between a migraine headache and the more common tension headache? Table 4.2 illustrates the how they differ.

Table 4.2. Characteristics Differentiating Migraines from Tension Headaches		
Characteristics	**Migraine Headaches**	**Tension Headaches**
Location	One or both sides	Both sides
Frequency	Intermittent	Intermittent
Duration	8 hours (2–72 hours)	Variable
Pain	Throbbing (50%)	Often Band-like
Severity	Moderate to Severe	Mild to Moderate
Associated symptoms	Nausea, Vomiting, Photophobia	Uncommon
Family History	Often Present	Present

Adapted from: S.D. Silberstein. 1990. "Advance in the Understanding the Pathology of Headaches." *Neurology.* 42(2):6–10.

Symptoms

Migraines are caused by a constriction of blood vessels in the brain, followed by dilation of these same vessels and then swelling of the vessel walls. The dilated vessels are painful, and the swelling prevents them from returning to normal size. Migraines often have an aura associated with them that coincides with the initial constriction of the blood vessels. Symptoms during the aura can include a particular smell, flashing lights, or any other unusual occurrence that doesn't makes sense in terms of what is actually going on. Following the aura, when the vessels dilate, a pounding headache begins. Other symptoms include nausea, vomiting, and photophobia (sensitivity to light). If you experience these symptoms, you end up in bed. They may be severe enough to keep you home for a couple of days. The special distinction of *menstrual* migraines, of course, is that they occur *every month*.

Prevention and Treatment

Let's take a look at some things you can do prevent and treat menstrual migraines.

- **Estrogen:** One of the theories about menstrual migraine is that it results from the change in the estrogen level as it drops just before a period begins. Some women avoid this drop and prevent a migraine with the estrogen skin patch. Patch use begins one week before a period is due. Oral estradiol is superior to other oral estrogens (see Chapter 8) for the treatment of menstrual migraines.

- **NSAIDs:** Some women do well with the antiprostaglandin effects of NSAIDs, which we talked about earlier in this chapter. NSAIDs are taken every six to eight hours for a week before a period is due and into the first two or three days of the menstrual period.

- **Vasoconstrictors:** Two commonly used constrictor drugs are DHE (dihydroergotamine) and sumatriptan succinate. Both are given by injection, though sumatriptan succinate is also available in pill form. The usual treatment is to take the first shot by self-administration at the first sign of the headache, and, if needed, to take a second dose one hour later. Only two shots can be used in a twenty-four-hour period. Because sumatriptan succinate can cause a heart spasm, it is first given in a hospital setting.

- **Prevention with Testosterone:** While the vasoconstrictors described above work quite well for migraines, you would probably prefer to prevent the headache than to treat the symptoms. Some success has been found clinically with the use of testosterone pellets injected beneath the skin (Lanka and Klingman 1997). With this method, the testosterone from the pellet goes directly into the bloodstream. Testosterone is converted into estrogen in a woman's brain (Leventhal 1997). The increased estrogen level in the brain may explain its effectiveness in some patients who have not been helped by other therapy (Lanka and

Klingman 1997). (Note: The new testosterone patch used by men for various reasons contains too high a dose for women. When cut in quarters, the patch may give relief to migraine sufferers and avoid the discomfort of an injection. Unfortunately, cutting the patch into quarters lessens its adhesiveness. See Chapter 8 for more about testosterone.)

- **Alternative medical therapies:** Alternative medical therapies can be remarkably effective in reducing migraine pain. These techniques can be the answer if you have been plagued by medication side effects or choose to use them instead of more conventional treatments. Biofeedback and acupuncture work quite well for many women. These programs usually require a series of treatments, but they are both good for stress reduction, and stress is a well-known migraine trigger. Hypnotherapy, massage therapy, and osteopathic manipulation can also be effective in moderating migraine pain, especially if you seek treatment at a time when you are vulnerable to an attack (such as premenstrually).

Summary

During perimenopause, PMS increases in severity and duration. Current treatment which works better than a placebo includes diuretics for physical symptoms and SSRIs for emotional ones. Physical and emotional symptoms are also mitigated by proper diet and exercise. For women who develop PMS for the first time late in their perimenopause, estrogen treatment may be sufficient. The good new is that PMS symptoms will disappear when you reach menopause.

○ ○ ○

5

Serious Changes: Cardiovascular Disease and Osteoporosis

The topics of this chapter, heart disease and osteoporosis, are late-appearing changes. If you are in the early stages of perimenopause, these problems, if and when they arise, will probably not come up for a number of years. You may be wondering why we've included a chapter on them in this book. The answer is that you are probably interested in making the next half of your life as vibrant and healthy as possible. During the approximately fifteen years of perimenopause, you have a good shot at averting the adverse changes these two conditions can wreak on your body later in life. The seeds for these conditions are being sown during your transition, but there is much you can do to avoid a harvest of ill health. Perimenopause is your wake-up call. Now is the time to learn about cardiovascular disease and osteoporosis so you can become proactive in preventing them. This chapter details the potential threat of each of these health problems and concentrates on preventive measures.

Cardiovascular Disease (CVD)

Alphabet Soup	
CVD	Cardiovascular disease
HDL	High-density lipoprotein
LDH	Low-density lipoprotein

Cardiovascular disease (CVD), which is a disease of the heart and/or vascular system (arteries, veins, and capillaries) is the leading cause of death for women in the United States. Dr. N. K. Wenger's 1993 study showed that every year, 550,000 people die because of CVD, and 250,000 of them are women. Compare that number to 60,000 annual cancer deaths in women over age fifty from all reproductive structures *combined*, including breast, uterus, ovary, cervix, and vagina. For women over fifty, CVD accounts for 53 percent of deaths, compared to 4 percent of deaths from breast cancer. CVD is an enormous public health problem.

The Numbers Are Amazing

Heart and vascular disease have traditionally been considered a male problem. A heart attack in a woman prior to menopause is not common; but men have them commonly in this under-50 age range. With diminishing estrogen, however, the risk of a woman's having a heart attack rises; and by age sixty to seventy, women have the same risk of heart attack as men. Between ages fifty to seventy-five, heart attack is the number one cause of death in women. Although you may be most concerned about breast cancer, Table 5-1 reveals that the risk of death from a heart attack is five times greater than death from breast cancer. It is ten times greater than from a hip fracture and fifty times greater than uterine cancer. The lifetime risk for developing CVD, which includes heart disease and strokes, is two women out of three. Not surprisingly, the nonfatal forms of CVD (heart attack, stroke) constitute a prominent cause of disability in women who have estrogen deficiency.

CVD is a major personal and public health problem for women in the United States, outranking any other disease you can name, yet it has not captured headlines or attracted significant research money. In CVD research studies, women have typically been underrepresented by a margin of 80 percent men to 20 percent women. Part of this gender discrepancy is accounted for by the fact that women tend to develop heart disease later in life than men and the studies usually focus on younger people. This effectively excludes women during their peak years of risk. Lack of these research studies has led to a gender bias that results in women being underdiagnosed and undertreated for CVD (Gurwitz 1992). That has begun to change for the better in recent years. The energy and drive of the "baby boomers" is likely to accelerate it even further. It's about time.

What do you suppose accounts for the gender-related difference in the prevalence of CVD? What is it that a premenopausal woman has, a post-menopausal woman does not, and men never did have? Estrogen, of course. Estrogen protects your heart. The evidence for this is not ambiguous; it is no longer scientifically disputable. Estrogen is one of the essentials for cardiovascular health. Many other avenues of protection exist, of course, and we discuss them as well, but estrogen protection is a major factor.

Table 5.1. Annual Deaths per 100,000 Women Age 50–75	
Condition	**Numbers**
Coronary heart disease	10,500
Breast cancer	1,875
Osteoporotic bone fracture	938
Endometrial (uterine lining) cancer	188

Adapted from: B.E. Henderson, et al. 1986. "Estrogen Use and Cardiovascular Disease," *American Journal of Obstetrics and Gynecology*. 154:1181

You're Not Menopausal—Why Worry?

You don't need to lose sleep over the possibility that you will develop CVD during your transitional years. Keep in mind, however, that estrogen is one of your guardians and that it begins decreasing significantly after your mid-thirties. Men are at far greater risk for CVD than you are during these years; but the gradual decline in estrogen begins to narrow the gap, so you are not immune to heart disease simply because you are still having menstrual periods. Prevention needs to start whenever the risk starts increasing; and for you, that is now.

Risky Business

Many of the risk factors for future heart disease are within your control. Take a look at Table 5-2, which lists risk factors for heart disease. Now is the time to get a handle on these factors and take charge of your own personal prevention program to help ensure a better long-term quality of life.

Estrogen Deficiency—Your Heart Is at Risk

During your perimenopausal years, one of the least evaluated risk factors for CVD is estrogen deficiency. Few women or their physicians think about this until menopausal symptoms appear or menstrual periods stop. Estrogen deficiency plays a much larger role during the transitional years than most women and health care providers realize. For example, it is obvious that loss of the ovaries for any reason (such as surgical removal, premature menopause, chemotherapy) will result in a dramatic decline in estrogen. But it is not widely known that many studies have shown a hysterectomy, even with conservation of ovaries, will result in menopause at an earlier age than would normally be expected. This happens as a result of disturbed blood flow to the ovaries from the surgery (Nachtigall 1995). If your uterus has been removed, be especially alert to symptoms of estrogen deficiency. If they appear, talk with your health provider about estrogen supplements or low-dose birth control pills.

If you are an overweight smoker with high blood pressure and an unfavorable lipid profile (high cholesterol, low HDL, high LDL, high triglycerides—more on these substances in a moment), you have a lot of CVD risk factors going for you. If estrogen deficiency symptoms are also present, serious consideration should be given to hormone supplementation. There is still time to implement lifestyle changes and start hormone supplements. Don't wait until you need cardiac rehabilitation.

Table 5.2.
Risk Factors for Heart Disease

Estrogen deficiency

Hypertension

Obesity: 20 percent more than recommended for your age and height

Sedentary lifestyle

Cigarette smoking

Diabetes

Family history of heart disease

Heavy stress in your life

Unfavorable lipid profile (cholesterol, HDL, LDL, triglycerides)

About Cholesterol

Cholesterol is a lipid (fat-like) substance that is synthesized by your liver. It is also present in animal fat, so the most common external source is from what you eat. Your body utilizes cholesterol for energy and as a precursor for hormones. *Lipoproteins* are the cholesterol carriers in your bloodstream, and estrogen has a potent influence on them. The two most important of these are *high-density lipoprotein* (HDL) and *low-density lipoprotein* (LDL).

Excess cholesterol can become deposited on the walls of the arteries, where it is called plaque. Plaque narrows arteries and restricts blood flow, which leads to *atherosclerosis* (hardening of the arteries), high blood pressure, heart attacks, and strokes. HDL carries cholesterol away from the artery walls and other tissues to the liver, where it is broken down and excreted from the body in bile. LDL also carries cholesterol in the bloodstream; but it allows the cholesterol to be deposited as plaque on artery walls. Normally, you have more "good" HDL than "bad" LDL. *Triglycerides* are a type of fat derived mainly from food. The exact role of triglycerides in causing CVD is not certain, but it is known that high triglycerides combined with low levels of HDL are associated with heart disease, especially in women.

According to a 1993 study by Dr. K. M. Bass and co-workers, there are some gender differences that affect the predictability of lipoprotein roles in causing CVD:

- Total cholesterol is a better predictor of CVD for men than for women.
- Low HDL puts women at greater risk than men.
- High LDL is a greater risk for men.
- High triglycerides combined with low HDL constitute an independent risk factor for women, but not for men.
- High triglycerides in diabetics raise the risk of CVD 3-fold in men, but 200-fold in women.

The "big three" risk factors are high total cholesterol, low HDL, and high LDL. This is true for both women and men, but the degree of risk is shaded by the gender differences.

Some Good News About Estrogen

Check this out: Estrogen *raises* "good" HDL and *lowers* "bad" LDL! It also lowers overall cholesterol levels. This is a major reason why you are protected (but not exempted) from cardiovascular disease during your reproductive years; and it explains why your risk for CVD begins to rise when estrogen declines. It also explains why women over fifty who are on HRT enjoy a *50 percent decrease* in heart attack deaths compared to nonusers of HRT. More than thirty published studies now document this reduced risk of CVD in estrogen users (Speroff 1994).

Your cardiovascular system enjoys a number of additional benefits as a result of estrogen. Dr. Leon Speroff, an internationally recognized expert in perimenopausal-menopausal issues and professor of Ob/Gyn at the Oregon Health Science University, summarized it better than any:

- Estrogen decreases total cholesterol blood level, lowers LDL, and raises HDL. (That's moving all three in the right direction.)
- Estrogen increases dilation of blood vessels, which improves flow of blood and lowers blood pressure.
- Estrogen has a direct strengthening effect on heart muscle (called an inotropic effect), which results in more efficient heart action, meaning that more blood is pumped per heartbeat.
- Estrogen prevents plaque deposits on artery walls, which avoids narrowing and helps to avert heart attacks and strokes.
- Estrogen increases antiplatelet aggregation factors, which means that estrogen reduces the risk of blood clots that can cause heart attacks and strokes.
- Estrogen improves proper metabolism of glucose so that less insulin is needed in circulation. Too much insulin is a major cause of hardening of the arteries.
- Estrogen inhibits the usual postmenopausal accumulation of central abdominal fat, which is associated with hardening of the arteries. With adequate estrogen, fat tends to accumulate about the hips, and a woman's body shape is typically pear-like. In estrogen deficiency, fat accumulates about the abdomen, and body shape more closely resembles an apple.
- Estrogen is an antioxidant. It prevents oxidation of LDL, so it will not get deposited on the walls of blood vessels and cause hardening of the arteries.

There you have it. The bottom line is that estrogen is crucial to your cardiovascular health, and lack of it is detrimental. Don't leave home without it.

Hypertension—It's Hard on Your Heart

High blood pressure results when there is an increased resistance to flow of blood through the blood vessels. More pressure is required to force blood through them. The most common cause of this situation is atherosclerosis, or hardening of the arteries from cholesterol deposits. If your arteries are narrowed by plaque deposits and the walls are inelastic because of them, your heart must pump harder to generate enough pressure to get the blood through them. Over time, the heart is adversely affected by this constant extra effort. In addition, there is always a risk that blood clots will accumulate on the plaque deposits and be dislodged, to then be carried to the brain and cause a stroke. It is easy to see that cholesterol control and maintaining a favorable ratio of HDL to LDL is important. Another factor in maintaining normal blood pressure is the effect of estrogen on keeping artery walls relaxed, thereby reducing the resistance to flow. A low-fat diet and adequate estrogen are both crucial to achieving this.

Obesity—Your Heart Hates It

Here, the big "O" does not refer the climactic point of sexual pleasure. If you are more than 20 percent over your ideal weight, you have crossed the line: It's not just an issue of physical appearance; it's a health risk. See Table 5-3 for healthy weight based on age and height. If you become overweight, your heart must work harder in every activity your body performs just to carry those extra pounds around. In addition, the extra body fat you accumulate will likely have resulted from a diet that is too high in fat. This raises your cholesterol level and puts you at greater risk for CVD. A healthy diet is not merely an option for you in your transitional years, it's a must. Slimming down for the long haul involves a permanent fitness program that stresses both a healthful diet and exercise. (Chapter 10 takes a close look at this topic.) A healthy heart will make the next half of your life a lot more livable for you.

Table 5.3. Guidelines for Healthy Weight		
Height	**Weight Without Shoes or Clothes**	
	Age 19–34	Age 35 and Over
5'	97–128	108–138
5'1"	101–132	111–143
5'2"	104–137	115–148
5'3"	107–141	119–152
5'4"	111–146	122–157
5'5"	114–150	126–162
5'6"	118–155	130–167
5'7"	121–160	134–172
5'8"	125–164	138–178
5'9"	129–169	142–183
5'10"	132–174	146–188
5'11"	136–179	151–194
6'	140–184	155–199

Source: U.S. Department of Agriculture, Health and Human Resources

A Sedentary Lifestyle Is Not Good for Your Heart

You've probably had it up to *here* with being reminded about the health risks of being a couch potato. Those TV ads showing slim, spandex-clad young women working out with permanent smiles plastered to their faces get to be a bit much. The kernel of truth in messages like those is that your heart does not tolerate low or nonexistent levels of exercise. Cardiologists and fitness experts throughout the world advise that cardiac fitness is essential, and you can achieve it with only moderate activity. Thirty to forty minutes of aerobic exercise, three to four times weekly, will keep your heart fit for the long term. It's a lot easier to do it now than later, when it is called cardiac rehabilitation. The formula for achieving and maintaining cardiac fitness is examined in Chapter 10.

Smoking—Bad News for Your Heart

Nicotine is a vasoconstrictor. It causes blood vessels to squeeze down, and more pressure is needed to force blood through them. Your heart must work harder. Inhaled tobacco smoke also damages the lungs, which reduces the amount of oxygen that gets into the bloodstream. This forces the heart to speed up blood circulation in order to deliver the oxygen your body's tissues need. Tobacco use also has a toxic effect on ovaries, leading to an earlier menopause and the risk of CVD from diminished estrogen.

If you smoke, your chances of dying from a heart attack are four times higher than if you do not. Even if you don't smoke, living with a smoker gives you three times more risk of a heart attack death. Lung cancer is also strongly associated with smoking and is the number one cancer-killer of women. Breast cancer makes all the headlines, but lung cancer is much more deadly. Heart disease or lung cancer will ultimately cause the death of 35 percent of smokers. There is some good news, though. The American Heart Association states that if you quit now, in ten years your risk of a heart disease death will diminish to the same risk level as for people who never smoked.

To quit smoking, you must deal with both of its two addictive components: Physical addiction to nicotine, and psychological addiction. It takes about one week to be relieved of the withdrawal symptoms of physical addiction if you quit cold turkey. Some people are helped by using a gradual nicotine withdrawal technique, such as nicotine gum or skin patches over several weeks.

The psychological addiction is more daunting because of the ingrained rituals of smoking: after a meal, on the phone, driving the car, having a drink, after sex. Your subconscious is programmed to respond to these triggers by lighting up, and failing to do so is stressful. If you got programmed to begin with, though, you can also be reprogrammed. As you know, there are loads of quitting smoking techniques out there. Consider the following:

- The most essential element to quitting smoking is that you must want to do so.
- Women often find considerable help in support groups or from a few close friends who can provide moral support.
- Biofeedback and hypnosis are beneficial.
- Quit after your menstrual period not before. Studies indicate that withdrawal symptoms are aggravated by premenstrual emotional changes.
- Exercise regularly while quitting smoking. A moderate program will help to relieve stress as well as the symptoms of withdrawal. Women who exercise during this time are far less likely to return to smoking.

As you read this book, you will notice numerous other references to the dangers that smoking poses for you. Your heart is only one of the beneficiaries of your being a nonsmoker.

Osteoporosis

Osteoporosis means porous bones. It is a condition that results from loss of calcium and bone protein, which causes weakened bones that fracture easily. Osteoporosis is mistakenly regarded as a problem of very old women. While it is true that the devastating effects on quality of life are primarily in postmenopausal women, osteoporosis has its beginnings in a woman's mid-thirties. In fact, you may even have set yourself up for osteoporosis in your teens and twenties. Osteoporosis is largely preventable, but to avoid it, you need to be able to recognize whether you are at risk. This section of the chapter takes a look at who gets osteoporosis, what happens and why, how to prevent it, how to diagnose it, and how it is treated. The underlying thread to keep in mind as you read is that while there are many things you can do to avoid osteoporosis, none is more important than having adequate estrogen (Prince et al. 1991). There are many factors intimately involved in maintaining bone density, such as weight-bearing exercise, adequate calcium intake, and elimination of risk factors, but estrogen is the single most important ingredient in preventing osteoporotic fractures.

Who Gets Osteoporosis

Twenty-five million Americans already have osteoporosis, and 80 percent of them are women. The National Osteoporosis Foundation estimates that half of all women over age fifty will suffer an osteoporotic fracture sometime during their life. Postmenopausal women sustain 250,000 hip fractures every year. As many as 20 percent are dead within three months from surgical complications and the heart and lung effects of the inactivity that results from fractures. Half of the survivors are never able to live independently again because of their inability to walk normally. Osteoporosis is a major factor in the rapidly rising number of women who require nursing home care. Indeed, 75 percent of nursing home residents over age sixty-five are women. The annual cost of medical care for osteoporosis is $10 billion, plus the appalling human toll.

This is an epidemic that can escalate to major proportions when the 38 million women of your baby boomer generation become postmenopausal. It does not have to happen, though, because osteoporosis is mostly preventable. The numbers quoted above should be dramatically improved when you baby boomers become sufficiently informed and motivated to "take charge" of this threat to your health and your quality of life.

Nuts and Bolts of Osteoporosis

Bone is a living, dynamic tissue. It is made up of protein collagen fibers, which are infiltrated with crystals of calcium phosphate. Bone tissue is constantly being added and removed, just like skin. Normally, bone removal and bone formation are in balance, and a sturdy skeleton is maintained. Osteoporosis results when bone formation falls behind bone removal. Loss of estrogen is a primary cause of this imbalance. Here's why. The cells that form bone are called *osteoblasts*. The removers are *osteoclasts*. And guess what? Estrogen receptors are known to exist on osteoblasts. This makes the presence of estrogen molecules plugged into those receptors a necessary condition for maintenance of healthy bones. Bone loss therefore begins when estrogen declines and the osteoblasts are not getting their job done.

As you already know, the onset of significant estrogen decline occurs in your mid thirties. You do not become ravaged by bone loss at this age. Osteoporosis is very slow and subtle, offering no particular symptoms to alert you to its presence. As a matter of fact, one of the reasons osteoporosis has been such a problem for women in the generations prior to yours is that its effects were often not recognized until about age seventy. A woman would do something as mundane as step off a curb and fracture her hip. An event like this, which can end up being fatal, is what established the diagnosis of osteoporosis. The point is that osteoporosis is a silent event, like the termites that work on your house until the family room falls into the backyard one afternoon. Fortunately, enough is now known about the causes and prevention of osteoporosis that you are not dependent upon a personal tragedy to alert you to your risk. You can learn whether you are at risk and take steps to avoid osteoporosis.

The Role of Progesterone and Progestins

Promoters of food supplements and "natural" hormonal products have been making a lot of noise recently about the use of natural progesterone cream for prevention of osteoporosis. It is true that natural progesterone and its synthetic form, called progestin, can reduce the rate of bone loss. They help, but they don't do a very good job of it. Estrogen is much better at it than progesterone. When these two hormones are combined, however, bone loss is not only stopped, there is a *small increase* in bone mass, which is certainly better than none. Because progesterone and progestins act as mild anti-estrogens, there was concern in the early 1980s that combining the two would inhibit estrogen's demonstrated beneficial effects. Fortunately, that turned out not to be true, and HRT that utilizes both hormones turns out to be quite beneficial.

Natural progesterone is produced from soybeans and wild Mexican yams and is therefore not regulated by the FDA. This form of progesterone has been used in Europe for many years, and use is now on the upswing in the United States. Don't take the claims of the cream promoters at face value, though; credible scientific studies have not been done that show the cream to be effective in prevention of osteoporosis. In spite of this, some claims imply that natural progesterone cream is adequate solely on its own for osteoporosis prevention, apart from other proven methods. (Note: In 1996, the laws were changed to prevent irresponsible promotion claims for nonregulated products, so the hype associated with the twenty-seven natural progesterone creams currently on the market may become muted.)

The Role of Testosterone and Estrogen

Testosterone? You probably think of it as "the male hormone," and yes, you're right. But don't worry that it will turn you into a middle linebacker if you take it in small doses. In 1996, Dr. L. G. Raesz published a study of osteoporotic women using both testosterone and estrogen. It was a small study, but it demonstrated increased bone formation, as compared to estrogen's ability to *limit* bone loss. For such a regimen to be accepted, it must be shown that the necessary dose of testosterone will not lower HDL, which would increase the risk of CVD. Clearly, more study is needed.

Let's Talk Calcium

Calcium is your body's most important mineral. As vital as calcium is to bone integrity, it is also necessary to proper functioning of your muscles, brain, heart muscle, blood-clotting mechanism, and many other bodily needs. Calcium is an ongoing, long-term necessity for bone strength; but for the other areas of calcium use, it is a short-term, daily need. Wide fluctuations of calcium levels are not tolerated for long, so an elaborate hormonal system exists to regulate calcium in your bloodstream. The system utilizes *calcitonin*, a hormone from the thyroid that stimulates bone production; reproductive hormones (estrogen, progesterone, and testosterone); corticosteroids from the adrenal glands, parathyroid hormone; and vitamin D. If your calcium intake or absorption from the intestinal tract is insufficient to maintain a normal blood level, the regulators get it from their handy calcium storage depot— your bones. In the next few paragraphs you will learn how to keep your calcium regulators happy and your bones strong.

The average American woman's diet is deficient in calcium. Because of the emphasis in this country over the last few decades on decreasing fat intake, consumption of dairy products has declined, and this has resulted in an insufficient calcium intake. Look over Table 5-4, which lists the calcium content of various foods. You will see that some of them are high in calcium but also high in fat and/or high in calories. With study and selection, you can achieve a diet with sufficient calcium. In 1994, The National Institutes of Health published the results of a Consensus Development Conference on Optimal Calcium Intake. (Note: You can get this pamphlet by calling 1-800-644-6627.) They found that the daily need for calcium in females from ages eleven to twenty-four is 1,200 to 1,500 mg, and from twenty-five to fifty years of age, it is 1,000 mg. During pregnancy and breast-feeding, the need goes back up to 1,200 to 1,500 mg. After menopause or during any other estrogen-deficient state, 1,500 mg are needed. During your transition years, you may not need a calcium supplement unless your bone density is already below normal or your diet is deficient in calcium. (The average American diet contains little more than 200 to 500 mg of calcium per day, so you may need a supplement now.) In later years, greater calcium supplements are needed because the intestine becomes less efficient in absorbing calcium. In addition, with declining estrogen, calcium utilization is impaired, so supplements are definitely important then.

Table 5.4.
Calcium Content in Various Foods

Food		Serving	Calcium	Calories	Fat Gms
Milk					
	Whole	1 cup	288 mg	150	8.1
	Skim	1 cup	296 mg	89	4.7
Cheese					
	Chedder	1 oz	204 mg	112	9.1
	Swiss	1 oz	260 mg	95	7.1
	Cottage, low fat, 2%	4 oz	78 mg	100	2.2
Yogurt					
	Whole milk	1 cup	274 mg	141	7.7
	Plain, low fat	1 cup	414 mg	143	3.4
Ice cream, 10% fat					
	Hard (vanilla)	1 cup	176 mg	270	14.1
	Soft serve (vanilla)	1 cup	236 mg	375	25.6
Ice milk					
	Hard, 4% fat (vanilla)	1 cup	176 mg	185	4.6
	Soft serve, 3% fat (vanilla)	1 cup	274 mg	225	8.6
Tofu					
	Firm curd	4 oz	6-100 mg	150	8
	Medium curd	4 oz	4-90 mg	90	6
Vegetables					
	Spinach, fresh, cooked, drained	1 cup	150 mg	40	0
	Broccoli, fresh, cooked, drained	1 cup	136 mg	40	0
	Lima beans, fresh, cooked	½ cup	81 mg	120	0

Continued on the following page.

Food		Serving	Calcium	Calories	Fat Gms
	Collards, fresh, cooked, drained	1 cup	357 mg	65	0
	Turnip greens, fresh, cooked	1 cup	252 mg	30	0
Seafood					
	Shrimp, canned, drained	3½ oz	115 mg	100	0.8
	Salmon, canned, with bones	3½ oz	183 mg	210	14
	Oysters, raw, 18 medium size	3½ oz	258 mg	160	2.0
	Sardines, canned, with bones	3½ oz	425 mg	311	24.4
Nuts and Seeds					
	Almonds, shelled, about 12 nuts	1 oz	45 mg	170	15
	Sunflower seeds, hulled	1 oz	35 mg	159	14

Adapted from: Osteoporosis Foundation table (1992).

What Are Your Chances for Osteoporosis . . . and Your Daughter's?

A 1992 study by Theistz established that the years most critical to bone accumulation are between the ages of eleven and sixteen. Bone mass peaks around age twenty-eight. Bone mass is constantly accumulating until that time if you are eating a healthy diet, getting lots of exercise, and have plenty of estrogen. In other words, a window of opportunity to build a sturdy skeleton exists between the ages of about eleven and twenty-eight. To accomplish healthy bone growth and bone mass accumulation during those years, girls and young adult women require four ingredients:

- 1200 to 1500 mg of calcium daily. A glass of milk or a plain nonfat yogurt has about 300 mg.

- 400 IU of vitamin D daily. A glass of milk has about 100 IU.

- Exercise.

- Adequate estrogen.

We can hear what you're thinking: "Did I just read *adequate estrogen*? I thought teenagers and young adults were awash in it." You're right, of course; but sometimes inadequate estrogen exposure results from delayed onset of menstrual periods past age sixteen, loss of ovarian function with eating disorders such as anorexia or bulimia, world-class athleticism, and other causes. Lloyd and colleagues reported in 1993 that birth control pill use during these years, if accompanied by adequate calcium intake, has the potential to increase a young woman's peak bone mass. This apparently does not hold true for young women with eating disorders, according to Klibanski's 1995 report. Severe dieting to comply with our cultural prescription that fashion-model thinness is the ultimate in attractiveness is damaging to bone mass accumulation. These situations can mean that a young woman will reach her life peak of bone density with inadequate bone mass. This young woman is at much greater risk for developing osteoporosis when her estrogen decline begins. A bean-pole thin young woman may appear in brimming good health; but there is a significant likelihood that her bone mass is below normal. Your children should be protected from this potential long term harm. You have the power and now the knowledge to help them. By the time you become perimenopausal, the window of opportunity for bone mass accumulation has largely passed. From this point on, your efforts need to be directed toward maintenance.

Many additional risk factors exist that you need to know about in order to avert osteoporosis. Some of these factors are not within your control to change, but many of them are.

- **Race:** Caucasian and Asian women are more at risk than African-Americans because African-American women produce increased levels of calcitonin. (Calcitonin is a hormone produced in the thyroid that stimulates bone formation.)

- **Family history of osteoporosis:** This is a strong indicator that you may be at risk.

- **Menopause prior to age forty-five:** This is a risk because you will have many more postmenopausal years to live with estrogen depletion. Early menopause can occur naturally, and it can also result from surgery and chemotherapy.

- **Skeletal size:** Small-boned women are more at risk. Having less bone mass makes a difference because your body uses the same amount of calcium each day, whether you have large or small bones. If your intake of calcium is inadequate, your body gets it from your skeleton.

- **Low body weight:** Underweight women are more likely to have osteoporosis. A weak form of estrogen called estrone is made from the conversion of body fat. Your body composition should be about

20 to 25 percent fat to avert loss of *estrone.* A "fashion-model" body is definitely under 20 percent.

- **Sedentary lifestyle:** A sedentary lifestyle allows bones to become weak. Weight-bearing exercise prevents this problem.

- **Low calcium intake:** If you had a low calcium intake in your past or if it is low now, you are at risk. During your transition, you need about 1,000 mg of calcium daily. If your diet doesn't give you that much, use a supplement. (Menopausal women need 1,500 to 2,000 mg unless they are on HRT, in which case 1,000 to 1,500 mg are enough.

- **Cigarette smoking:** This is a double whammy. First, nicotine interferes with the ability to absorb calcium. Second, tobacco smoke has a toxic effect on the ovaries, leading to earlier menopause and major estrogen depletion. Half a pack a day is all it takes.

- **Alcohol:** Alcohol interferes with calcium absorption from the intestine. The risk level is exceeded by more than two alcoholic beverages per day.

- **Caffeine:** Caffeine interferes with calcium absorption. More than two caffeine beverages, such as coffee or cola drinks, are enough to increase risk.

- **Phosphate-containing carbonated sodas:** These can be a problem. Too much phosphorus stimulates the parathyroid gland to become more active in removing calcium from your bones. Red meats and processed foods often contain phosphates as well. Moderation is advisable.

- **Absence of menstrual periods:** If you haven't had a menstrual period for an extended time (except during pregnancy) low estrogen levels result. Anorexia, bulimia, excessive exercise and prolonged severe stress can cause your periods to stop.

- **Fad dieting:** If you are on a high-protein/low-carbohydrate diet now or have been in the past, your risk for osteoporosis is increased. High-protein/low-fiber diets interfere with calcium absorption by speeding up the transit time of food through the intestine. There is less time to absorb calcium.

- **Hyperthyroidism or hyperparathyroidism:** These conditions both result in calcium loss at the expense of the bones.

- **Long-term corticosteroid use:** Corticosteroid (such as cortisone and prednisone) use in a long-term regimen can deplete bone mass by 30 percent in as little as six months.

- **Depression of long duration:** This puts you at higher risk for osteoporosis at any age. Dr. Philip Gold, chief of neuroendocrinology at the National Institute of Mental Health, showed that women with depression had 10 to 15 percent lower bone density in their hips than normal for their age. The average woman in his study was age forty-one, but with a bone density level equivalent to that seen in seventy-year-old women. The cause was felt to be elevated levels of the stress hormone cortisol. This finding was confirmed in a separate 1996 study by Michelson.

Are you wondering why you didn't know all that? One answer is that the end results of osteoporosis occur in elderly women, who have not had a loud voice when it comes to bringing women's health problems to the attention of medical researchers. That should change with women in your generation, however, who show an admirable tendency to resist, tooth and tong, giving up independent living as the result of a problem they can prevent.

Minerals and a Vitamin You Should Know About

Magnesium has a function similar to calcium in maintaining proper contracting ability of muscles and transmission of nerve impulses. A little-known fact about magnesium is that an excess of it can inhibit calcium utilization and thereby adversely affect bone density. Ironically, high doses of magnesium in the range of 1,000 mg are beneficial for PMS. If you are treating PMS with this level of magnesium, it should be as short a course of therapy as possible. Ordinarily your intake of magnesium should never be more than half that of calcium. If you estimate the calcium in your daily diet to be 500 mg daily, magnesium should be no more than 250 mg. If you are taking a 500 mg calcium supplement for a total of 1000 mg daily, magnesium can be 500 mg. Magnesium food sources include nuts, green leafy veggies, legumes, and seafood.

Phosphorus is a major component of bone, but an excessive intake leads to bone loss. The parathyroid gland is a major regulator of calcium, and high levels of phosphorus cause the parathyroid to remove calcium from bones. As mentioned above, carbonated sodas, red meat, and processed foods are loaded with phosphates.

Vitamin D receptors exist in the intestinal tract and enhance the absorption of calcium. That would seem to be good for bones. On the other hand, enhanced calcium levels in the bloodstream do not in themselves lower the fracture rate in postmenopausal women. It takes estrogen to do that. About 400 IU per day of vitamin D are needed to maintain optimum calcium absorption. Exposure to sunlight is another source of vitamin D, and people who have no sun exposure may need 800 IU.

"Tell Me If I've Got It"—Diagnosis

The early stages of osteoporosis are free of symptoms, so this is a blind alley for diagnosis. Routine X-ray is nearly useless because it does not disclose osteoporosis until bone mass loss approaches 30 percent. By that time it is usually too late to completely replace lost bone. The most reliable test is *dual energy X-ray absoptiometry* (DEXA). It can detect as little as a 1 percent loss. This is a low-dosage X-ray technique that takes about three to five minutes to measure bone density. The cost is $175 to $200, but this is declining as more and more DEXA machines become available. DEXA evaluates your spine, wrists, and hips, which are the most common sites for fractures. Computed tomagraphy (CT scan) has also been used for diagnosis; but it is more expensive, uses more X-ray irradiation, and does not evaluate the hip very well.

Ultrasound may have a future role to play as a screening technique. Ultrasound scans of the heel and kneecap have been shown to correlate well with DEXA results in evaluating bone density. The advantage of ultrasound is that it does not utilize X ray and is less expensive than DEXA.

At present, DEXA is the gold standard for evaluating bone density. If you know you are at high risk for osteoporosis, you should have a DEXA at about age forty. Assuming your bone density is normal, it can serve as a baseline for future comparison after your menstrual periods have stopped. On the other hand, if your DEXA reveals a lower-than-average bone density prior to menopause, you should start an aggressive prevention program immediately. In addition to changing the risk factors that are changeable, you should consider estrogen supplements during perimenopause if you have deficiency symptoms. The low-dose birth control pill works well for this, and you can take it right to menopause. In fact, it serves not only as prevention, but as treatment as well.

Treating Osteoporosis

Until recently, "treatment" for osteoporosis consisted of little more than an aggressive prevention program, as we discussed above. Few of you will require treatment during your transition, but let's take a look at some of the breakthroughs that have been made in treatment, in case you need it further down the line. Prevention of osteoporosis has been called the *only* game in town; but now that some treatments are available, prevention can be thought of as the best game in town.

Bisphosphonates are a nonhormonal class of drugs that have been shown to be helpful not only in prevention of osteoporosis, but also in retrieval of lost bone density. The new second generation of these drugs (*alendronate* and *pamidronate*) increases bone density and strength if taken with calcium and vitamin D. (Speroff 1994)

Another form of treatment is use of calcitonin, a hormone produced by the thyroid gland that reduces bone loss and may cause an increase in bone mass. It is synthesized from salmon and is available in an injectable form and a nasal spray. Daily use combined with adequate calcium will increase bone density in vertebrae; but there is no significant benefit to hips or wrists, which are common fracture sites. In advanced osteoporosis, salmon-calcitonin may be of considerable help in chronic pain.

Estrogen and testosterone taken together have been shown to increase bone density, but as we mentioned earlier, this form of treatment requires more research before it can be widely advocated.

Sodium fluoride may be a new method in the wings for treating osteoporosis. Dr. Charles Pak, director of the Center for Mineral Metabolism Research at Texas Southwestern Medical Center, has studied this method. He reports that a slow-release form of sodium fluoride, when accompanied with calcium citrate, can build new bone and prevent spinal fractures. In the past, fluoride was shown to build bone, but it did not reduce the fracture rate. This method also builds bone but, apparently, stronger bone (Eastman 1997).

You are probably getting the impression that no one has a good handle on treating osteoporosis. That's about right. Fortunately, research on this issue is continuing in view of the large number of women of your generation who may be at risk.

Summary

This is the time in your life to assess your personal risk for the future development of cardiovascular disease. If you can identify certain CVD risk factors that apply to you, give them the serious consideration they deserve. Most of the risks listed above in Table 5-2 are amenable to change if you become proactive in managing them.

Osteoporosis must be avoided if you are to enjoy a full life after you become menopausal. If you and the rest of your boomer cohorts live en masse into your eighties as predicted, osteoporosis is one of the major threats to your maintaining the ability to live independently. Now, before you have to experience it, is the time to take the steps necessary to avert this devastating incursion on the second half of your life. The bottom line is that while calcium, vitamin D, cessation of smoking, moderation of alcohol use, limitation of caffeine and phosphorus intake, and weight-bearing exercise are all important to maintaining bone density, estrogen is the underlying necessity for prevention of fractures. Be alert to the signs and symptoms that your estrogen levels may be declining. If they are, consider starting an estrogen supplement, and jump all over a prevention program now.

Discuss your concerns about cardiovascular disease and osteoporosis with your doctor, and establish a plan for altering the risks in your favor. With your commitment and the support of an informed physician, you can implement changes now that will improve your chances for a better quality of life in the best half of it.

O O O

6

The Great Imitator: Thyroid Change Can Fool You

In transitional women, thyroid disease can mimic many of the symptoms you have been learning to associate with estrogen decline. Fatigue, sweating, disturbed concentration, short-term memory loss, depressed mood, irritability, and diminished sexual desire all may result from thyroid disease of one type or another. It's best that you know about this, because abnormal thyroid function is commonly missed by health care professionals. For transitional women, thyroid symptoms more frequently trigger a suspicion of ovarian hormone decline. If female hormones are prescribed for these symptoms and they fail to improve, testing for a thyroid abnormality should be the next step. For women in whom thyroid disease is not considered and recognized, the symptoms may acquire a psychiatric label, such as anxiety or depression; psychiatric hospitalizations have even been prescribed for severe unrecognized thyroid disease. This chapter describes the signs and symptoms that can alert you to a thyroid problem and concludes with diagnosis and treatment.

The Thyroid Foundation of America (see Appendix A) says that by age fifty, 10 percent of women will suffer from *hypothyroidism*, which means the thyroid gland is underactive. As many as half don't even know they have a failing gland. *Hyperthyroidism,* which means an overproduction of thyroid hormones, is much less common. If all types of thyroid disorders are included, the frequency is up to twenty times more in women than in men. The incidence in women peaks during the forties and continues well into old age. For these reasons, it's important to know that your perimenopausal symptoms may not be entirely a result of estrogen decline.

What Should You Look For?

Thyroid disease can imitate many illnesses, including major depression, heart disease, arthritis, and even cancer. In addition, the symptoms of an overactive or underactive gland can simulate many of the complaints commonly seen with estrogen decline in perimenopausal women. Some have called thyroid disorders "the great imitator," and with good cause. We compiled Tables 6-1 and 6-2 to illustrate the similarities between abnormal thyroid function and perimenopausal changes.

Table 6.1.
Comparison of Complaints Common to Hypothyroidism and Estrogen Deficiency

Complaint	Hypothyroidism	Estrogen Deficiency
Fatigue, sluggishness, no energy	Persistent	May wax and wane
Depression	Very persistent	May wax and wane
Menstrual change	Irregular to absent	Same
PMS symptoms	Aggravated or initiated	Same until mid- to late forties
Decreased sexual desire	Common	Same
Difficulty becoming pregnant	Common	Same
Short-term memory loss	Common	Same
Diminished concentration	Common	Same
Loss of hair	Common	Late forties and beyond
Brittle hair	Common	Maybe
Dry skin	Common	Same

Table 6.2.
Comparison of Complaints Common to Hyperthyroidism
and Estrogen Deficiency

Complaint	Hyperthyroidism	Estrogen Deficiency
Increased sweating	Common	Hot flashes are similar
Scanty menstrual periods	Common	Common
Irritability and moodiness	Common	Common
Heat intolerance	Common	Common
Trouble sleeping	Common	Common
Pounding of heart	Common	Common

These tables show why thyroid disease can be easily missed in peri-menopausal women. It is important not to miss this diagnosis, however, because thyroid disease is easily treated and resolved. If you do have thyroid disease but you or your doctor is misled into an investigation of diminished sex hormone levels, a trial of estrogen supplements will not improve your symptoms. If your FSH and estradiol blood levels are checked, they will be normal. At this point, don't throw up your hands in despair at failing to find the cause of your symptoms. The next step in diagnosis is thyroid testing.

Table 6-3 is a listing of additional hypothyroidism and hyperthyroidism symptoms that are not comparable to transitional changes. If you have some combination of these noncomparable changes plus estrogen deficiency–like symptoms, a thoughtful evaluation of them may suggest thyroid disease and lead to an earlier diagnosis; but your doctor must be a skillful listener. In addition, you must be aware of the changes that have happened in your body and communicate them accurately to your doctor. Once suspicion of thyroid disease has surfaced, laboratory testing will give you the answers. The appropriate tests are discussed later in this chapter. First, let's take a look at how your thyroid gland works.

How Your Thyroid Gland Works

Your thyroid weighs about one ounce, but it is a powerhouse. It is butterfly shaped and straddles the trachea (windpipe) at the base of your neck. Its function is to regulate the body's metabolism, which means it has major control of chemical and physical changes throughout your body. It influences

---

Table 6.3.
Additional Thyroid Symptoms

Hypothyroid	Hyperthyroid
Weight gain and difficulty in losing it	Nervous energy, inablity to sit still
Dry scaly skin and scalp	Rapid resting pulse rate
Brittle hair and nails	Unexplained weight loss
Cold intolerance, inability to get warm	Increased appetite
Sleeping more than usual	Buttoned collars fit too tightly
Slow heart rate	Eyes bulge slightly
Sluggish tendon reflexes, knee jerk	Frequent diarrhea
Puffiness of face, ankles	Frequent indigestion
Tingling in wrists and hands	Swollen ankles
Aching muscles and cramps	
Multiple joint aches	

---

growth and development of every body tissue and organ, it regulates how much oxygen cells consume and how much energy is expended. As you can see, this gland is a real *player*. The thyroid accomplishes its regulatory function by manufacturing and releasing its hormones into the bloodstream, which carries them to every tissue and organ—even your fingernails!

Your thyroid produces two hormones: triiodothyronine (T3), which is the biologically active hormone, and thyroxine (T4). Once T4 is released into your bloodstream, it is converted into T3. Your pituitary gland monitors and controls the amount of thyroid hormone in the bloodstream. The pituitary works with your thyroid in much the same way it does in regulating the pro-

Alphabet Soup

SHTH	Subclinical hypothyroidism (SHTH)
T3	Triiodothyronine
T4	Thyroxine
TSH	Thyroid stimulating hormone
TSI	Thyroid stimulating immunoglobulin

duction of estrogen and progesterone by the ovaries (see Chapter 2). The pituitary releases a hormone called *thyroid stimulating hormone* (TSH), which is carried in the bloodstream to your thyroid and directs it to deliver just the right amount of T3. When T3 is too low, an increase in TSH causes your thyroid to replenish the supply; when T3 is too high, TSH is lowered. If your thyroid cannot produce enough T3 to satisfy the pituitary, more TSH is sent to it, and then more, and maybe still more. This forms the basis for thyroid testing. A high TSH blood level confirms an underactive gland, and hypothyroidism. The reverse situation is seen in hyperthyroidism.

Hypothyroidism—Underdoing It

Ninety percent of hypothyroidism occurs in women. (It hardly seems fair, does it?) The gender difference is not well understood as yet; but it is reasonable to assume that a disparity this large must be related to a quintessential female feature that women have and males do not have—estrogen! Hypothyroidism seems to be associated with women who are overweight and have an early onset of menstrual periods, a large number of full-term pregnancies, and a late menopause. In women between the ages of forty and sixty, 3 percent will develop clinically demonstrable hypothyroidism, and another 10 percent will develop a *subclinical* form of it, which means that the thyroid hormone is a little low, but not enough to produce the usual signs and symptoms.

The predominant cause of hypothyroidism for 90 percent of women who have it, is the development of antibodies that attack the thyroid tissue and the hormones the thyroid produces. This is called an *autoimmune* reaction. If you have a reaction like this, your thyroid gland becomes inflamed, and tissue damage renders it unable to produce enough thyroid hormone. Your pituitary then generates more TSH, causing the thyroid to work harder. This works for a while, but at the expense of the thyroid cells multiplying and becoming larger. (An enlarged gland is called a goiter.) Ultimately, your thyroid can't keep up with hormone demands. Your pituitary's TSH is whipping a tired horse, however, and, thyroid hormone eventually drops low enough to cause the classic symptoms of hypothyroidism shown in Tables 6-1 and 6-3.

Hyperthyroidism—Overdoing It

Hyperthyroidism is most commonly seen in the thirties and forties. It affects about 2 percent of women. There are several forms of this disease, the most common being Graves' disease. Graves' disease is caused by a rogue antibody called *thyroid stimulating immunoglobulin* (TSI). When TSI plugs into thyroid receptor sites ordinarily occupied by TSH, it causes the thyroid to produce more hormone than normal.

This condition speeds up heart rate, steals sleep, causes a fine hand tremor to develop, increases appetite, and causes eyes to protrude slightly. Blinking the eyes becomes less frequent, and the skin is warm and moist most of the time. Menstrual periods may stop, which triggers concerns of pregnancy at first, and then premature menopause when an "emergency pregnancy test" is negative. Women who already have coronary artery disease may develop angina or have a heart attack. If you have it, you may feel weird, act fidgety, and feel as though you're about four inches off the ground all the time.

Your doctor can confirm a diagnosis of hyperthyroidism by hearing your story, doing a physical examination, and ordering lab tests. The tests will reveal a high thyroid hormone level and elevated TSI. TSH will be low or even undetectable.

The Ovary/Thyroid Connection

The ovaries and thyroid interact with each other in terms of hormone production. Estrogen and progesterone receptors exist in the thyroid, and T3 receptors are in the ovaries. Not surprisingly, then, a diminished female hormone effect may cause your thyroid to function sluggishly. Your perimenopausal symptoms from lessened estrogen may then be exaggerated by the additional symptoms of hypothyroidism. A confusing array of symptoms may be present. If you are on HRT but find that relief has not occurred for such things as a depressed mood, short-term memory loss, or difficulty in concentration, a thyroid check may be in order. If both glands are malfunctioning, supplementing both hormones can be magic.

The other side of the coin is this: Thyroid disease can cause a malfunction of the ovaries. Hypothyroidism or hyperthyroidism can be the root cause of several significant health problems for women:

- **Menstrual irregularity:** Irregularity in the form of lighter flow and a prolonged cycle is commonly seen with hypothyroidism. Menstrual periods may be skipped altogether. On the other hand, hyperthyroidism may cause heavier flow and shortened cycles initially; left untreated, though, it ultimately causes scanty flow or absence of bleeding. Thyroid malfunction may fool you into thinking you have become prematurely menopausal. In the prolonged absence of menstrual bleeding, however, laboratory testing quickly distinguishes between menopause and hypothyroidism. The important point is that you and your doctor must first *think* about the thyroid possibility. It is a good idea for transitional women with menstrual irregularity to insist on a thyroid check before agreeing to a surgical investigation like a D&C or surgical treatment such as a hysterectomy for uncontrolled bleeding.

- **Loss of sexual desire:** One of the less frequently recognized causes of loss of sexual desire is an overactive or underactive thyroid. Nearly 90 percent of hypothyroid and 50 percent of hyperthyroid women have loss of sexual desire (Eskin 1995). The causes vary all the way from vaginal dryness to depressed mood to overpowering fatigue. Happily, when thyroid disease is identified and treated, the problem usually disappears.

- **Infertility:** Infertility is a common accompaniment of hypothyroidism. Ovulation fails to occur because of inadequate levels of thyroid hormone. This situation is easily treatable, which is why a thyroid check should be part of every infertility investigation. Once you become pregnant, you need to track your thyroid function closely; pregnancy demands *much* more thyroid hormone. If the condition is undertreated in pregnancy or, worse yet, untreated, your risk of miscarriage rises. In addition, lack of maternal thyroid hormone may result in an enlarged thyroid in your baby. This can present a problem at full term; the enlarged thyroid may prevent your baby's head from flexing into the best position for a safe delivery.

- **Postpartum blues:** This situation is difficult to deal with for new mothers with new babies and who have partners who are new fathers. As many as 40 to 60 percent of women suffer from postpartum blues. For most, it is mild and self-limiting. However, estimates are that about 10 percent are actually suffering from an inflammatory condition called thyroiditis (Hayslip 1988). This is an autoimmune problem caused by antibodies that attack the thyroid, causing an inflammatory reaction. Thyroid-related postpartum blues generally occur six to twelve weeks after delivery, unlike typical postpartum blues, which start within a few days. It may be caused by a previously unrecognized viral infection in the thyroid.

The bottom line for you in thyroid disease is the importance of being aware of it as a possible cause of your symptoms. Once suspicion is aroused, a trip to the doctor should be next on your agenda.

What Your Doctor Will Do—Diagnosis

The symptoms and signs may not be obvious at first. As their severity increases, however, the initial subtleties become easily recognizable changes. Your doctor must take a number of factors into account in determining your diagnosis, including your own report of what has been happening, a physical exam, and testing.

Your Story

Whether you perceive your body's altered status as feather-like or sledgehammer-like, it's important to report these changes to your doctor, who will then take a medical history. You can help by being prepared to answer questions such as these:

- What is happening?
- When did the symptoms start?
- Have you ever had these symptoms before?
- Are they getting worse, better, or staying the same?
- How bothersome are they to you?
- What do think is causing it? (Every wise health care professional knows that this question may elicit invaluable information.)

It is unlikely that your history alone will nail down a diagnosis, but a skillful listener will be able to eliminate all but a few culprits.

Your Body

Physical examination plays an important diagnostic role in establishing thyroid disease and in distinguishing whether it is a *hypo*thyroid or *hyper*-thyroid problem. Table 6.4 lists some key observations.

The physical signs of hypothyroidism are usually late in appearing. This means that in the early stages of an underactive thyroid gland, physical examination may not be particularly revealing of your condition.

Table 6.4.
Physical Symptoms in Hypothyroidism and Hyperthyroidism

Physical Examination of	Symptom in Hypothyroidism	Symptom in Hyperthyroidism
Resting pulse	Too slow	Too fast
Blood pressure	Lowered	Raised
Reflexes (knee jerk)	Slow and sluggish	Brisk and intense
Eyes	Slow lid movement	Eyes may bulge slightly; infrequent blinking
Thyroid gland	May be enlarged	May be enlarged

Your Lab Results

Many decades ago, thyroid disease was diagnosed and treatment initiated on the basis of history and physical findings alone. Mistakes were common, of course. Fortunately, current laboratory testing is much more sophisticated. A blood sample is all your doctor needs.

Both thyroid hormones, T3 and T4, can be measured in blood tests, but the pituitary hormone, TSH, is a more sensitive indicator of thyroid function. For this reason, most doctors skip the T3 and T4 tests. If you have an underactive gland, your pituitary attempts to spark it up with more TSH. If your thyroid is overactive, the pituitary cuts back on TSH stimulation.

Small lumps, or nodules, are common in the thyroid. A small percentage of them can be detected by physical exam, but with an ultrasound scan, about one third of women can be shown to have one or more small nodules. They are usually harmless, but it is important to have them evaluated; they have been associated with hypothyroidism, hyperthyroidism, and cancer. Several methods exist for evaluating lumps, as well as for testing a diffusely enlarged thyroid without lumps. These include ultrasound, needle biopsy, radioactive iodine uptake, and thyroid scan.

Treating Thyroid Disease

Let's take a look at the treatments available for hypo- and hyperthyroidism.

Treatment of Hypothyroidism

The best treatment for hypothyroidism is simple hormone replacement, and that is a happy thought because there is no cure. Thyroxine, or T4, is your native hormone, and this is what you will be taking. Thyroxine is a safe, inexpensive, and reliable treatment. The correct daily dose will require some adjustment from time to time until you hit upon the right one for your particular needs. Monitoring your TSH level is a reliable method to assess the effectiveness of your dose. The correct thyroxine intake will gradually bring your TSH back down to normal.

A controversy exists among the giants of the thyroid world as to whether subclinical hypothyroidism (SHTH) should be treated. On the surface of it, you can understand the reluctance to treat a symptomless condition. The problem is that up to 25 percent of SHTH eventually progresses to full blown hypothyroidism (Danese 1996). Nearly one in ten of you who are walking around with antithyroid antibodies in your system will become actively hypothyroid each year. In addition, some evidence exists showing that women with SHTH are more at risk for coronary artery disease and subsequent heart attacks because of unfavorable lipid profiles. Since treatment

is simple, safe, and inexpensive, a good case can be made for utilizing it.
Some advice and precautions about thyroxine use:

- Aluminum-containing antacids (Gelusil, Amphogel, Tempo, Maalox Plus in tablets, and Mylanta liquid) adversely affect absorption.

- Iron adversely affects absorption. Take thyroxine and iron at different times of the day.

- Take *only* the amount prescribed as necessary to keep your TSH level normal. Overdoses cause bone resorption and puts you at greater risk for osteoporosis. In addition, overdoses cause symptoms of hyperthyroidism, such as sleepless nights, nervousness, pounding heart, and diarrhea. It can even damage your heart muscle.

- Take thyroxine the *same time* every day. If the dose varies from day to day, you will have fluctuations in your blood level, and uneven effectiveness. Morning is the best choice because thyroxine can keep you awake if taken too late in the day.

- Get a TSH blood test once or twice a year after your thyroxine dose is stabilized. Your thyroid function may drift lower as time passes; and you must stay on top of maintaining the right dose.

- If you become pregnant, be certain your obstetrician is aware that you are taking thyroid hormone replacement. Your requirements for thyroxine supplements will often fall in the first trimester but rise in the third trimester. Therefore, your TSH should be checked several times during pregnancy. The correct dose must be maintained to protect your baby.

Treatment of Hyperthyroidism

Prior to starting treatment for hyperthyroidism, a beta blocker medication is usually prescribed. This type of drug strengthens the heart muscle and lowers blood pressure. Hyperthyroidism can seriously damage the heart muscle, so this is an important first step. Two most commonly used beta blockers are *propranolol* and *atenolol*.

Three methods are currently in use to manage an overactive thyroid.

- **Antithyroid medication:** This is usually the first line of treatment. Drugs in this category prevent your thyroid from making all that extra hormone. The two most commonly prescribed are propylthiouracil (PTU) and methimazole. They are taken in a tablet form once daily for six months to a year. Over several months of treatment, you will gradually revert to normal from the "look weird, act fidgety, nervous wreck" you used to be.

- **Radioactive Iodine Therapy (RAI):** If drug treatment fails, RAI may be the next best form of controlling your runaway gland. RAI is taken orally. Your thyroid selects the radioactive iodine from the bloodstream and concentrates it in the overactive cells, which are then destroyed. The net result is that your thyroid can't produce as much hormone as it had been doing, and things settle down. And no, you won't glow in the night, because the radioactivity disappears from your body in a few days.

CAUTION! RAI therapy must be avoided if you are pregnant because it can have an adverse effect on a developing fetus. Dr. Bernard Eskin reports (1995) that the ovaries may absorb some of the RAI, so he recommends avoidance of this therapy if you are planning a pregnancy in subsequent years.

- **Surgical removal:** Sometimes, surgical removal of all or part of your thyroid is necessary. If you have only a single overactive nodule, simple removal of that nodule may be all you need. Most of the time, the entire gland is too active, and a total, or near total, thyroidectomy is necessary.

Any of the treatment methods we just described for an overactive thyroid can result in an underactive gland; so it is important for you to have annual thyroid evaluations.

Summary

Thyroid problems are often subtle and easily overlooked. This is especially true for perimenopausal women. You or your doctor may be misled by symptoms that are more commonly attributed to decline in female hormone production. Thyroid disease is one of those conditions that you just have to think about as a possibility when your body wisdom starts telling you that changes are taking place. It is worthwhile to have a TSH blood test every two years after age forty. This ensures that abnormal functioning of your thyroid will be picked up early; and you can avoid the weirdness that severe thyroid dysfunction can wreak in your life. An underactive thyroid is the most likely thyroid dysfunction, and its treatment is simple, inexpensive, and safe. Vigilance and awareness are your best friends in identifying thyroid problems.

○ ○ ○

7

Frightening Changes—Cancer

Cancer risks are not high for you in your transitional years. Why, then, discuss them in this book? First of all, your chances are not zero either, as you no doubt know, so a discussion of these potential threats is appropriate to arming you with information about your health after thirty-five. And, as you'll learn in this chapter, there are steps you can take during the transitional years to reduce your chances of getting cancer. This chapter covers the four most common female cancers: breast, uterine, cervical and ovarian. In addition, because they are also common (in both women and men), we take a look at lung and colon cancer. You will also learn what cancer is, what your risks are for getting it, how it is diagnosed, the all-important prevention methods available to you, and current treatments.

What Changes?

In cancer, cells change. Each of your several trillion cells has genes that control all aspects of cell life. The genes determine what chemicals are manufactured, when the cell reproduces itself, and how long each cell lives. As time passes, genes may be changed by the aging process and by the effects of outside agents you consume or to which you are exposed, such as pesticides, preservatives, tobacco smoke, alcohol, fat, various foods, and other environmental carcinogens (cancer-causing agents). These genetic changes are called *mutations*. After a mutation has taken place, the altered gene operates the cell in a different fashion. Most of the time, the change is relatively inconsequential, but sometimes the mutation produces a cancer-causing gene called an *oncogene*. All subsequent generations of that cell possess the oncogene and have the potential to become cancer cells if the oncogene is activated by one of the influences mentioned above. Some people are born with oncogenes that they inherit from their parents and that lie dormant unless or until activated later in life. Cells also have tumor suppresser genes that control how a cell grows. If the tumor suppresser gene is damaged, it can no longer control the growth rate, and the cell takes off on its own to produce a cancerous growth.

Once the oncogene is active, the cell it controls no longer behaves in a normal way. It becomes a rogue cell, producing an anarchy of uncontrolled growth and invasion of neighboring cells, tissues, and organs. Cancer cells cannot perform the same functions as normal cells, and the body suffers as these functions are lost. If the cancerous tissues are not removed or their growth halted, the body in which they exist will not survive.

According to a recent Associated Press article, scientists worldwide have made huge gains behind the scenes in working on methods to identify oncogenes and neutralize them with genetic engineering. Immunologists are making progress in using vaccines and using the body's own immune system to halt malignant cells. In recent years, cancer biologists have identified a protein called *telomerase*. It is a chemical produced by cancer cells that confers immortality upon the cancer cell. With telomerase, cells can divide over and over without succumbing to aging and cell death, as normal cells do. Telomerase can be detected in about 85 percent of cancers. In breast and lung cancer, it can be detected even before the tumor has started to spread. The problem so far is that telomerase can be detected only from the tissue cells themselves, so a biopsy is needed, rather than a simple blood test; for this reason telomerase testing is not appropriate as a mass screening tool. About a dozen pharmaceutical companies are working on drugs to shut down telomerase, which would starve the cancer cells of a chemical they need to survive. This is exciting news. The future appears promising, but it makes it no less important that we stay vigilant in terms of prevention, early diagnosis, and treatment methods, which are steadily improving.

The risk of your developing a cancer is not dependent upon a sole factor, such as the presence or absence of an oncogene. Other factors include the state of your nutrition, the competence of your immune system to combat abnormal cells, your genetic makeup, and uncounted external hazards to which you may be exposed. Cancer development is the sum of diverse circumstances and conditions that are brought to focus on regulation of cellular growth. Some of your risk for cancer is based on the shuffle of the genetic deck, and some of it is luck. The good news is, some of it is under your direct control.

Breast Cancer

Alphabet Soup	
BSE	Breast self-exam
HDI	High-definition imaging
MRI	Magnetic resonance imaging
PET	Positive emission tomography

The topic of breast cancer is a hot-button issue if there ever was one. Breast cancer is the second most common cause of cancer death in women. (Lung cancer is first.) Breasts are an important feature of femininity, so it is not surprising that the thought of breast cancer should strike such concern and fear in women. You should know as much as you can about breast cancer because you may need to make some important decisions during perimenopause that hinge on accurate information.

First, Some Numbers

Currently, 182,000 American women develop breast cancer annually, and this results in 46,000 deaths each year. Of all cancer sites in women, breast cancers constitute 32 percent (ACOG 1995). An often-quoted figure is that since 1950, the rate of breast cancer has increased by over 50 percent, from 1 in 12 to the current figure of 1 in 8. This statistic is misleading, though; it applies only to women who are currently age 20 and will live to age 85. You have a better chance of understanding your own risk for breast cancer by looking at Table 7-1. The odds of getting breast cancer increase as you age; by age 40 they are 1 in 217, for example, but by age 65, they are 1 in 17. Many women (and their physicians) actually believe that one in eight American women now living will develop breast cancer. It simply is not true. The 1 in 8 figure mentioned above is true only if you are a 20-year-old woman who will live to age 85. But you are perhaps forty, not twenty, and your risk is much lower.

What Are Your Risks?

Aside from the age factor, a number of other conditions influence development of breast cancer.

Family History

If your mother or sister (these are called first-degree relatives) has had breast cancer before age fifty, your risk is double that of someone without that history. If the cancer occurred after fifty, your risk is less high, but still 1.4 times more than usual. If two or more relatives (mother, sister, aunt, grandmother) have had breast cancer, especially before menopause, you are also at higher risk. This is called familial breast cancer, and it may be inherited. (Colditz 1993).

Table 7.1. Odds of Developing Breast Cancer by Age	
By age 25	1 in 19,608
By age 30	1 in 2,525
By age 35	1 in 622
By age 40	1 in 217
By age 45	1 in 93
By age 50	1 in 50
By age 55	1 in 33
By age 60	1 in 24
By age 65	1 in 17
By age 70	1 in 14
By age 75	1 in 11
By age 80	1 in 10
By age 85	1 in 9
Lifetime	1 in 8
Source: 1987–1988 data, SEER Program of the National Cancer Institute and the American Cancer Society	

Two genes (called BRCA1 and BRCA2) have now been identified that can predispose their carriers to breast cancer. There may be others. When these genes are normal, they have a protein that functions as a tumor suppresser. It is estimated that mutation of these genes (into oncogenes) accounts for 10 percent of all breast cancer. The mutated gene has abnormal or nonfunctional tumor suppresser protein and may fail to prevent normal cells from overgrowing. When activated by other influences, the breast cells these genes control are no longer prevented from unrestrained growth, and a cancer starts. More than one hundred mutations of BRCA-1 are now known; and it is possible to identify them with DNA testing. A woman with a mutated BRCA-1 gene has an 87 percent lifetime risk for breast cancer and a 63 percent risk for ovarian cancer (Shattuck et al. 1995, Hoskins et al. 1995). Each of her children of either sex has a 50 percent chance of inheriting BRCA-1 from her. Her male children who inherit a mutated BRCA-1 gene are at threefold increased risk for prostate and fourfold for colon cancer. Estimates are that 1 in 800 American women may be carriers of a mutated BRCA-1 gene. Carriers of a mutated BRCA-2 gene have an 80 percent lifetime risk for breast cancer and a 20 percent risk for ovarian cancer. (Male carriers of BRCA-2 have a 20 percent risk of breast cancer, plus increased risk for colon and prostate cancer.) What this means is that assessing your risk for familial breast cancer must include evaluation of both the maternal and paternal sides of your family. (Note: DNA testing for these genes is possible, but it is very complex and expensive. At present, it is not recommended except for families with a strong history of these cancers.)

Smoking

And you thought the cancer risk of smoking was to the lungs. That's still true, of course, but the complex toxins in tobacco smoke are apparently causing cancerous changes in breast cells also, because smokers have more breast cancer than nonsmokers (Bennicke 1995). Just another good reason to be a nonsmoker.

Estrogen

Life situations that result in prolonged and uninterrupted cyclic estrogen exposure, as well as situations that cause estrogen exposure without the protective effect of progesterone, seem to predispose women to breast cancer. Table 7-2 lists these factors.

Hormone replacement therapy is a complex issue in regard to breast cancer and is thoroughly discussed in Chapter 9.

Obesity and High Fat Diet

Japanese women, whose diet traditionally includes only 10 to 20 percent of calories from fat and animal protein, have 75 percent less breast cancer than American women. However, when Japanese women convert to a typical *Western* diet, their rate of breast cancer increases, in one generation, to that of American women (Notelovitz and Tennessen 1993). The typical American diet (if such a thing truly exists) averages 30 to 40 percent of calories from animal fat and another 12 percent from protein.

Whether or not dietary fat plays a significant causative role in breast cancer has not been firmly established. A pool of data exists that suggests fat does indeed play a role (Willet et al. 1992), but the published studies have used retrospective analysis, which is not the most reliable scientific method. A major ongoing prospective study called The Women's Health Initiative is looking at this relationship and should provide definitive answers about 2005 (Seltzer 1996).

Alcohol

A variety of studies have reported on this issue, and they published varying results. What they mostly agreed on is that alcohol consumption is associated with an increased risk for breast cancer. They diverged when it came to how much, how often, and how much higher the risk. The "how much" ranged from three drinks per week to three per day, and the risk increase varied from 50 to 250 percent over average risk rates. The Harvard Nurses' Health Study reported in 1987 that perimenopausal women were at a four times higher risk of breast cancer with one or more drinks per day than postmenopausal women. (This study, which has been in progress since 1976, continues to collect data every two years on the 121,700 women enrolled in it.) On the other hand, a large epidemiological study conducted in Wisconsin, Massachusetts, Maine, and New Hampshire reported in 1995 no significant increased risk for breast cancer in women taking estrogen who had varying alcohol consumption (Newcomb et al. 1995).

Table 7.2.
Risk Factors

Factor	Result
Early onset of menstrual periods (before age 12)	More lifetime years of monthly estrogen cycles and monthly changes in the breasts
Late menopause (after age 54)	More lifetime years of estrogen cycles
Having a first baby after age 30 or having no pregnancies	More uninterrupted years of estrogen cycles
Prolonged infertility from lack of ovulation	If ovulation is not occurring, progesterone's anti-estrogen protection is lost
Obesity (more than 20 percent above ideal weight)	Excess estrogen results from conversion of fat to estrogen
Prolonged perimenopause with absence of ovulation	Causes unopposed estrogen exposure
The woman's birth weight	A birth weight over 4,000 grams (8 lbs., 8 oz.) seems related to high estrogen exposure during fetal life (Michels 1996)
History of several pregnancies	Multiple pregnancies are protective, apparently because they interrupt the monthly breast changes caused by the normal hormonal cycle

None of these studies could explain why alcohol increases the risk for breast cancer, but speculation centered around adverse effects on estrogen levels, liver function, the immune system, and altered DNA. Since the jury is still out on this issue, abstinence may be the best policy, with moderation in definite second place.

Prior Abortion and Breast Cancer

In 1996, Newcomb reported some additional information from his study—that it found a small positive association between early pregnancy terminations and breast cancer. Approximately seven other studies have also shown a slight positive relationship between induced abortion and breast cancer, while nine have failed to find any association (Speroff 1996). However, what is called recall bias seems to have been a factor in the results of the studies showing an increased risk—it turns out that breast cancer patients are more likely to report having had an abortion than those who were free of breast cancer. Other studies, including a huge (1.5 million women) one in Denmark (Melbye et al. 1997), have concluded that the risk of breast cancer is identical in women who have had one or more induced abortions.

Exercise

The effects of exercise in reducing breast cancer have been studied for premenopausal women to date; but postmenopausal exercise research is just now under way. The Harvard Nurses' Health Study found that breast cancer risk was reduced by 50 percent if women exercise about four hours per week (Thun 1997). The risk was even lower if regular exercise had been part of your lifestyle dating back to the teens and twenties. Be sure to share this information with your daughters, and consider joining them if you are not already an exercise devotee. (Exercise is covered in Chapter 11.)

Screening for Breast Cancer

The traditional screening methods for breast cancer have been breast self-examination and physician exams; in recent years, mammograms have become a regular part of the mix. Other more sophisticated, and sometimes more expensive, methods are also emerging.

Breast Self-Examination (BSE)

Self-breast examination is an important element of breast cancer detection. Keep in mind, though, that self-examinations, and those by a health provider, can detect only relatively large breast lumps. This means that by the time you or your doctor can feel a cancerous lump, it may have been present for a considerable period of time—possibly more than two years. Regular mammograms, on the other hand, can detect lumps that are too small to feel by BSE, and they are being relied on more than BSE to detect new lumps. However, it is not yet time to abandon BSE. Mammograms miss about 10 percent of breast tumors because some of them do not contain calcium, an important identifying sign of cancer.

It's important to know what to look for when examining your breasts. (You may be reluctant to do this exam because of cultural perceptions that it's improper to touch certain parts of your body, but it really is important to do the exam.) Check with your health provider for the correct information. Remember to press firmly as you do the exam. After a few exams you will have become acquainted with your breasts, becoming the single most quali-fied expert on what they feel like. The advantage for you is that with this internal database established, you then are acutely aware if there is a change.

Change is what you are looking for. It is difficult, but possible, to detect lumps much smaller than one half inch in size; but the more expert you become, the better your chances of recognizing a small one. The earlier you find it, the better.

The best time to do BSE is just after your period, because there is less congestion and less tenderness in your breasts. You can examine your breasts firmly without it being painful, and with lessened glandular swelling, you are more likely to recognize a new lump. If your periods have stopped, just select a regular date each month that you are likely to remember, like the first or last day.

Physician Breast Examination

A thorough breast exam should be part of any physical exam and gy-necological checkup. Your doctor's exam should be regarded as part of your backup system. Although you are the established expert on what your breasts feel like, an experienced physician has felt many more abnormal lumps than you. If you are concerned about a difference you have noticed, this is the person whose opinion you should solicit. Once you know that what you are feeling is not suspicious, you can be less concerned. If, on the other hand, you are both in agreement that something suspicious is indeed present, an investigation will be set in motion. The next exam will likely be a mammogram.

The above has been the traditional thinking; but this is beginning to change also. Nearly half of our population is now enrolled in HMO health coverage. In this system, it can take several weeks to get an appointment to see your primary health provider. When your breast lump is confirmed by your regular doctor, you are then referred to a surgeon to be evaluated for a possible breast biopsy. This can take additional time. Some HMO physicians are now urging that you make an appointment directly with a surgeon, and avoid wasted time. This is the doctor who will be handling your evaluation, so you might just as well eliminate an unnecessary step.

Mammography

The survival rate for women with early breast cancer that has not spread has risen in the past fifty years from 78 percent to 93 percent. (ACOG 1995). Dr. Robert Tarone of the National Cancer Institute's Biostatistics Branch reported in 1996 that since 1987 there has been a continuing decline in the death rate from breast cancer. This is attributed to earlier diagnosis as the result of screening mammography and to improved treatment. Mammograms can detect tumors of less than 1 centimeter in size. This is about one quarter of the size found by the average woman's self-exam. Since early detection is a major key to surviving breast cancer, it is obvious that mammography plays an important role.

The examination is done with an X-ray machine that passes radiation through your breasts after they have been compressed to a flatter shape. This can be uncomfortable, so be sure not to get it done in the latter half of your cycle, when your breasts may be naturally tender. The X-ray film shows the general architecture of the breasts and any abnormal densities within them. Cancer densities are different in character than others, and they usually have a certain type of calcium flecks that can be recognized by a skillful radiologist.

TIP! Be sure to avoid using body powder before a mammogram; the powder granules may be misleading on the X-ray film, masking calcium flecks in a tumor.

About one in ten screening mammograms discloses an abnormality. In this situation an additional magnification view may be necessary. An ultrasound exam may also be done to get a better look at a suspected cyst. One or two in ten of these exams may lead to a recommendation for a biopsy of the suspicious area.

Like many women, you may have some worries, fears, and cost concerns about mammography. Let's take a look at some of the things you may be thinking:

- **It hurts:** Yes, it is uncomfortable to have your breasts squeezed. Fortunately, the exam is brief, and the pressure is tolerable.
- **Too much radiation is bad for you:** That is also true, but the exposure you get from a mammogram is 0.2 rads to each breast. This is less than you get from background cosmic radiation in a round-trip transcontinental plane flight. It's very small.
- **It is unnecessary:** Wrong! Neither you nor your doctor can detect a tumor as small as the mammogram can, so you may be sacrificing the distinct advantage of early detection. Mammograms have already been credited with reducing the death rate from breast cancer by 25 percent because of early identification.

- **They are too expensive:** The cost of a mammogram ranges from $75 to $150, and there isn't any low-cost alternative. Treating advanced breast cancer, though, costs from $25,000 to $150,000.

A big question is how often to have a mammogram. The long-term survival studies of breast cancer recently showed that women in their forties who have had mammogram screening survive their breast cancer better than women who did not have mammograms (ACOG 1997). However, mammograms in women under age 50 produce a higher percentage of false positive readings. They also resulted in four times as many biopsies as in women over fifty. The reason is that younger breasts are denser, and this results in more suspicious shadows on the X-ray film. As a matter of fact, until recently, most experts believed that mammography in women under thirty is useless unless there is a strong family history of premenopausal breast cancer. In 1993, the National Cancer Institute (NCI) withdrew its endorsement for screening women under fifty. They adopted a neutral stance, suggesting that you should "decide for yourself." However, more recent studies have shown that cancer grows more rapidly in younger breasts, and annual mammograms are indeed justified in women under fifty. Two separate studies showed that mammograms reduced breast cancer deaths of women in their forties by 44 percent and 35 percent (ACOG 1997). In light of this and the new school of thought about the value of BSE, the thinking has changed. Leaders in the field now recommend annual mammography for all women starting at age 40. In March 1997, the American Cancer Society revised their recommendation to include annual mammograms starting at age forty, and the National Cancer Institute reversed their 1993 decision; they have suggested a compromise recommendation of mammograms every one to two years over forty.

We know what you're thinking: "Rats! How can I decide if you doctors can't agree?" (Well sometimes you can't get agreement from a group of doctors on whether or not to leave a burning building.) This particular controversy seems to be getting settled, though, as a national consensus is emerging on annual mammograms for everyone over age forty. Mammograms of younger breasts may lead to unnecessary biopsies; but early detection of cancer by means of a mammogram may pay off by saving your life. If you run into opposition from your health insurance carrier or HMO on the issue of annual mammograms, don't take it lying down. If you get turned down, write a letter pointing out the national consensus on annual mammograms, any risk factors you may have; and ask for their denial of this service in writing. There's a good chance you will receive prompt approval for annual mammograms.

TIP! Augmentation breast implants may somewhat diminish the effectiveness of mammography. (Scar tissue around the implant may hinder the breasts from being compressed adequately.) Most X-ray facilities have special techniques for dealing with this, so ask them about it when you make your appointment.

Ultrasound

Ultrasound is a useful backup tool for mammography. The sound waves pass *through* structures if they are composed mostly of water, but they are bounced back if they strike something solid. This creates an image on a monitor that can then be interpreted and evaluated. Ultrasound is not a good primary screening tool for breast cancer because it will not pick up lumps smaller than 1 to 2 centimeters. In addition, ultrasound cannot distinguish the tiny calcium flecks that are so important in recognizing early cancer. Its main usefulness is in distinguishing between breast masses that are cystic (fluid filled) and those that are solid. Mammograms do not make this distinction. If a lump is cystic, it may not be necessary to do more than drain the cyst with a tiny needle. A solid mass is more ominous and usually requires biopsy or removal. Ultrasound saves a lot of biopsies.

New Developments in Breast Cancer Screening

Let's look now at some new ways that are being developed to detect breast cancer.

In 1996, the FDA approved an advanced high definition ultrasound machine designed to distinguish between benign and malignant breast lumps. Conventional ultrasound produces a rather grainy image, but a process called high-definition imaging (HDI) is much more distinct. In several other countries where HDI has been used for some time, studies showed that it is 99 percent accurate in predicting that a breast lump is noncancerous, but it is only 60 percent correct when it predicts cancer. This means a 40 percent false positive cancer prediction; but it has the potential to reduce by 40 percent the 700,000 breast biopsies that are done each year. This can represent a huge advantage in reducing the pain, inconvenience, and expense of diagnosing or ruling out cancer by biopsy.

Magnetic resonance imaging (MRI) is another option. It is expensive and can be a daunting procedure—the patient must lie still in a narrow tube for thirty minutes or more. A horseshoe-shaped open MRI tube has been developed to alleviate this claustrophobic effect, but they are not yet widely available. MRI offers these advantages in breast screening:

- It can aid in deciding whether a breast lump is benign or malignant, possibly avoiding an unnecessary biopsy.
- It can detect whether a cancerous lesion is the sole tumor or in multiple locations.
- It utilizes no radiation.
- It can detect a leaking silicone breast implant.

A disadvantage is that MRI will detect breast lesions that are noncancerous and yet still lead to needless biopsies. It is not a practical tool for primary screening, but it can be useful as a mammography backup.

Another scanning process, called positive emission tomography (PET), measures the uptake of a radioactive sugar by a cancerous breast tumor. Because cancer cells have a high metabolic rate, they need more sugar for energy, and they concentrate the radioactive sugar more than normal cells. This creates a "hot spot" on the scan. The cost is quite high, so PET is not a first-line-of-defense screening device. The National Cancer Institute has recently funded a study to see whether PET can identify cancer cells in lymph nodes. If it can reliably do this, it will save painful lymph gland surgery in women with proven breast cancer, if the glands can be shown to be free of cancer cells.

As mentioned earlier in this chapter, it is now possible to identify the mutated forms of BRCA1 and BRCA2 genes that raise the risk for breast cancer to over 80 percent. The DNA screening technique for identifying these genes is becoming more available in research centers; but it is labor intensive and quite expensive. The question arises as to who should be screened. Shattuck-Eidens (1997) and Hoskins (1995) believe that a strong family history of breast and ovarian cancer justifies screening of any woman with that background. If genetic screening by DNA analysis reveals you have the mutated form of the gene, your family should also be screened. The American College of Obstetricians and Gynecologists Committee on Genetics (1996) believes that in the future, testing will become more reliable and practical.

Difficult questions arise as to how the information from such tests should be handled. If you are cancer-free and discover you carry the mutated gene, you must take many things into consideration: Should you have both breasts and your ovaries removed? What should you do about getting married? Does your fiancé have a right to know you may face a serious health threat at some future time? Should you plan a family? Does your employer have a right to know? How will this affect your health insurability? Must future disease potential be disclosed if it becomes known? You can see where this is leading. A mountain of genetic information is about to descend upon us in the next few years, and we are not prepared to handle it medically, morally, ethically, or legally. Science is beginning to outdistance the wisdom necessary to utilize its discoveries. There are no easy answers to these questions. However, the American Society of Clinical Oncology (ASCO) is working to keep on top of these issues. Guidelines were issued in May 1996 to help physicians advise their patients regarding breast cancer prevention, recognition of risk factors, early detection, counseling about familial cancer, and utilization of genetic screening (Gershenson 1996).

Treatment of Breast Cancer

The topic of treating breast cancer is too broad to be covered completely here. A great many options are available with regard to management. This means, of course, that if you are diagnosed with breast cancer, you have a great many decisions to make. Your best decisions will come from a base of good information about treatment. You can gather information from breast surgeons, plastic surgeons, radiation therapists, oncologists (cancer specialists), and a broad choice of literature (see Appendix B). Check for a local support group in your area. Enlist the support of your family and close friends. It isn't easy to make important decisions when you are under the stress of contemplating survival issues; a compassionate partner, friend, physician, or counselor can be of immense help.

Current surgical treatment of breast cancer with "lumpectomy" manages to avoid over two thirds of complete breast removals (mastectomies). Surgical reconstruction of a new breast is available if your breast must be removed. Radiation therapy and chemotherapy are extending lives by reducing the recurrence of tumors.

Tamoxifen Treatment for Prevention of Breast Cancer Recurrence

Tamoxifen, a weak estrogen, is being used as a follow-up treatment in women who have been treated for breast cancer. It is molecularly similar enough to estrogen that it can occupy estrogen receptor sites on breast cells and thus prevent estrogen from stimulating cancer growth in any residual cells. It is especially valuable if the breast cancer has estrogen receptors. For the first five years of use, it lowers the cancer recurrence rate by 25 to 35 percent. Tamoxifen was at one time being considered as a method of preventing breast cancer in women who are at particularly high risk for it. Because of the potential increased risk of uterine cancer and small intestine cancer with Tamoxifen use, it is no longer seriously considered for breast cancer prevention. This drug also helps prevent osteoporosis, and has a positive effect on cholesterol and lipoproteins. What a great drug, right? That was the good news.

The bad news is that when Tamoxifen occupies the estrogen receptor sites on the cells of endometrial glands, it stimulates the glands to overgrow and causes *hyperplasia* (an increase in cell growth). This can lead to endometrial cancer. The risk is about the same as in women who use unopposed estrogen (hormone replacement of estrogen with no progesterone). So what is a body to do? The best course for Tamoxifen users is to use periodic ultrasound scanning of your uterus to detect any thickening of the endometrium. If thickening is detected and hyperplasia is proven by endometrial biopsy (an office procedure), a course of progesterone therapy will reverse it. If not, you can have your uterus removed, which will cure it.

Summary of Breast Cancer

Breast cancer is a frightening prospect. It may not be an everyday worry for you as a transitional woman, but it is important to assess your personal risk factors for breast cancer and let this information help chart your life course. Prevention techniques, in those areas you can control, are important. In addition, new discoveries about breast cancer continue to be made that promise to enhance the available methods of prevention, early diagnosis, and treatment.

Endometrial Cancer

Cancer of the endometrium (uterine lining) is the most common genital cancer in women over forty-five (ACOG 1993). It is primarily a disease of post-menopausal women. Approximately 33,000 cases are diagnosed each year, and almost 6,000 deaths result. The annual risk rate is almost 2 per 1,000 women. Endometrial cancer ranks as the fourth most common female cancer of any type. (Lung, breast, and colon cancer are the first three, in that order.) In recent years, the frequency of this cancer's death rate has been diminishing. Speculation is that the decrease is due to better recognition of the disease in its early stages, as well as from the practice of adding progestin (synthetic progesterone) to the regimen of women who use estrogen replacement.

Hormones and Endometrial Cancer

In 1975, two studies reported that the frequency of endometrial cancer was increased in women on hormone replacement therapy (HRT) who used estrogen with no added progestin. Unfortunately, this use of unopposed estrogen had been the common practice for the previous two decades. Further research by numerous investigators confirmed the increase in endometrial cancer, indicating that this form of HRT causes an increased cancer risk of five to eight times the normal range (Gershenson, 1997). More important, the research also showed that if progestin is added to the HRT, the increased risk was reversed to the same level as in those women who took no hormones at all.

The protective mechanism of progestin is based on the effect that your natural, native progesterone (what your body produces) has on endometrial cells. Estrogen causes growth of endometrial cells, and progesterone inhibits and limits the extent of the growth. This is the same way your menstrual cycle works. At the end of a menstrual period, the endometrium has been shed and estrogen initiates new growth. After ovulation, at mid-cycle, progesterone comes into play and makes the endometrium more vascular and receptive to implantation of a fertilized egg. If a pregnancy is not initiated, estrogen would just continue the growth stimulus if it were not for progesterone, which stops it. This is because progesterone is an anti-estrogen. Progesterone protects the endometrium by reducing the number of available estrogen receptors on the cells and by inducing enzymes in the cells to convert estrogen from estradiol, the most potent form of estrogen, to estrone, the least potent. This reduces the degree of estrogen stimulation and, in turn, the risk of abnormal growth. Later in the cycle, both hormones decrease, and the endometrium is shed in a menstrual period. In hormone replacement therapy using both hormones, the protective effect of progestin (synthetic progesterone) works in the same fashion.

The net effect of too much estrogen stimulation, whether from unopposed estrogen replacement or from life events, is that the endometrial glands become enlarged, and the endometrium thickens (called hyperplasia). Over time, the excess stimulation results in distorted glands, called atypical hyperplasia, which is a precancerous condition.

Are You at Risk?

The risk factors for endometrial cancer are increased by estrogen stimulation without the modulating effect of progesterone. The following are known risk factors.

Absence of Ovulation

Most of the progesterone you produce occurs after ovulation. A variety of situations can result in failure to ovulate, called *anovulation*, and underproduction of progesterone. This can occur during the perimenopausal transition; if you are having irregular menstrual cycles, there may be prolonged periods of anovulation. This can lead to hyperplasia and abnormal bleeding. Be sure to get a consultation for any change in your bleeding pattern.

Failure to ovulate can also occur as a result of infertility from a hormonal cause. Another condition, polycystic ovary syndrome, can result from abnormal estrogen production, an increase in male hormone, and irregular or absent ovulation. Women with this condition are also at increased risk for endometrial cancer.

Obesity

A process called *aromitization* converts fat to estrone, the weak form of estrogen. This estrogen source is constant, rather than cyclic like the estradiol produced in your ovaries. After years of extra stimulation from estrone, an endometrial cancer can finally result. The more overweight a woman is, and the longer that condition exists, the greater the risk.

Diabetes and High Blood Pressure

Many diabetics are overweight and at risk from the extra estrone. Even diabetics of normal weight, however, are at risk because diabetes itself is an independent risk factor; diabetes plus obesity is a double whammy. Many diabetics are hypertensive from hardening of the arteries. If high blood pressure is also added to the mix, endometrial cancer is even more likely.

Hormone Replacement With Unopposed Estrogen

This was discussed above, but it bears repeating. Newer techniques for monitoring the endometrium of women who use unopposed estrogen are available. This is discussed in Chapter 8.

Screening and Diagnosis

How does your doctor detect endometrial cancer? Abnormal bleeding is the single most important clue. When this occurs, ultrasound and tissue sampling are the primary means of evaluating it.,

Ultrasound to the Rescue

If the endometrium becomes thickened by hyperplasia, ultrasound can detect, and even measure, the thickness. (The procedure involves inserting a specially designed probe into your vagina.) Your ovaries can be evaluated at the same time. If the endometrial thickness is 4 mm or less, everything is okay. If the thickness is 5 mm or more, a sample must be taken for microscopic analysis. Vaginal ultrasound saves a lot of endometrial biopsies for women who have abnormal uterine bleeding.

Tissue Sampling

When ultrasound findings and/or abnormal vaginal bleeding suggest that endometrial tissue must be evaluated, tissue sampling is the next step. Several methods are available to accomplish this:

- **Dilation and curettage (D&C):** The traditional method of obtaining tissue samples until the last decade or so. It involves dilating the canal of the *cervix* (the opening of the uterus) sufficiently to introduce instruments for scraping a sample of the uterine lining. It is a blind procedure—the tissue being removed cannot be seen. As you might surmise, a D&C has built-in inaccuracies. Polyps, fibroids and cancers can be missed. Polyps are pieces of endometrial tissue that hang by a stalk and are not shed by a menstrual period. They tend to cause a prolonged trickling pattern of bleeding. Fibroids are benign (noncancerous) muscle tumors in the wall of the uterus that can cause abnormal bleeding. Fibroids are discussed in Chapter 15.

- **Endometrial biopsy:** A simplified version of the D&C. A tiny tube, called a canula, is inserted through the canal of the cervix into the uterine cavity. Dilation of the cervix is not required because the canula is about the same diameter as the cervical canal. This is an office procedure, and it takes only seconds to obtain a tissue sample. The disadvantage is that, like a D&C, it's blind, and it hurts.

- **Hysteroscopy:** The hysteroscope is a hollow metal tube with an eyepiece and internal fiber-optic lighting. When inserted into the uterine cavity, it offers a view of the entire endometrial surface. Abnormalities can be pinpointed and accurately biopsied.

Preceded by ultrasound, hysteroscopic evaluation and tissue sampling represent a giant step forward in endometrial assessment.

Prevention of Endometrial Cancer

What can you do to prevent endometrial cancer? Let's take a look at the options.

Be Alert to Your Bleeding Pattern

Abnormal bleeding is a convenient (yes, we really mean that) marker for endometrial disease. Hyperplasias and cancers bleed easily and early. Knowing this can get you under care promptly and increase your chances for a complete cure. If hyperplasia is present, it can be reversed with progesterone therapy (see the next section), and a potential cancer can be avoided. Early treatment of endometrial cancer approaches a 100 percent cure rate.

CAUTION! Do *not*, repeat not, ignore an abnormal pattern of vaginal bleeding.

Hormones

Proper and timely administration of progesterone can reduce your risk for endometrial cancer. Absence of progesterone puts you at risk. The less you are exposed to unopposed estrogen stimulation during your lifetime, the less your likelihood of this cancer. The low dose birth control pill, which uses small doses of estrogen and synthetic progesterone, can provide what you need. Anytime you are anovulatory for a period of many months or years, the Pill can help. This can occur in the early teens, when anovulation is common, and in the perimenopausal years as well. We can hear what you're thinking: "Do you mean I should put my fourteen-year-old on the Pill? Gulp." We recognize the anxiety you may feel about your young daughter becoming prematurely sexually active if on the Pill. It would involve a certain amount of trust, but it will protect her endometrium if she is not ovulating.

As you know, during your perimenopausal transition, failure to ovulate can be sporadic or prolonged. Taking the low-dose Pill during this time affords you a number of advantages, including contraception, protection against cardiovascular disease, and osteoporosis, and a reduction in the risk of ovarian cancer. Add one more to that list: a decreased risk for endometrial cancer. Studies show that for women on the Pill, the endometrial cancer risk is lower by more than half compared to those who never used it. If the Pill use continues for ten years or more, the risk reduction is 80 percent, and the protection continues at a 30 percent reduction for about twenty years after the

Pill is discontinued (Reichman 1996). The take-home message is that if you have risk factors for endometrial cancer such as diabetes, obesity, and anovulation, taking the Pill in your forties protects your endometrium into your fifties and sixties. Other forms of progesterone are available for you if you cannot or must not take estrogen.

Treatment of Endometrial Cancer

An abdominal hysterectomy is usually required to treat endometrial cancer because lymph glands in the pelvis must be removed. A newer alternative to this surgery involves using a *laparoscope* to detach the uterus from its surrounding structures, followed by its removal through the vagina. The laparoscope is a hollow tube with a fiber-optic lighting system, which can be inserted into the abdomen through a small incision to view internal organs. Operating instruments can be inserted to perform surgery. A video camera can be attached for viewing the operation on a TV monitor. This operation, called laparoscopically assisted vaginal hysterectomy, or LAVH, is explained in Chapter 15. The pelvic lymph glands can also be removed with this technique. The advantage is a shorter hospitalization and quicker recovery as a result of smaller incisions. When endometrial cancer is diagnosed early, the cure rate is 95 to 98 percent. In more advanced stages, post-operative radiation and chemotherapy may be needed.

Summary of Endometrial Cancer

Endometrial cancer death is mostly preventable. Recognition of your risk factors and becoming proactive in altering them favorably is crucial to avoiding this disease. All that is necessary is to get a consultation if you have abnormal vaginal bleeding, be aware of the risk factors your may have, and have the diagnostic studies your doctor suggests. If you catch it early on, you can be cured.

Lung Cancer

Lung cancer is numero uno. Every year there are more than 72,000 new cases. Since 1987, more women die of it than of any female malignancy. Breast cancer causes 46,000 deaths annually, but the American Cancer Society says that lung cancer kills 59,000 women each and every year. And the numbers are continuing to rise. It is much less curable than breast cancer, with an overall five-year survival rate of only 13 percent. Even if caught early, the five-year survival rate with intense treatment is still only 37 percent. Lung cancer symptoms are usually a late-in-the-disease event. Screening with routine chest X-rays has little positive value in early detection. It may not make front page news, but the current means of diagnosis and treatment of lung cancer are clearly inadequate.

Risk Factors

In a word ... smoking. The "smoking gun" that links tobacco use to lung cancer—an ingredient of tobacco tar called benzo(a)pyrene—has been identified. The experts agree that cigarette smoking accounts for 85 percent of lung cancer cases. The converse is therefore obvious, that you can eliminate 85 percent of your risk for the most common cancer you face by being a nonsmoker. That's the end of the story, right? Yes—that is, if you have always been a nonsmoker and you were never exposed to secondary tobacco smoke.

The fact is, second-hand tobacco smoke causes 3,800 lung cancer deaths annually in nonsmokers. Nonsmoking women who live with smokers have a 1.5 times increased risk for *any* kind of cancer. If you were raised by smokers, your lung cancer risk is already 17 percent higher than if you were not. Ex-smokers still have double the risk of nonsmokers, even after many years of having quit. Still, that's better than the thirty-five-fold increased risk of long-term smoking.

What other factors play a part in lung cancer? One of them is fat. The National Cancer Institute found in a study of nonsmokers that a high saturated fat intake increases the risk of lung cancer by six times. Other diseases, such as chronic bronchitis, tuberculosis, asthma, and emphysema, add to the risk as well.

Environmental pollutants are also a factor. Be sure your house is free of asbestos, a well-established carcinogen. The same for radon gas. Atmospheric smog has not been linked to lung cancer, but it seems to have an additive effect if you are a smoker.

Lung cancer is a discouraging disease because there are no early symptomatic markers, there is no effective screening tool, and treatment does not result in a favorable survival rate. The best we've got is prevention; don't smoke, and don't hang out with smokers. Keep in mind, too, that one of the best services you can do for your children is to set an example by being a nonsmoker.

Colon and Rectal Cancer

Colon and rectal (colorectal) cancer is the number three cancer killer of women. Actually, it's about the same in both genders. In the 1990s, about 75,000 women are being diagnosed with colorectal cancer yearly, and 28,000 deaths have been recorded. Your lifetime chances of *getting* a colon cancer are about 6 percent, but with early pickup and effective treatment, your lifetime chances of *dying from it* are only about 3 percent. The chances of getting colorectal cancer are 11.5 times greater after age fifty than during your perimenopausal years. Why talk about it now? Because there are some changes you can make now that will decrease your personal risk later on.

Speaking of Risks, What Are They?

Would you guess that factors influencing the risk of cancer in the digestive tract would turn out to include food? You'd be right. Dietary components can be both positive and negative factors. Let's take a look at some of them:

- **Animal fat:** This is the primary risk in your diet, and red meat consumption is the major culprit. The Harvard Nurses' Health Study followed 90,000 women for six years and found two and a half times more colorectal cancer in red meat eaters than for women who ate fish or skinless chicken. That's pretty strong evidence. Dairy products appeared to have no influence on the incidence of colorectal cancer. If animal fat consumption is reduced to 20 percent of total daily calories, colon cancer is reduced by two thirds and rectal cancer by one third. (Reichman 1996)

- **Inadequate fiber:** A lack of fiber in your diet predisposes you to colorectal cancer. (Willet 1994) If you have a high fiber intake (25 to 30 grams a day), your risk for colorectal cancer is reduced by over 40 percent. The average American diet has only 10 to 15 grams a day. (See Chapter 10 for more on fiber.)

- **Heredity:** Heredity also influences cancer. Your risk is increased 1.7-fold if a first-degree relative has had colorectal cancer under age fifty-five, and 2.7-fold or higher if two or more have had it. When colorectal cancer is a familial trend, there is a greater likelihood that women will develop it in their thirties and forties than after fifty. (Note: A genetically induced condition called inherited polyposis syndrome causes 1 percent of colorectal cancer. The gene has been identified, so if this is in your family, get a consultation from a gastroenterologist (intestinal tract specialist).)

- **Colon polyps:** If you have had polyps identified in your colon, your risk of colon cancer is higher, even if the polyps were removed. You can get more of them, so periodic colonoscopy, explained in the next section, is important for you.

Screening—No Fun at All

There's nothing elegant about any of the screening methods for colorectal cancer. They all involve poking around a rather sensitive area of your body and doing perfectly revolting things like stool examinations. Keep in mind, though, that this one is the number three cancer killer for you. Let's take a look at the advantages offered by screening for colorectal cancer.

Digital Rectal Examination

A digital rectal examination is a necessary and important component of your annual pelvic exam. It is awkward and uncomfortable, but so is the rest of a pelvic exam, so why not put up with a few seconds more of that for an important check? Polyps, tumors, hemorrhoids, rectoceles (bulging of the rectum into the vagina), and abnormalities on the back of the uterus, as well as ovarian problems, can all be detected by a rectal-vaginal exam. If your annual exam does not include a rectal, ask for it to be done.

Screening for Fecal Occult Blood

Occult blood refers to invisible traces of blood in your stool. Bleeding anywhere in the gastrointestinal tract, from the mouth to the anus, can produce a positive occult blood test. The test for occult blood has been useful in detecting colorectal tumors (and for polyps over 1 centimeter in size).

You can do the test in the privacy of your home or take stool samples to the laboratory. Several things can trigger a false positive test, so for seven days before you collect a stool specimen, you must avoid red meats, raw fruits (especially melons), raw vegetables (especially radishes, turnips, and horseradish), aspirin, nonsteroidal anti-inflammatory agents (like ibuprofen), and vitamin C. The dietary restrictions must continue during the three days of stool sample collection. Vaginal bleeding can contaminate a stool specimen, so be certain to avoid collection during your menstrual period.

A positive test requires a more thorough investigation. One study (Reichman 1996) of over 21,000 people showed that the mortality from colorectal cancer was reduced by one third in people with positive tests, if colonoscopy (which we explain in a moment) was done and the responsible polyps removed. The American Cancer Society suggests that occult blood testing be done annually on women (and men) over age fifty.

However, fecal occult blood screening is starting to go the way of the dinosaur. It is cumbersome and inconvenient, so strict compliance is difficult for most people. Newer thinking, backed by newer technology, is resulting in abandoning this time-honored screening test. Colon cancer experts now feel that integrating family history of colorectal cancer with examination through the use of two techniques, flexible sigmoidoscopy and colonoscopy, are better screening methods. Colonoscopy is an examination of the entire interior length of the colon with a flexible fiber-optic tube. Flexible sigmoidoscopy is similar, but only about one third of the colon is examined. The newer recommendation to replace occult blood screening is this: If you have first or second-degree relatives who have had colon cancer under age fifty-five, you should have a colonoscopy at an age ten years younger than your relative's age when it was discovered in that relative. If everything is normal, your colonoscopy should be repeated every five years. If there is no colorectal disease in your family, a colonoscopy or flexible sigmoidoscopy should be done every ten years starting at age fifty. At this point in time, these exams are not available in all communities. In this situation, the three-day test for fecal occult blood should be done annually starting at age fifty. The occult blood test done at the time of a rectal exam has been abandoned because of too many false positive results.

Another screening procedure for colorectal cancer is the barium enema. Barium shows up on X-ray, so filling the colon with it outlines the walls of the rectum and entire colon. Barium enemas disclose about three-quarters of tumors or polyps larger than 1 centimeter. Colonoscopy and trained colonoscopists may be in short supply in some areas, so a barium enema may be the first test done when the occult blood test is positive. If a tumor or polyps are found, the next step is direct visualization and biopsy with sigmoidoscopy or colonoscopy.

Prevention

We've already looked at diet (low animal fat intake and high fiber levels) and screening methods as the two most important preventive methods for colorectal cancer. There are a few more you should know about:

- **Beta-carotenes:** Beta-carotenes play a role in preventing colorectal cancer. These are food pigments that are converted to vitamin A. You will find them in green and yellow vegetables such as carrots, squash, sweet potatoes, pumpkin, spinach, broccoli, and cantaloupe. Consumption of a diet rich in these foods results in less colorectal cancer when compared to those who eat little of them.

- **Exercise:** As a preventive measure for colorectal cancer, exercise may surprise you, but consider this: Exercise increases the production of prostaglandins, which stimulate involuntary muscle activity. (See Chapter 4 for more about prostaglandins.) The theory is that prostaglandins decrease the chance of colorectal cancer by speeding up the propulsion of food wastes, thereby reducing the amount of time the colon walls are in contact with any carcinogens that were consumed.

- **Aspirin and other nonsteroidal anti-inflammatory drugs (NSAIDs):** These inhibit a type of prostaglandin (PGE2) that is overproduced by colorectal cancers; it is this form of prostaglandin that enables the cancer to promote its own growth into surrounding tissues. The Harvard Nurse's Health Study found that long-term (twenty years) use of four to six aspirin tablets a week reduced the cancer risk by 50 percent. NSAIDs such as sulindac are also beneficial (Calle and Thun 1997).

- **Estrogen:** Calle and Thun reviewed twenty-three studies on colorectal cancer and estrogen use. They found than estrogen reduces your risk of getting colorectal cancer by 20 to 60 percent.

Summary of Colorectal Cancer

Your risk for colon and rectal cancer is much higher than for any of the female genital cancers. As the third most common malignancy you face as a woman, it deserves your attention. This may sound like an old song in this chapter, but let's sing it again: This disease is largely avoidable if you know your personal risks, include the recommended preventive measures in your life, and take advantage of available screening methods. Just as for other tumors, you must become informed and proactive to be in control of this type of cancer.

Cervical Cancer

Since 1950, cervical cancer deaths have been reduced by more than 70 percent. Something to crow about, right? No, not yet. If routine screening were available to all women (and unfortunately, it is not) and women took advantage of that screening (and they don't always do so, for a number of reasons), deaths from cervical cancer might be reduced up to 90 percent. Every year 13,500 women still develop invasive cervical cancer, and 4,400 die mostly needless deaths. Cervical cancer is a young woman's disease. About 75 percent of cases are at an age less than sixty-five, and most are premenopausal (ACOG 1993).

Alphabet Soup	
ASCUS	Atypical squamous cells of undetermined significance
HPV	Human papilloma virus
HGSIL	High-grade squamous intraepithelial lesion
LEEP	Loop electrosurgical excision procedure
LGSIL	Low-grade squamous intraepithelial lesion
STD	Sexually transmitted disease

Cervical cancer is quite slow to develop. It is estimated that in 95 percent of women with a high-grade cervical lesion (the most severe noncancerous cellular abnormality), it takes eight to twelve years from the time it appears to the development of invasive cancer. In 5 percent, however, a much faster progression, of 6 to 24 months, may occur. (Celentano 1989)

What Puts You at Risk?

In a word, sex. And no, this doesn't mean you have to stop it. In recent years, sexually transmitted diseases (STDs) have been linked to cervical cancer. This has given additional meaning to the term "safe sex." Several factors are known to play a role.

Human papilloma virus (HPV)—The Main Player

Like other cancers, the causes of cervical cancer are not yet completely understood. But it is known worldwide that the human papilloma virus (HPV) is present in about 95 percent of all cervical cancers. The virus has more than seventy known strains, twenty-four of which are known to infect the genitals of both sexes. As additional types of this virus are discovered, its presence in cervical cancer approaches 100 percent (Bosch 1995). Researchers now feel that certain strains of HPV, called *oncogenic HPV*, are necessary to the development of cervical cancer, but that they in themselves are not completely sufficient to cause cancer. Other factors, which we'll look at in a moment, can also influence your risk.

The health risk of HPV is not a serious one—except in women! If you are infected, the risk of high-grade cellular abnormalities in the cervix increases by as much as 25 percent. The risk is especially high for twelve specific strains of HPV (Braly 1997). Most women who have been infected with HPV do *not* develop cervical cancer or precancerous changes in the cervix *unless* they have one of the cancer-causing strains. HPV is also linked to vaginal and vulvar cancer.

A mutually monogamous relationship appears to be the best protection from HPV. If your Pap smear shows evidence of an HPV-induced cellular abnormality, a colposcopic exam (exam with a binocular magnifying instrument) with appropriate biopsies may need to be done, and treatment initiated. The colposcopic exam should also include your vagina, vulva, perineum (area between vagina and anus), and the anus. Regular follow-up Pap screening is a must.

Now let's look at a few other factors that influence risk:

- **Multiple Partners:** The most significant risk factor for your developing cervical cancer is whether or not you have had multiple sex partners. The more you have had, especially if a barrier contraceptive method was not used, the greater is the likelihood that you will have acquired HPV. The second most important determinant is whether your partner(s) have also had multiple sex partners.

- **Unprotected sex at an early age:** The earlier you started having sex unprotected by condoms, the more at risk you are for cervical cancer, simply because HPV will have been in your cervix a greater number of years. Multiple partners and unprotected sex add to the risk for teens, just as for anybody else.

- **Herpes virus:** Herpes is a virus that is readily transmitted sexually. It causes very painful skin ulcerations on the vulva (a woman's outer genitals), as you will well remember if you have been infected. Herpes can be a life threat to a newborn infant; but in adults it rarely is a serious problem. Nevertheless, women who carry the virus are known to have a higher incidence of abnormal Pap smears. Herpes virus can lead to precancerous abnormalities.

- **Cigarettes:** Cigarette smoking is recognized as a cofactor for cervical cancer. It doubles your risk. Nicotine has been found in the vaginal secretions of smokers at concentrations forty times higher than the bloodstream (Notelovitz 1993). If you smoke, it is just as important for you to have regular Pap smears as for any of the situations already mentioned.

- **Genetic susceptibility:** A 1995 Japanese study report by Nawa indicated that heredity may also be a factor.

Screening—The Pap Smear

The Pap smear is easy, painless, and affordable; insurance covers it. It is done during a pelvic exam. A speculum is placed in your vagina so your cervix can be seen, and then some cells are collected and placed on a slide for analysis. Getting a Pap smear doesn't take long, and it might save you from getting a cancer.

The lab looks for specific changes in the cervical cells that are the precursors of cancer cells. These changes occur well in advance of cancer, and this is the advantage the Pap smear gives you. It can take eight to twelve years for cervical cells to be transformed from normal to cancerous. When precancerous cells are found, they can be easily and completely removed, preventing the development of a cancer.

A new method of evaluating cervical cells in liquid (called Thin Prep) is emerging that can also test for HPV and other sexually transmitted diseases, which in itself is a big step forward. With this method, more cells are available to study. Studies of the liquid method indicate it is more accurate in determining not only the presence of abnormal cells, but also the likelihood of whether abnormal cells will go on to become a cancer. In addition, compared to the standard dry slide technique, there are far fewer cellular abnormalities that are deemed to be of an "undetermined significance."

When Should You Get a Pap Smear, How Often, and for How Long?

The conventional wisdom for many years was to do the initial Pap smear by age eighteen (or at any younger age for those who were sexually active) and then every year after that. The National Cancer Institute, American Cancer Society, and American College of Obstetricians and Gynecologists, on the other hand, currently recommend the starting age just described but indicate that after three consecutive normal smears have been taken annually, a Pap every three years is adequate for protection. But new evidence coming from studies in Canada, Denmark, Norway, and the United States shows that lower levels of cervical cancer are seen when the screening interval is every two years. There appears to be no significant difference between one- and two-year intervals, but according to these studies, the cancer rate is up to four times higher if the test is done every three years.

It is now known that some HPV infections can cause a severe cellular abnormality in the cervix, called *high-grade squamous intraepithelial lesion* (HGSIL), which in about 5 percent of instances can progress to an invasive cancer within six to twenty-four months (Koutsky 1992). This is why Pap screening must begin as soon as sex begins. It was formerly thought that these abnormalities went through a multiyear process of progressive worsening from low-grade to high-grade precancerous lesions, but this is not the case. In fact, it is possible to have a *low-grade squamous intraepithelial lesion* (LGSIL) coexisting with HGSIL. On the other hand, LGSIL is not typically a precursor of cancer and it usually does not even progress to HGSIL. LGSIL often disappears without treatment. But a Pap is necessary to tell what may be happening in your cervix.

There is a variation in opinion as to the age at which Pap screening can be discontinued. For women who have had a high-grade cellular abnormality or cervical cancer, Pap testing should continue indefinitely, even if the uterus has been removed. (It is possible to develop a vaginal cancer after the cervix has been removed if high-grade cervical disease was present.) Aside from that situation, an emerging policy in large clinics like Kaiser Permanente and others is to stop screening in the late sixties to early seventies if there have been three normal Paps at intervals of at least one year over the prior ten years. However, gynecologic oncologist Dr. Walter Kinney (1997) feels Pap screening should continue indefinitely for most women. He notes that 25 percent of cervical cancers and 40 percent of deaths from cervical cancer are in women who are over age sixty-five, and many women by this age have had multiple sex partners and or partners with multiple other partners, which puts them at risk. He recommends, for this reason, that Pap smears be done throughout a woman's lifetime.

Changing Names for Precancerous Cervical Abnormalities

The names for precancerous abnormalities have been undergoing gradual change over the years. We are striving for a system that will describe the degree of severity and mean the same thing to every doctor. The ancient *Class I* through *Class IV* Pap smear report gave way to: *mild dysplasia, moderate dysplasia, severe dysplasia,* and *carcinoma-in-situ.* This final term means a cancer that has not begun to spread. Next came *cervical intraepithelial neoplasia* (CIN), which meant all of the above expressed as *CIN I, CIN II,* and *CIN III.* More recently, all of the above were replaced by the *Bethesda System* for reporting pap smears. As we mentioned earlier, low-grade or high-grade squamous intraepithelial lesion (LGSIL or HGSIL) is now used. LGSIL is the same as the former terms for mild dysplasia and CIN I, while HGSIL covers moderate to severe dysplasia, or CIN II to CIN III. When your cells are not normal, but it isn't clear what's going on, it's called *atypical squamous cells of undetermined significance* (ASCUS). When atypical glandular cells are seen, they call it AGCUS. Don't worry about these terms; there won't be a quiz. Doctors are just trying to learn how to talk to each other about this disease in uniform terms that are meaningful to all of us. We just wanted to familiarize you with the Bethesda System so you will be less surprised when your doctor talks to you about pap results.

Computer Screening of Pap Smears

You will probably not be surprised to learn that the FDA has approved two systems that use high-resolution digital scanners to record images of cells and feed them into a computer. The computer is programmed to distinguish between normal and abnormal cells. Neither system (they are known as AutoPap and PapNet) is licensed to do more than retrospective screening of Pap smears. This means that Pap smears that have already been read as negative by conventional methods can be reviewed by the computer method. They are strictly a quality-control mechanism for laboratories, in spite of what you may have read or heard. As these tests are presently used, your Pap smear will not be read by either of these computerized programs unless it was normal to begin with. Dr. Kenneth Noller, chairman of the Ob/Gyn department at the University of Massachusetts, believes that if they prove themselves to be reliable and valuable, their future use for initial interpretation of Pap tests may become a reality. Even if that comes to pass, any abnormal results by a computer will be rechecked by human experts.

Now let's get back to more practical information.

Evaluating Your Abnormal Pap

Pap screening is your entrée to diagnosis. If it is abnormal, the next step will depend upon what the Pap report says. Generally it sorts itself out into either of two recommendations. For a high-grade abnormality, cervical biopsies using a colposcope are needed. Low-grade abnormalities are not regarded as serious and immediate risks. One option is to do a colposcopy. A second choice is to simply repeat the Pap three times at six-month intervals. If all three repeats are normal, routine screening intervals are resumed. If a second abnormal Pap shows up, a colposcopy and biopsies must be done. ASCUS reports are handled the same way as LGSIL.

The Pap smear to test for cervical cancer is not perfect. Failure to detect an abnormality happens about 10 percent of the time, which makes it fortunate that the 95 percent of cervical cancers develop slowly. If you are getting regular Pap screening, however, the likelihood of a developing cancer being missed on every Pap smear is quite small.

Treatment of Precancerous Cervical Abnormalities

The principle involved in treatment of precancerous cervical lesions is to destroy or remove the abnormal cells so that they can be replaced with normal cells. This can be accomplished in several ways:

- **Cryocautery:** A method of freezing the targeted tissue with specially designed probes. Extreme cold kills cells just like extreme heat. This method is usually restricted to low-grade lesions that are not very large or extensive. It is an inexpensive office procedure that does not require anesthesia.

- **Surgical removal:** Surgery involves cutting out the abnormal tissue. The tissue is removed intact for microscopic examination to be certain all the abnormality is contained within its borders and to check for involvement that might not have been revealed by smaller biopsy samples. One type of procedure, called LEEP (loop electrosurgical excision procedure), uses electrical current to remove the tissue. It can be performed in a doctor's office. Another, surgical conization of the cervix, is a hospital procedure. It is performed when the abnormal tissue has extended into the canal of the cervix or there is a suspicion of more advanced disease, such as an invasive cancer.

(Note: The method of laser vaporization was used for a few years but has largely been abandoned. In this procedure, the laser beam causes water in the cell to boil and the cell literally explodes. This process releases DNA material from the human papilloma virus into the atmosphere and thus poses a risk to anyone in the vicinity.)

After treatment for high-grade cellular abnormalities, it is very important to have Pap screening at increased intervals. A 1990 study by Gemmell demonstrated that recurrence or progression of cervical disease is most commonly detected in the first years following treatment, even if it was a hysterectomy. Therefore, Gemell's recommendation is for rescreening at six, twelve, and twenty-four months. If everything stays normal, a normal interval of every two years is then appropriate.

Summary of Cervical Cancer

Cervical cancer can and should be prevented. The simple Pap smear has a pretty good fifty-year track record in reducing the deaths from this disease by 70 percent; but it is still not good enough. Modern techniques and tools are very effective in preventing invasive cancer of the cervix, but getting a Pap is the first step.

Ovarian Cancer

Of all gynecologic cancers, ovarian cancer is the most difficult to diagnose, most unlikely to be cured, and therefore the most deadly. Luckily, it is also the least common. In every 100,000 women, 15 will develop ovarian cancer each year. Your lifetime risk for getting this cancer is 1.4 percent (1 in 70); but if you are unlucky enough to develop ovarian cancer, your chances of surviving five years are just 40 percent. The death toll is 14,000 women each year (ACOG 1993). This terrible track record stems from the fact that there are no early symptoms for ovarian cancer and that no effective screening methods are available. As a result, about 70 percent of women are already far advanced in the disease when the diagnosis is finally established. Unless you have a strong family history of ovarian cancer, the likelihood of getting this cancer during your perimenopausal years is quite small. Most of it occurs in the sixties and then diminishes in advanced age.

For a more detailed discussion of ovarian cancer see chapter 15 where it is discussed in the section regarding ovarian removal with a hysterectomy.

Summary

If you've made it all the way through this chapter about cancer, congratulations. It isn't pleasant to read about this type of disease. Still, if you made it this far, it means you have improved your fund of information about a disease process that frightens most of us.

Let's review the most important issues surrounding cancer:

- Cancer is not a high-risk disease for you as a perimenopausal woman, but you must not ignore it as a possibility.
- Many of the risk factors for these cancers can be altered it your favor, but you need to start changing them now, while you are young and there is plenty of time.
- Most, but not all, cancers have effective screening techniques that are readily available.
- Certain body signs and symptoms can tip you off that you may be entering a cancer danger zone. Knowing them can save your life.

As a young woman, you may feel distanced from the diseases discussed in this chapter. For the most part, if they occur at all, they are still well down the road. We hope cancer is not a part of your future and that this chapter assists you in avoiding it.

◯ ◯ ◯

Section II:

Changing the Odds

8

You Can Change Your Hormones: The Case for Hormone Replacement Therapy (HRT)

Chapters 1 and 2 explained how estrogen and progesterone are produced, where they are produced, and changes that happen to you when their production slows down. This chapter is about some steps you can take to manage hormone deficiency. It covers the use of estrogen, progesterone, and androgens (male hormones)—their appropriateness, risks, and side effects, their dosage, and regimens for effective use. (Chapter 9 takes a look at alternatives to hormone replacement therapy.)

The first decision facing you is whether or not to *replace* estrogen and progesterone. This can be a dilemma of the first magnitude. It can hardly escape your attention that the issue of hormone replacement (hormone supplementation for perimenopausal women), is a polarized field. You hear "take 'em" and "don't take 'em" advice with equal fervor from divided camps.

The news media, unfortunately, tend to focus on negative news: "Estrogen Implicated in Breast Cancer." What little positive news is published has a negative spin: "Estrogen May Decrease Heart Attacks" (note the "may"). Only 20 percent of American women who use estrogen take it long term and consistently (Ettinger 1996), and that may be in part because useful information about it is hard to come by.

Dr. Daniel Mishell, chairman of the OB/Gyn department at the University of Southern California, has been a strong advocate of low-dose hormone replacement for perimenopausal women for many years. His experience, and that of many other physicians—generally ignored in the media—has been that the symptoms of hormone decline are reliably controlled with hormone supplements.

The case has already been well made for the dominant role of hormone use to prevent cardiovascular disease and osteoporosis. Also, there is striking new evidence that estrogen reduces and prevents the devastation of Alzheimer's disease, increases blood flow in the brain, and improves short- and long-term memory. And there is now general agreement that estrogen alleviates the symptoms of hormone decline.

Hormone Replacement Therapy (HRT) with Estrogen

Several hormones can be used in HRT, including estrogen, progesterone, and testosterone (male hormone). They are usually used in combination, but we will talk about each of them separately. Let's first look at the use of estrogen.

Benefits of Estrogen Use

Estrogen use offers a number of benefits:

- **Control of symptoms:** Hot flashes, sleep disruption, short-term memory loss, impaired concentration, moodiness, vaginal dryness, diminished sexual sensitivity, and all the other disturbances of perimenopause are not life threatening, but they can threaten your quality of life. Replacing estrogen reliably and quickly controls estrogen deficiency symptoms.

- **Cardiovascular protection:** The risk of death from coronary heart disease for women over age 50 is 31 percent (Cummings et al. 1989). Almost three dozen studies in the past quarter century have uniformly shown the extraordinary benefit estrogen has on the heart. The death rate from heart attacks is reduced by 50 percent if estrogen deficiency is corrected (Judd 1996). Estrogen has beneficial effects on all aspects of your cardiovascular system. As we've discussed elsewhere in this book, it lowers cholesterol, improves lipoprotein ratios of good HDL and bad LDL, lowers blood pressure, strengthens heart muscle, and reduces plaque formation in arteries. A recent analysis of CVD death rates from the Harvard Nurses' Health Study revealed a refinement of the 50 percent figure quoted above (Grodstein et al. 1997). They found hormone users who had the largest reduction in the risk to be women who had high risk factors for CVD. (See Chapter 5 for CVD risk factors.) High-risk women had a 49 percent reduction in CVD deaths, but in low-risk women it was 11 percent. This suggests, of course, that if you are in good health and you stay that way, estrogen replacement may not be as important to you for prevention of CVD.

- **Osteoporosis prevention:** Adequate calcium, weight-bearing exercise, vitamin D, a good diet, and avoidance of alcohol and tobacco are beneficial in prevention of osteoporosis, but they can't get it done as well without estrogen. Bone density can be improved by these other methods, but bone strength sufficient to lessen the fracture rate doesn't occur without estrogen (Felson et al. 1993, Cauley et al. 1995).

- **Better brain function:** Estrogen receptors in your brain cells receive estrogen molecules, which then improve the transmission of impulses from one neuron (nerve cell) to the next. Memory and other thought processes depend on adequate estrogen levels. In addition, estrogen use increases the number of functioning nerve cells. The more neurons you have, the larger the network of functioning nerve cells, and the better your brain functions. Estrogen supplements in elderly women have now been shown to decrease the incidence of Alzheimer's disease by 40 to 60 percent (Henderson 1995, Birge 1996). Estrogen also removes cholesterol plaques from the blood vessels in the brain, smoothing the walls of the vessels and allowing an increase in blood flow to those important little brain cells.

- **Vaginal dryness and thinning (atrophy):** Estrogen can not only prevent these problems, it can clear them up if you already have them. Advanced atrophy, with thinning of the vaginal walls, loss of their elasticity, and painful sex, is unlikely to happen to you during perimenopause, but it's important to stay alert to estrogen deficiency symptoms.

- **Prolapse of pelvic organs:** Loss of elasticity in the supporting structures of your uterus, bladder, and rectum may allow them to sag so far out of position that they protrude through your vagina. Childbearing and aging both play roles, but loss of estrogen is a facilitator (Cutler et al. 1992).

- **Urinary incontinence:** As in prolapse, loss of elasticity and atrophy can cause urinary incontinence; but estrogen depletion may contribute to both. Estrogen replacement does not restore lost tone, but use of estrogen before a surgical repair promotes more rapid healing (Fantl 1994).

- **Cancer prevention:** *Prevention?* Yes; evidence is accumulating that estrogen significantly reduces the incidence of colorectal cancer, your number three cancer risk. Drs. Eugenia Calle and Michael Thun of the American Cancer Society reported in 1997 that in as many as eighteen separate studies since 1989, the reduction ranged from 20 to 60 percent for women on estrogen replacement therapy. They found three additional studies that showed no association between estrogen use and colon cancer and three studies in which a small but statistically non-significant increase was suggested. (In other words, the number of cases observed was not sufficient to have reliable predictive power.)

- **Better skin:** Estrogen is necessary to maintaining normal collagen and elastin in skin. These two connective tissues are responsible for keeping your skin smooth and pliable. When estrogen declines, you start losing both collagen and elastin. If skin thickness diminishes from loss of collagen and skin elasticity declines from loss of elastin, guess what you get? Wrinkles. Estrogen is not a fountain of youth for skin, but it helps.

If you add all this up, you can see that estrogen can have a beneficial effect on your heart, blood vessels, bones, brain, vagina, bladder, colon, and skin. It also controls deficiency symptoms. Before you back the truck up to your pharmacy for a load of estrogen, though, be sure to read the next section.

Estrogen Risks

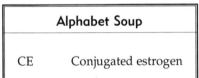

Alphabet Soup	
CE	Conjugated estrogen

If all the good news about estrogen were the complete story, the decision to use HRT would be a snap. Like most medical regimens, though (and like life in general, for that matter), the good news must be tempered by the downside: risks. To be effective and to avoid side effects and risks, estrogen must be used in appropriate situations and in appropriate doses. Both you and your doctor need to know your personal risk factors and the role estrogen may play in influencing them.

Estrogen risks are at the top of the list for most women when the subject of HRT comes up. A commonly expressed fear is, "They say it causes cancer." Of course you don't want a malignancy, so let's address that issue first.

Endometrial Cancer Risk with Estrogen Replacement

If a woman takes unopposed estrogen, her risk of endometrial cancer goes up 5 to 8 times compared to nonusers. The magnitude of the increased risk depends on the dose and duration of use. In a 1995 meta-analysis (review of all published studies), Grady and colleagues (1995) found that as little as six months of unopposed estrogen use increases the risk of endometrial cancer fourfold, and the increased risk lasts for several years. Even with the addition of progesterone after unopposed estrogen use, the risk is lowered only to twofold. It is now well established, however, that combining estrogen with progesterone reverses the cancer risk to the same level as for women not on HRT. One recent study in England cast some doubt on this when it reported that the combination of estrogen and progesterone does not completely reverse the risk to the same level as nonusers (Beresford et al. 1997). For such a report to be generally accepted, it must be confirmed by additional studies, such as the Women's Health Initiative, which we discuss a little later in this chapter. Meanwhile, if you decide on combined hormone HRT, which we describe later in this chapter, you are relatively free to concentrate on the remaining risk factors for endometrial cancer: obesity, diabetes, and high blood pressure.

Breast Cancer Risk with Estrogen Replacement

Researchers studying estrogen today think that in the few instances where an increased association of estrogen replacement and breast cancer exists, it is related to the total length of time breast cells are exposed to estrogen molecules (Zhang 1997). (Note: Numerous studies put this risk at about 5 percent.) This is based on the observation that there is a slightly greater association of breast cancer with native (produced by the body) estradiol replacement (Estrace) than with conjugated estrogen (CE) derived from animal sources.

The most commonly used conjugated estrogen is widely known by its brand name Premarin. It is derived from the urine of pregnant mares. CE has now been synthesized but has not received FDA approval. Premarin has been on the market since 1941 and is regarded as the "gold standard" for hormone replacement. Nearly every American study of long-term estrogen effects on hearts, bones, brains, and longevity has used Premarin. Other estrogen products relate their effectiveness to whatever a given dose of Premarin will do. It has a good record of effectiveness, which is why it is so widely used.

Conjugated estrogen molecules can occupy breast cell receptor sites for about three months at a time. This displaces estradiol and reduces the total amount of time breast cells are exposed to the native hormone. In other words, different types of estrogen have differing effects on the breast cells and other estrogen-sensitive tissues.

The evidence to date strongly suggests that estrogen may worsen an existing cancer. What most women fear, though, is that estrogen will *cause* cancer if they use it for replacement or supplementation. This fear was dramatically accentuated by broad coverage in the American media of a Swedish study (Bergkvist et al. 1989) that linked long-term estrogen use (over ten years) to an increased risk for breast cancer. Over the next several years (and without major media coverage), major flaws in this study were discovered. In their final article, published in an obscure medical journal in 1992, the authors corrected their erroneous 1989 data and found that estrogen did not cause an increase in the incidence of breast cancer (Adami 1992). This was ignored by the media, however, and the public fear generated by the original article persists.

More than fifty studies have now been published on the issue of breast cancer and estrogen (ACOG 1994). An analysis of all of them by researchers does not show convincing evidence that there is a causal relationship between estrogen and breast cancer (Dupont and Page 1991, Speroff 1995). Some of the studies (less than five) report increased risk, but the large majority do not. Another 1997 report, from the large Harvard Nurses' Health Study (which we described in Chapter 7) has shown an increase in breast cancer deaths in hormone users (Grodstein et al. 1997). Like other similar studies reporting increased breast cancer risk, it received national media attention. The study found that the risk of dying from breast cancer is increased by 43 percent in postmenopausal women who take female hormones for over ten years. Women between the ages of 50 and 94 who do not take hormones have a risk of 2.8 percent (Cummings et al. 1989), and the Grodstein study found that long-term hormone users have a 1.2 percent increase in risk, for a total of 4 percent. The Grodstein study also found that short-term hormone users (fewer than ten years) actually have a reduced risk of breast cancer death; and for all women studied, whether short-term or long-term hormone users, the overall mortality rate from breast cancer dropped. This means the reduced risk in short-term users more than offset the increased risk in long-term use of hormones.

The implications of this recent study are that a reappraisal must be made of whether lifetime use of hormones should be advocated. It certainly suggests that the decision for or against hormone replacement must be individualized. For many women, the benefits of hormone use may not compensate for the fear of acquiring breast cancer and having to live with the resulting bodily and emotional changes. For women with low risk factors for heart disease and osteoporosis but at high risk for breast cancer (see Chapter 7 for risk factors), the benefits of hormone replacement may not outweigh the risks. (Note: One exception to hormone use and risk factors for breast cancer found by the 1997 Grodstein report is that hormone users with a family history of breast cancer are not at any more risk of breast cancer than nonusers.)

Some epidemiologists (researchers who study large population disease trends) say that there is actually some reassurance in the fact that these studies

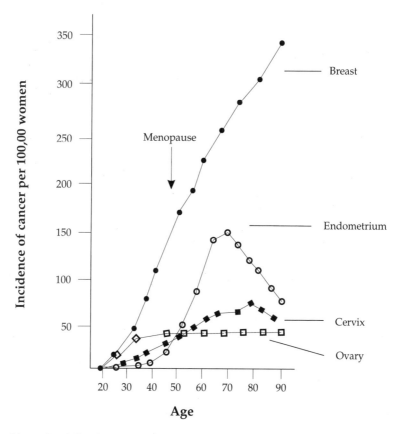

Adopted from: Grombell et al. 1983.

Figure 8.1. Female Cancer Rates in Nonhormone Users

disagree. They point out that if there were a close relationship between breast cancer and estrogen use, the studies would all have been in agreement. These scientists reason that if there is such a relationship, it is in a specific subset of women that is too small for current methods of investigation to reveal.

There is one more reassuring point about estrogen and breast cancer. Look over Figure 8-1. It demonstrates the incidence of female cancer in women who are *not* taking estrogen and shows that the incidence of endometrial cancer (which, it has been established, can be caused by hormone use) decreases after menopause, but the incidence of breast cancer *increases*. If estrogen is a factor in causing breast cancer, it would make sense for its incidence to decrease after menopause, when estrogen production is lost, but it does not. This strongly suggests that estrogen is not a major risk factor.

An additional point this diagram demonstrates is that breast cancer is not a disease of young women; eighty percent of it is in postmenopausal women. The definitive answers are not in. In other words, the two most significant risk factors for breast cancer are: being a woman and aging.

Widely publicized articles containing negative information about estrogen, such as the Swedish study we mentioned earlier, have resulted in uncounted numbers of women discontinuing their estrogen and have discouraged others from starting it. The definitive answers will come from the Women's Health Initiative (WHI), a prospective study of massive proportions sponsored by The National Institutes For Health that is currently under way. WHI is the largest study of women's health ever undertaken. One of the issues WHI is examining is the relationship of estrogen use to breast cancer. Their results will not be known until about 2005. Meanwhile, your best bet is the credible sources of information available from current studies, the preponderance of which do not show that estrogen causes breast cancer.

Gallstone Risk with Estrogen

Formation of cholesterol stones in the gallbladder is a small risk associated with estrogen. Estrogen enhances the level of HDL (high-density lipoproteins), which brings cholesterol to the liver. The cholesterol is then concentrated in the gallbladder and excreted in bile. (Bile is an intestinal aid in the digestion of fat; it passes out of the body in bowel movements.) If cholesterol concentrations are high while bile is being stored in the gallbladder, stones can be formed. Small ones are passed into the intestine with liquid bile, but larger stones remain in the gallbladder. The problem with gallstones arises when they start irritating the gallbladder or one of them gets stuck in the bile duct. Pain and vomiting after eating fatty foods results.

Risk factors for cholesterol gallstones are closely related to situations that produce high levels of estrogen in the bloodstream, such as pregnancy. The higher the level, the greater the risk. Other factors are also related to stone formation:

- **Dosage and potency:** The estrogen risk from HRT or birth control pills is related to dose and potency. Conjugated estrogen is sometimes prescribed in higher-dose tablets for special situations. The higher the dose, the greater the risk of gallstones, by as much as 50 percent. Transdermal (skin patch) estrogen enters the bloodstream directly through the skin and bypasses the liver. If you have some or all of the risk factors listed below for gallstones, the patch is probably the best route of administration.

- **Pregnancy:** Pregnancy raises the estrogen level to about 100 times the normal level. Gallstone problems are common during and just after a pregnancy, or after multiple pregnancies (twins).

- **Obesity:** Obesity results in more estrogen from the conversion of fat to estrone, the weak estrogen. This estrogen source is constant, not cyclic like ovarian production of native estradiol.
- **High-fat diet:** A diet high in animal fat puts more cholesterol into the bloodstream to cause not only problems like plaque formation in arteries, but cholesterol gallstone formation as well.

In the past, surgery to remove an inflamed gallbladder full of stones was a difficult operation from which to recuperate because of the large incision and long hospital stay needed. Now the operation is being done through a laparoscope, utilizing tiny incisions and a brief hospitalization.

Estrogen Side Effects

Side effects of estrogen range from breast tenderness and enlargement to headaches, nausea, and bloating. They are not serious health threats, but they certainly influence quality of life. For most women, side effects appear soon after starting estrogen replacement. They tend to diminish or disappear as the body becomes accustomed to the new estrogen level. This is similar to the way a woman gets used to the huge estrogen increases during pregnancy.

If you are experiencing side effects, it may be necessary to change the dose of estrogen, the type you are taking, the route of administration, the schedule of taking it, or all of the above. For example, women with headaches and nausea problems do better on the skin patch or oral native estradiol. Bloating and PMS-like symptoms are improved with a continuous schedule, rather than a cyclic regimen. More than half a dozen types of estrogen are available, so switching can be the answer. In other words, hormone replacement must be individualized for you. A "one size fits all" mind-set simply does not work. The bottom line is this: Don't give up on this important health benefit because of side effects. A caring physician who is knowledgeable about hormone replacement and perimenopausal changes can help you.

Types of Estrogen

There are several types of estrogen, available in a variety of forms from a number of manufacturers. They sort themselves into three categories: native (human) estrogen, animal-derived estrogen, and plant-derived estrogen. We'll take a look at each of them here.

Human Estrogens

The amount of each of the human estrogens present in your body at any given time is determined by a variety of life situations, including age, pregnancy, diet, amount of body fat, lifestyle habits that can affect your ovaries, and your genetic make-up. These are the three types:

- **17-beta estradiol:** For simplicity, we will refer to this type as estradiol. It is the predominant form of estrogen in your body from puberty through menopause. Produced in the ovaries, it is the biologically active form of estrogen that acts at the cell receptor sites throughout your body. It influences over 400 of your body's functions. This is the form of estrogen that starts declining after age thirty-five and finally reaches very low levels after menopause. It affects your heart, blood vessels, bones, brain, skin, hair, vagina, bladder, and other organs. It would seem the logical choice for hormone replacement, but conjugated estrogen, described in the next section, has been the predominant choice for decades in the United States. The commercial brands of estradiol are molecularly the same as what your ovaries produce, but they are derived from plants and *micronized* (broken down to fine particles) for better absorption. They are available as tablets, a vaginal cream, a vaginally inserted ring, and skin patches.

- **Estrone:** The predominant estrogen after menopause, following the decline in estradiol. Estrone is produced by conversion of body fat and by the ovaries. It is also made in the liver, which converts estradiol to estrone. Since estrone can be converted back into estradiol, estrone serves as a reservoir the body can use for its primary form of estrogen. After menopause, body fat continues as a source of estrone, so it wins the estrogen race by default. Estrone is a weaker form of estrogen than estradiol, so it takes a higher dose to be effective in hormone replacement. It has been known for many years that postmenopausal obese women, when compared to slender women, are less likely to develop osteoporosis but more likely to develop endometrial cancer, breast cancer, and gallbladder disease. Speculation among some researchers is that excess estrone may be the source of the increased risk. Estrone is commercially available as Ogen and Ortho-Est.

- **Estriol:** The biologically weakest estrogen. It is not present in measurable amounts normally, but it is produced in large amounts during pregnancy. Estriol has been tried for estrogen deficiency, but it has not been shown to be as protective as estradiol for the heart, bones, brain, and other organs. Some symptom relief occurs, but it has little beneficial effect on moods, memory, and fragmented sleep. Estriol is not commercially available, nor is it FDA approved for use as hormone replacement.

Conjugated Estrogens

Conjugated estrogens (CE) are derived from pregnant mares' urine, so they are also called conjugated equine estrogens. They are actually a group of ten estrogens rather than a single hormone. Some of these estrogens have a greater ability to attach to estrogen receptor sites than estradiol, so they may in effect displace human estradiol. This may be the reason for a lower association of breast cancer with CE than estradiol. Some women, especially the elderly, show improved memory with conjugated estrogen—even women with Alzheimer's disease (Henderson 1995). Conjugated estrogens are not uniform in their effects on various tissues. Some symptoms may be relieved and others not. Conjugated estrogens stay in the body for two to three months after the last dose, compared to less than twenty-four hours for estradiol, so an adverse effect may be prolonged. On the other hand, recent research has shown that some conjugated estrogens are less frequently associated with breast cancer than estradiol (Cutler and Garcia 1992). This may be related to their prolonged duration of effect. If CE is occupying the breast tissue receptor sites, estradiol is prevented from doing so. Conjugated estrogens also are more potent than native estradiol in improving lipoproteins by raising HDL and lowering LDL (low-density lipoprotein). If this form of estrogen doesn't work for you, don't despair. Other forms of estrogen and other routes of administration are available.

Synthetic Estrogens

The term *synthetic* refers to manufactured estrogens that are chemically *different* from your native hormone. By contrast, Estrace, for example, is a manufactured form of 17-beta estradiol, which your body produces; it is molecularly the same as your native hormone and therefore is considered a "natural" hormone.

Three representative examples of synthetics are

- **Ethinyl estradiol:** This synthetic estrogen is most commonly found in birth control pills. It is much more potent than native estradiol and provides more estrogen than is needed for hormone replacement, so it is little used for that purpose in the United States.

- **Estradiol valerate:** About 100 times more potent than native estradiol, so it is rarely used in the U.S.

- **Estrone:** A semisynthetic in its brand-name forms (Ogen and Ortho-Est) because piperazine is added to pure estrone to enhance absorption into the body.

Plant-Derived Estrogens

Phytoestrogens are compounds that act as precursor molecules from which estradiol is manufactured inside your body. They are found in a variety of plants, including soybeans, wild Mexican yams, ginseng, dong quai and black cohosh. These latter three are herbs widely used by herbalists to treat symptoms of estrogen decline, such as hot flashes and mood swings. However, ginseng, dong quai, and black cohosh have not been shown to be potent enough to prevent osteoporosis and cardiovascular disease. How do dong quai and black cohosh, the favorite of Native Americans, work? They are vasoconstrictors, which means that they cause the blood vessels in the skin to constrict. When you have a hot flash, the blood vessels in your skin dilate, or enlarge. Both dong quai and black cohosh prevent this from happening.

CAUTION! A high soy diet acts like unopposed estrogen, and abnormal uterine bleeding can sometimes result. Plant sources vary widely in the amount and potency of their estrogenic effects. In China and Japan, where diets are typically high in phytoestrogens, hot flashes are uncommon for peri-menopausal and postmenopausal women. (Landau 1994)

Estrogen Skin Creams

Estrogen creams are sometimes applied to the skin of the body. Let's take a look at a couple of them.

European women have been using estradiol cream for estrogen replacement in a gel form they rub into the skin once daily. After drying in a few minutes, the invisible residue is contained in the skin and acts as a time-release mechanism for the estrogen. The blood levels achieved are similar to the skin patch, but without the skin irritation problems. The cream is not yet available in the United States; but some specialty pharmacists can formulate a similar product (see Appendix A).

Another skin cream, estriol-progesterone, is made from soybeans and the wild Mexican yam, so it contains estriol, the weakest estrogen, and natural progesterone (which we talk about later in the chapter). Some researchers are investigating the possibility that estriol may have anti-breast cancer properties. The research is based on the observation that Asian women, who have a low incidence of breast cancer, excrete large amounts of estriol in their urine. This suggests that they have more estriol in their blood, and maybe that is why they have less breast cancer. In a giant leap of faith, promoters of this cream claim it will help prevent breast cancer and, further, that the progesterone will stop osteoporosis from advancing. Neither of these claims has valid scientific backup, although it is known that progesterone, in adequate oral or injected doses, will indeed halt bone loss. There have been no major studies of osteoporosis prevention by progesterone delivery in a cream, so use of the cream is still a shot in the dark.

Estrogen Vaginal Creams, Tablets, Liquids, and Rings

Conjugated estrogen, and estradiol are available in a vaginal cream. Their primary use to date has been to prevent or reverse atrophic changes (thinning) in the vulva, vagina, and bladder. If you find sex painful because of estrogen deficiency or you are suddenly plagued with recurrent bladder infections, you may benefit from vaginal estrogen. If you have decided to start hormone replacement with oral tablets, the use of a vaginal estrogen cream can "jump-start" vaginal rehabilitation—it works faster than the oral route. When your vagina is back to normal, you can stop the cream, and the oral tablets will keep things balanced.

In more frequent andor larger doses, estrogen from vaginal cream enters the bloodstream in measurable amounts, usually about one half to one quarter of the equivalent dose taken orally. There is interest among some researchers in whether this might be an effective route for estrogen replacement. At the present, no products are available to use this route as a sole source of HRT. It seems that micronized estradiol suspended in saline (salt water) and placed in the vagina by douching results in a blood level four times higher than the cream route. Micronized estradiol vaginal tablets are also well absorbed, and can be a convenient method for those who have side effects, such as nausea, from oral tablets (Reichman 1996).

An estrogen-containing vaginal ring, called *Estring*, first appeared on the market in 1997. (This is currently the only brand available.) It is inserted much like a diaphragm and constitutes a continuous-release estrogen source that lasts three months. Its primary use is for restoring vaginal and urinary tract thinning (atrophy). A small amount of estrogen gets into the circulation; but not enough to influence the uterine lining, so progesterone is not needed. Dr. Rosemary Ayton and co-workers reported in 1996 that the vaginal ring is better tolerated than estrogen cream, and the continuation rate of usage is much better since it is convenient to use.

The creams and the vaginal ring work well for treatment of estrogen deficiency of your vagina or bladder, but they do not deliver adequate dose levels for other estrogen deficient parts of your body. To accomplish that, you need the oral tablet form or the skin patch.

To Pill or to Patch, That Is the Question

The differences between the Pill and the patch have to do with how the body handles them. The oral estrogen pill is absorbed into your bloodstream from the intestine. Then it passes through the liver (called first-pass metabolism) where it is reconfigured largely into estrone for safekeeping, as we described earlier in the chapter. Estrogen's first pass through the liver also has a beneficial effect on your lipoproteins, raising HDL and lowering LDL. Triglycerides, a form of fat derived from food, are an independent risk factor for heart disease in women; they are sometimes elevated by oral estrogens, which is undesirable. Other first-pass metabolic changes are the production of certain liver proteins that bind some of the estrogen and make it less useable. Oral estrogen increases blood-clotting factors, a risk if you have a prior history of a blood clot in your legs or lungs. Oral estrogen also increases the risk for cholesterol gallstones, and it can raise blood pressure in about 5 percent of users (Wild 1996).

In contrast, estrogen delivered by patch initially bypasses the liver and immediately starts being used in tissues. There is a delayed beneficial effect on lipoproteins of three to six months, but it eventually kicks in. Because estrogen in this form initially bypasses the liver, triglycerides are not elevated by the patch. Estrogen from the patch does eventually pass through the liver, but there are advantages to avoiding first-pass metabolism. There is less negative effect on the liver's functioning, and the liver has less negative effect on the estrogen. (Note: If you are also using progesterone, you must still take it every day in pill form; the progesterone patch is not yet available in the United States. It is being used in Europe, so it may soon become available here.) Here are some factors to help you decide whether the Pill or the patch is the right choice for you.

Consider the Pill if:

- The patch fails to deliver acceptable estradiol blood levels. This is especially important if you have risk factors for heart disease or osteoporosis, because you may fail to receive estrogen's beneficial effects under these conditions. Skin thickness, which varies from one woman to the next, influences how well estrogen is delivered into your bloodstream.

- Your lipoprotein profile is unfavorable, and you do not wish to risk the three- to six-month delay in improving your HDL and LDL levels. Knowing your cardiovascular disease risk factors is important to this decision.

- The patch won't stick because you live in a hot climate or sweating is a problem.

- The patch causes intolerable skin irritation.

- You are taking progesterone pills and prefer to take both hormones at the same time.

Consider the patch if:

- You have high triglycerides.

- You took oral estrogen and it raised your blood pressure. The patch does not do this.

- You have gallbladder disease or are at risk for it.

- Taking the Pill causes nausea.

- You have had abnormal clotting disease in the past such as a blood clot in a leg or in the lung (called a pulmonary embolus).

- Taking the pill aggravates your migraine headaches.

- The pill does not maintain a steady enough estrogen level to relieve your estrogen deficiency symptoms, such as hot flashes, mood swings, and short-term memory loss.

- You are a poor pill-taker and often forget to take them.

Other Options

Two methods of estrogen supplementation that we haven't mentioned are estrogen pellets placed under the skin and estrogen shots. Pellets provide steady estrogen levels for three months, when new ones must be added. They have the same advantages as the patch in terms of avoiding the first-pass effect. The disadvantage of pellet use is that they must be placed under the skin with a large bore-tube called a trocar. This requires local anesthesia and stitches afterward. It's easy to see why they are not in widespread use. Estrogen shots are generally discouraged because they can cause up and down estrogen levels from one shot to the next. Nevertheless, estrogen shots may be the only option for women whose bodies do not absorb oral preparations and who have reasons not to use the patch. And the highs and lows that occur with injectable estrogen can be reduced by more frequent, smaller injections.

On the Horizon—Customized Estrogen

What if you could take an estrogen that would work to prevent osteoporosis and cardiovascular disease but had no adverse effect on your uterus or breasts? Research is currently being done on a drug that may do just that (Brody 1997). Called *raloxifene*, it avoids adverse effects by more specifically targeting the tissues and organs in the body and avoiding those areas where it can cause problems such as the breasts and uterus. This drug is in the final stages of testing and could be available in the next year or so. Such drugs (there are several in the research pipeline) are an astonishing breakthrough that can perhaps lay to rest the concerns you may have about the ill effects of estrogen replacement.

Estrogen with Progesterone

Now let's take a look at another female hormone, progesterone. The main reason for adding progesterone to estrogen in HRT is to protect the uterus from developing endometrial cancer. As we mentioned earlier in this chapter, use of unopposed estrogen increases the risk for that type of cancer between five and eight times. When progesterone, is added, however, the cancer risk is reduced to about the same level as in nonusers (Gershenson 1996). If your uterus has been removed, progesterone is not needed in hormone replacement.

Progesterone has, until recently, been used exclusively in the synthetic form called progestin (see Chapter 2). There are a variety of progestins. Natural progesterone is now available as well. Natural progesterone supplements are inactivated in the intestine and poorly absorbed, so it originally was not useful in hormone replacement. That problem has been solved in recent years by micronization, which, as it does for estrogen, breaks natural progesterone into very fine particles that are easily absorbed. Both forms of progesterone are quite useful in hormone replacement.

What Does Progesterone Do

You know that progesterone protects the lining of your uterus from overstimulation by estrogen because it is an anti-estrogen. But what about estrogen's role in prevention of heart disease and osteoporosis? Does progesterone prevent the prevention? As it turns out, for the most part, it doesn't. Let's see what effects it does have in terms of risk factors.

Cardiovascular Disease

An established benefit of estrogen is that it lowers cholesterol, raises HDL, and lowers LDL. The question is whether progesterone might negate estrogen's good deeds. It does, but not much. When progesterone is combined with estrogen, the net effect is that the rise in your good HDL is slightly less than with unopposed estrogen and has no effect on bad LDL.

Progestins and natural progesterone have been found to lower triglycerides (Writing Group for the PEPI Trials 1995). That is a welcome benefit because high triglycerides are closely related to heart disease in women. Although progestins slightly diminish the beneficial effect of estrogen on HDL, the benefit is not negated. There is no effect on total cholesterol levels and no adverse effect on LDL. Even the slightly adverse HDL effect diminishes with time. It is not believed that this attenuation of HDL benefit will make a clinically significant difference in cardiovascular protection (Speroff 1994). One 1995 report from the Harvard Nurses' Health Study showed that a reduction in coronary heart disease among users of estrogen combined with progestin was equal to or greater than the benefit with estrogen alone (Folsom et al. 1995). The final answers will come upon completion of the Women's Health Initiative referred to previously.

Osteoporosis

When progesterone is combined with estrogen, the positive effect of estrogen is not lost. As a matter of fact, new bone formation is enhanced slightly (Cauley et al. 1995). Even used alone, progesterone stops bone loss, but it is not nearly as effective as estrogen in this regard.

Depression and Mood

Progesterone lowers serotonin, one of your "feel good" brain chemicals, and decreases the absorption of its precursor, tryptophan. Both of these effects cause an increase in the frequency of feeling mildly depressed when progesterone is in your bloodstream. You can probably confirm this yourself if depression is a common emotion in the latter half of your menstrual cycle, when progesterone levels are normally highest. These effects occur in some women using HRT when either natural progesterone or progestins are used. It is estimated that between 5 percent and 10 percent of women have depressive feelings or other adverse side effects (mentioned below) as a result of using any form of progesterone. Some women become severely depressed (dysphoric) when exposed to progesterone. These are women who could not take birth control pills when they were younger and find that they cannot use progesterone replacement therapy as they age. (Leventhal 1997)

Breast Cancer and Combined HRT

Several studies have been published on combined estrogen-progesterone HRT and breast cancer; but so far, the results have not been in agreement. In 1995, an analysis of the Harvard Nurses' Health Study was published in the *New England Journal of Medicine* and gained national headlines (Colditz et al. 1995). That study showed a 30 to 40 percent increase in breast cancer for women over 55 who had been on combined HRT more than five years. The study predicted that in following 200 such women over a period of ten years, instead of the seven breast cancers that would be expected, there would be ten if all 200 had been on HRT more than five years. A month later, a study from the University of Washington was published in the *Journal of the American Medical Association* citing more statistically significant (meaning scientifically reliable) figures, and they found no increase in breast cancer for women taking combined HRT (Stanford et al. 1995). As a matter of fact, the women in their study who had used HRT for eight or more years had a *decreased* risk for breast cancer, although the media ignored this.

Are you confused? The point we are making is that the links between combined HRT (using progesterone) and breast cancer have not been adequately studied. The current consensus among researchers on estrogen and breast cancer after dozens of studies is that if a risk for breast cancer exists, it is in a small segment of the female population that has not yet been identified, and the same may be true when estrogen and progesterone are combined in HRT. The Women's Health Initiative, mentioned earlier in this chapter, is studying this issue.

Types of Progesterone and Progestins

A number of types of progesterone and the progestins are available, and we take a look at them here.

Medroxyprogesterone acetate (MPA)

MPA (Provera, Cycrin) is a progestin, or synthetic progesterone. The Women's Health Initiative is using it in their study. Most other progestins are derivatives of testosterone; but MPA is derived from progesterone. It is available in a variety of doses for flexibility in using it in cyclic or continuous HRT regimens. Side effects such as moodiness and bloating may occur with MPA, so the lowest dose possible should be used. Researchers have found over past years that we can safely lower the dosage of progestins to reduce side effects and still maintain endometrial protection (Woodruff and Pickar 1994). MPA and other progestins do prevent good HDL from rising to as high à level as it would with unopposed estrogen; but there is no effect on bad LDL. There is no apparent long-term adverse effect on heart disease (Speroff 1994).

Norethindrone Acetate

Norethindrone acetate (Aygestin), a progestin, is derived from testosterone by changing the molecule chemically. It produces no male-like effects. Norethindrone acetate behaves much like MPA in the bloodstream, declining after about twenty-four hours. The tablets are scored so they can be broken in half for lower dosages. Side effects are about the same as for MPA, or perhaps a little less. The effect on lowering HDL is the same as for MPA.

Norethindrone

Norethindrone (Micronor, Brevicon) is the "Mini-Pill." It is similar to norethindrone acetate. It provides a very low dose compared to norethindrone acetate. The primary use for this hormone has been as a progestin-only (no estrogen) birth control pill. It is currently being used with estrogen in the continuous HRT regimen (taking a pill every day, 365 days a year). It is too soon to say how effective this very low dose of progestin is in protecting the endometrium from developing hyperplasia. For this reason, if you are taking this pill, it is a good idea to monitor the thickness of your endometrium by having a vaginal ultrasound once yearly.

Natural Progesterone

Natural progesterone, unlike progestin, is derived from Mexican yams and soybeans. It is micronized for easy absorption from the intestine. It has not been marketed by any pharmaceutical companies, and many doctors have little experience with it. However, it is available from specialty pharmacies in 25, 50, 100 and 200 mg capsules (see Appendix A).

Natural progesterone is metabolized more rapidly than progestin, so it must be taken twice daily to maintain the same blood levels as progestin, once in the morning and again, possibly in a higher dosage, in the evening. (Since it may produce drowsiness, the higher dose should be reserved for around bedtime.) (Writing Group for the PEPI Trials 1995)

Many women describe fewer side effects with natural progesterone than with progestin. The Postmenopausal Estrogen/Progesterone Interventions

(PEPI) trials (1995) compared natural progesterone and progestin. PEPI found that natural progesterone does not inhibit estrogen's beneficial effect on HDL as much as progestins, but the differences were not statistically significant. The PEPI study found that natural progesterone is a safe product to use in combined HRT.

Megestrol Acetate

Megestrol acetate (Megace) is a progestin that has been used primarily for treatment of recurrent cancer of the breast and endometrium. It is a very potent progestin, supplied in 20 and 40 mg tablets. For women who cannot take estrogen or who are having hot flashes from tamoxifen use in breast cancer (see Chapter 7), megestrol acetate can relieve hot flashes with a dose of 20 mg twice daily. This progestin has also been shown to increase bone density at these doses, which is a plus (Reichman 1996). A minus is that it may have an adverse effect on lipids if used long-term. Megestrol is a special-use drug, and more research needs to be done on it.

Side Effects?

Taking progesterone can make some women feel awful. Progesterone is the hormone that reaches high levels in the second half of the menstrual cycle, and it can give you sore breasts, lower your energy level, cause water retention, increase your appetite, make you feel bloated, and get you depressed. (This is the same thing that happens in the first eight weeks of pregnancy and again at about the 34th week—do the symptoms sound familiar?)

Not all women experience these side effects with progesterone use. If you do have adverse side effects, they can probably be managed by changing the type of progesterone you use, the schedule on which you take it, or the dosage itself. It may take a while to find the right combination, but hang in there.

Androgens (Male Hormones)

Alphabet Soup	
T	Testosterone
ASD	Androstenedione
DHEA	Dehydroepiandrosteron
DHEAS	Dehydroepiandrosterone sulfate

Guess where your estrogen comes from. Give up? Male hormones. Your ovaries, as well as your adrenal glands, start with *androgens* (male hormones) and the follicles in your ovaries convert them to estrogen. The same thing happens in fat cells: Cholesterol is converted first to an androgen and then to estrogen. Both genders make female and male hormones. The fundamental difference is that one of them is very dominant in each gender.

There are five different androgens. Your ovaries make two of these five: testosterone (T), a strong androgen, and androstenedione (ASD), a weak one. Both T and ASD are made in the interior cells of the ovary, called the *stroma*. They are then converted to estrogens by the follicle cells near the surface of the ovaries as they mature every month and prepare an egg cell. Small amounts of the androgens remain unchanged, however, and enter your circulation. There they perform certain important functions, such as maintaining your energy level, improving your sense of wellness, and activating the sexual circuits in your brain. Your adrenal glands also produce ASD, as well as dehydroepiandrosterone (DHEA), another weak androgen, which enter your bloodstream. Your ovaries can pick them up and convert them to estrogens too (a sort of back-up supply source). Some of these androgens remain unchanged by your ovaries, though, and make their rounds in your body, where they may be later converted to estrogens by whatever tissue they visit: fat cells, muscles, skin, brain, kidneys, and others.

Estrogen-Androgen Ratios

The net result of all the reconfiguration and conversion we just described is that a stable ratio between blood levels of estrogen and androgen is maintained in your body from puberty to menopause, but estrogen levels exceed androgen by a huge margin. With time, ovarian follicles diminish in number, as you know from Chapter 2, so production of estrogen and androgen both decline. By menopause your follicles are sufficiently diminished in number that estrogen declines sharply, by 80 to 90 percent. Androgen levels only go down by about 50 percent, however, because the cells in the stroma of your ovaries can still make androgen, as can your adrenal glands (Rosenberg et al. 1988). There are just not enough follicles left to convert the androgen to estrogen, and this distorts the ratio of estrogen to androgen: There is a net loss of both hormones, but there is relatively more androgen than before.

At this point, androgen is less suppressed by estrogen, and it may express itself in male-like ways. You may notice more facial hair, a deeper voice, and a changed body fat distribution. Body fat distribution changes from a "pear-like" female concentration about the hips, to the "apple-like" male shape around the waist. Weight gain in mid-life is *not* from estrogen use as the popular myth would have you believe. It is from the changed balance of estrogen and androgen, with the assistance of reduced physical activity and increased food consumption to more than a lowered metabolic rate justifies. It has been known for decades that the rate of metabolism slowly declines during aging. This means that less food is required to sustain your body, so continuing the customary eating habits of youth gradually results in weight gain. (See Chapter 11 for more about weight control.) The androgen imbalance also creates a risk for other, unfavorable male-like changes, such as rising blood pressure, higher cholesterol, lowered HDL, and raised LDL. These changes can start in your forties; as a transitional woman, you should know some things about recognizing the imbalance and correcting it if needed.

Symptoms of Androgen Deficiency

Male hormones have important functions in terms of maintaining muscle tissues, building bone, and keeping an optimal energy level, but they also have potent influence on how your brain works. Too much testosterone can cause hyperactivity, a shortened attention span, scattered thoughts, aggressive, violent dreams, and abnormally increased sexual desire. When male hormone levels decline, you may experience a deterioration in these areas. Also, loss of muscle mass may be noticeable in the unwelcome appearance of flabby arms and other parts of your body. Your skin may become dry and your hair thinned. You may notice that you just don't have your customary get-up-and-go. Your interest in sex may have slipped several notches on your agenda of "great things to do at every opportunity." Or you may simply feel that "something is wrong," but you just can't put your finger on it. If symptoms of estrogen decline are also present, such as hot flashes, sleep disruption, disturbed concentration, moodiness, and so on, then think about the possibility that your body is experiencing not only an estrogen decline; but a low testosterone level as well.

Should You Really Take Male Hormones?

Not every woman needs to take male hormones, but a number of situations might justify your considering it, usually in combination with female hormones:

- **Both ovaries surgically removed:** This procedure immediately drops the bottom out of androgen and estrogen production. According to a 1985 study (Sherwin and Gelfand), if symptoms from sudden estrogen loss (hot flashes, moodiness, short-term memory loss) are combined with the symptoms of androgen deficiency (loss of energy, slowed thinking, absent sexual desire, diminished sense of well-being), you may need both hormones to get back on an even keel. Dr. Robert Greenblatt (1987), a pioneer in HRT, found that androgens in women are basically psychotropic (affecting the mental state) hormones that influence the way you feel: They act as an antidepressant. This is consistent with the observed effects of androgen deficiency. These studies concluded that estrogen replacement therapy should be the first treatment for estrogen deficiency symptoms. Then, if symptoms of androgen deficiency persist, male hormone replacement should be added.

- **Hysterectomy:** If your uterus is removed, even if the ovaries are not taken out, you have a thirty percent chance of becoming menopausal within four years (Cutler 1990). It has to do with compromised blood supply to the ovaries as a result of the surgery. Estrogen replacement is, of course, important for all the reasons we've discussed. Male hormone replacement is an option if **androgen** deficiency symptoms are also present.

- **Loss of sexual interest:** There is no longer any question that the major hormonal influence on female sexual desire derives from maintaining a normal level of male hormones. Estrogen is primarily involved with sexual responsiveness, such as lubrication, arousal, and orgasm, but testosterone is the engine of desire, fantasies, and the motivating forces that make you want to have sex. It is true that sexual interest can be blunted by estrogen deficiency symptoms such as hot flashes, moodiness, and vaginal dryness. If your loss of interest in sex does not improve with estrogen replacement, though, and is not related to other problems like hypothyroidism, depression, or relationship problems, adding testosterone can make the difference.

- **Loss of energy:** A general loss of energy may well be from things like anemia, hypothyroidism, other chronic diseases, or just a frantically busy lifestyle. If these aren't factors, supplements of male hormone may put the zing back into your life.

- **Vertebral osteoporosis with compression fractures:** This is a problem seen in postmenopausal women who have done little to prevent osteoporosis. Adding testosterone to HRT can help prevent more fractures but a good prevention program starting now is a much better option.

- **Breast tenderness:** Women taking female hormones often complain of breast tenderness. If you have been hormone deficient for several years, your breasts may be more sensitive when you start HRT. (A good "eight point hug" may be out of the question.) Adding testosterone helps reduce the pain.

There are a lot of negative myths about androgen use in women: You'll get a mustache and a beard plus acne, you'll look like a muscle-beach volleyball player, your voice will deepen, you'll get liver damage, you'll become a sex-starved maniac. Like most myths, there is a kernel of truth in them, but problems like these are related to the *dose* and *type* of male hormone used. Androgen sensitivity varies from woman to woman, and its use in therapy must be individualized.

Types, Dosages, and Administration

Several types of preparations of male hormones are available. They come in varying dosages, and they are administered in a number of ways.

Types of Preparations

Synthetic hormones are chemically compounded in a laboratory to resemble what the body naturally produces. Testosterone can be made exactly the way your ovaries make it, but it is not well absorbed from the intestine. To get around this, what is called a methyl group is added to the molecule. This makes it more potent than natural testosterone, so small doses are necessary. Methyltestosterone (Android, Estratest) is being used less and less in recent years. Fluoxymesterone (Halotestin), another synthetic, has largely supplanted it. Fluoxymesterone is better tolerated, lasts longer in the body and has fewer side effects. Synthetic preparations are commercially available in tablets, pellets, patches, and injectables. Several products (Estratest, Depo-Testadiol) are now available that combine estrogen and methyltestosterone in a single tablet or injectable. With a prescription, a knowledgeable pharmacist can prepare skin creams, skin gels, and vaginal suppositories.

Natural testosterone from soybeans and Mexican yams is poorly absorbed, so it is micronized in the laboratory. It is available in tablets of varying strength from specialty pharmacy companies (see Appendix A).

Dosage

Proper dose is important in the use of androgens. This is another situation where one dose *doesn't* fit all. Each woman's dose should be individualized and fine-tuned as necessary. Typically, treatment starts with a low daily dose and gradual increases over time until your androgen deficiency symptoms improve. If symptoms (lack of energy, slowed thinking, absent sex drive, depressed mood) are unimproved with a moderate dose, you probably don't need the testosterone you are taking, and another source of your persisting symptoms should be investigated. Indeed, before agreeing to a higher dose, you should insist that your blood level of testosterone be checked first. An adequate blood level of testosterone indicates that a higher dose is not the way to proceed.

Testosterone testing is expensive. This is probably a factor in the emerging practice of giving a trial dose of androgens at first, rather than checking blood levels in the laboratory. If the desired benefits are not obtained with a trial of use, tests can then be ordered.

Routes of Administration

Androgens are usually taken orally. Tablets were originally designed for men, in doses generally too high for women, but lower-dose tablets are now available. A good way to get androgens into your system is by letting the tablet dissolve under your tongue. Lozenges are available; but the smallest one contains way too much testosterone for a woman. Skin gels are being tried, but not much is known about them as yet. Many women find a combination estrogen-testosterone tablet the most convenient way to take both hormones.

CAUTION! If you are taking estrogen-testosterone in combination, you still need progesterone; androgen does not protect your endometrium from the unopposed effects of estrogen.

Injectable preparations cause wider fluctuation in blood levels than tablets, which makes it more difficult to keep your symptoms controlled. Unwanted side effects are more common because it is more difficult to find the right dose. Too much male hormone can result in the development of coarse facial hair. Once a hair follicle is stimulated by male hormone, it continues to be dark and coarse, even after the hormone is stopped. Electrolysis is then required to remove the unwanted hairs. (No amount of plucking or waxing will get rid of them.) Injectables sometimes wear off without notice, causing significant fluctuations between there being too little and too much male hormone in your system. On the other hand, injectables have the advantage of bypassing the liver and intestinal tract, which avoids the potential for partial hormone inactivation. Long-acting injectables (Depo-Testadiol) may be useful once an appropriate dose has been established through the use of tablets.

Androgen pellets are also available. Placed under your skin, pellets provide a constant male hormone level, without the ups and downs of oral or injectable testosterone (Notelovitz and Tonnessen 1993). The dosage is always within the normal testosterone range, so excessive hair growth and acne are rarely a problem. The disadvantage of this method of male hormone administration, however, is a big one: placement of new pellets to keep the hormone level constant requires a small incision and stitches every three months. Biodegradable pellets are being developed for other hormone supplementation and may be a future source for androgens. A recent study of pellets used to increase sexual desire showed that it returned to normal within three months compared to no improvement in women who used placebo pellets (Leventhal 1997).

The testosterone skin patch is available for men, but it delivers far too much testosterone for use in women.

If you decide to take androgens, keep in mind that your body is different from that of every other woman. Your symptoms and needs are yours alone. You are the only one who knows how you feel and the only one who knows when you feel better. Androgen use requires a close working relationship with your doctor , and individualization of your dosage. Don't settle for less.

Other Androgens: DHEA and DHEAS

Some links have been drawn between DHEA (dehydroepiandrosterone) and the aging process. This hormone is produced by the adrenal gland, as we mentioned earlier in the chapter. Some of it circulates in the bloodstream in its free form, but most of it is bonded to a sulfate, becoming DHEAS. This weak androgen can be converted to testosterone if needed. Some recent studies have suggested that DHEA has another role, in addition to acting as a reservoir for conversion to testosterone.

Humans and other primates are the only species capable of making large quantities of DHEA and DHEAS. At birth, we all have high levels of these hormones. Then they decline until puberty, when they begin to rise again, reaching a peak in the late twenties. From that time on, a slow steady decline ensues, and about 80 percent of DHEA and DHEAS is gone by the seventies.

Given in large doses to laboratory mice and rats, DHEA and DHEAS produced some surprising health benefits (Schwartz 1995):

- They prevented diabetes.
- They slowed weight gain, even if the animals were overfed.
- They prevented auto immune disease (when the immune system attacks the body).
- They protected killer cells, which destroy abnormal cells, from being inactivated.
- They inhibited the development of breast cancer.
- They helped resist genetic mutations from carcinogen exposure.
- They increased the life span.

The question arose as to whether the human aging process is influenced by the steady drop that occurs in these hormones. Low levels of DHEA and DHEAS in men have correlated with an increased risk for heart disease, but an apparent gender difference exists because in women, the highest risk for CVD was in those who had the *highest* levels of DHEA and DHEAS. People with Alzheimer's disease were observed to have a 50 percent decrease in their expected levels of both forms of the hormone (Nestler 1995).

Researchers next turned to the question of whether supplements of these hormones would act as an anti-aging drug. Men and women were given a high dose on a daily basis. The men did fine, with improvement in their lipoproteins; but women did poorly. Women had worsened lipid profiles with lower HDL, they became insulin resistant, which caused weight gain, and they developed the "apple body" male pattern of obesity.

Then, a small group of women and men were given a significantly smaller amount daily, just enough hormone to restore the DHEA and DHEAS to the levels of their youth in about two weeks. In women, male hormone levels doubled, and they had slightly lower HDL; another study is being conducted to see whether an even smaller dose lessens this adverse effect. Other positive benefits noted with this study and others in both women and men were as follows:

- No decrease in insulin sensitivity, a common trait of aging (Bates et al. 1995)
- Increased activity of natural killer cells, suggesting that immune competence was improved (Araneo 1995)
- Improvement in major depression (Wolkowitz et al. 1995)
- Better sleep, memory, and mood (Baulieu 1995)
- Increased energy
- Improved ability to handle stress

These were all small studies, but the prospect of slowing the adverse effects of the aging process is exciting. If DHEA and DHEAS supplements can be shown to prevent the usual age-related loss of immune competence, a reduction in the cancer rates associated with aging can be expected. More will, of course, be needed. Since there have been no large, long-term clinical trials to back up these claims, there is no approval for using DHEA in humans for any reason. Even though there is no scientific evidence indicating that it should be a part of the human diet, this hormone is currently being sold without prescription as a food supplement (Skolnick 1996). It will be interesting to see what further research reveals.

Hormone Replacement Regimens

We've taken a pretty detailed look at the effects of taking estrogen, progesterone, and androgen. Now you are ready to understand how they are put together in a treatment plan. There are several approaches, and none of them works for everyone; the one that works for you may be quite different from that of other women you know. Your decision on whether to take HRT and, if so, in what form, should be based on your understanding of why it is recommended and the form in which you are comfortable using it.

A national study of women who received prescriptions for HRT revealed that 20 to 30 percent never even got their prescriptions filled (Reichman 1996). Another study found that 38 percent discontinued HRT in less than a year. Within six months of starting HRT, 63 were using the hormones "from time to time," and this spotty use was up to 90 percent after two years After seven years, only 10 percent were still taking hormones. (Berman 1996)

There are many reasons for such low numbers:

- On the part of women, fear of cancer and irregular bleeding were the most frequently cited reasons for declining HRT (Speroff 1994).

- Side effects (bleeding, bloating, fluid retention, sore breasts) are intolerable.

- Physicians and health providers of all stripes have failed to educate American women about hormonal decline in general and on the value of HRT. Part of this is because perimenopausal and menopausal understanding is not widespread enough in the medical community. Part is because we haven't made a strong enough effort.

- Preventive health care is a hard sell. Until confronted with an adverse health problem (obesity, heart disease, osteoporosis, high blood pressure, cancer), many people are not motivated to do much of anything about averting the problem.

- Fear of aggravating prior health problems (breast cancer, uterine cancer, blood clots in legs or lungs).

- Some women decide that HRT is unnatural and regard it as experimenting with their bodies.

The regimens we describe in the following sections are those currently in use. It cannot be said that one is superior to the others; there are reasons for using each. One of them will likely meet your hormonal needs, your life schedule, and your comfort zone.

Unopposed Estrogen

We discussed the risks of unopposed estrogen use earlier in this chapter. It has practically disappeared as a way of treating women, except for those who do not have a uterus. Today, a common source of unopposed estrogen is herbs, such as ginseng, dong quai, and black cohosh, which contain phytoestrogens. It is not yet known whether consuming these herbs increases cancer risk. If you use unopposed estrogen or herbs with phytoestrogens, it is important to monitor the thickness of your endometrium. This is done with ultrasound and is a painless office procedure.

Recently there has been a rising interest in and use of estrogen only; but with the addition of progesterone for two weeks every three months. This method is actually quarterly *cycling* rather than unopposed estrogen. This regimen could be a reasonable accommodation for women who are turned off by the monthly bleeding of cyclic regimens. A few physicians are returning to the old estrogen-only regimen to accommodate women who just can't tolerate progesterone. These women are being monitored with ultrasound measurements of the endometrial lining.

CAUTION! Chances of developing an endometrial cancer are quadrupled with as little as six months of unopposed estrogen use (Grady et al. 1995).

Cyclic HRT

There are two methods for accomplishing cyclic HRT. The classic regimen uses both estrogen and progesterone in a cyclic fashion, with five days off each month. The other is to use estrogen continuously but progesterone cyclically. The cyclic methods may be the best to use for women who are estrogen deficient but still having menstrual periods or for women who have just recently become menopausal.

Cyclic Estrogen and Progesterone

In a course of treatment involving cyclic estrogen and progesterone, you typically take estrogen each month from day 1 through day 25. Progesterone is added for the final twelve to fourteen days of estrogen use. Then both are stopped until day 1 of the next month. During the five or six off days (depending on what month it is), you have a menstrual period.

With this method, menstrual periods continue as always, which can be either reassuring or a nuisance, depending on your point of view. A further disadvantage for some women is that during the five or six days off, estrogen deficiency symptoms may return, such as hot flashes, mood fluctuations, and fragmented sleep.

Cyclic HRT may be the best method in late perimenopause or early menopause because less breakthrough bleeding occurs than with the continuous method (see the next section). Nevertheless, it can take three to four months for your body to fall into the rhythm you are imposing on it. During this time you may have episodes of light breakthrough bleeding. For the large majority of women, this situation resolves itself. If the bleeding is heavy or continuous, though, be sure to contact your doctor. You could have an endometrial problem.

Continuous Estrogen and Cyclic Progesterone

In the second cyclical treatment plan, estrogen is taken continuously, 365 days per year. Progesterone is added for twelve to fourteen days of each month. It is a popular method for HRT because it eliminates the "off" days experienced with the first method. With this method, it also takes three to four months for your body to become accustomed to the cycle. Once that has happened, bleeding should occur only when you are off progesterone. Any other type of bleeding should be reported to your doctor.

Continuous HRT

With continuous HRT, both estrogen and progesterone are taken daily, 365 days per year. The progesterone dose is half that used for the cyclic methods. The rationale for continuous progesterone is that it provides continuous protection of the endometrium. With this method, the uterine lining eventually becomes thin, and the glands inactive. With nothing to shed, there is no more uterine bleeding. That sounds like good news, but 30 to 40 percent of women will have breakthrough bleeding at unannounced intervals for about the first four months. After a year, 80 to 90 percent of women using this method will have stopped all uterine bleeding (Reichman 1996). This pattern (or more accurately, "no-pattern") of bleeding is most likely to occur in women who are fewer than three years past their menopause. The cyclic regimens tend to work best during these years. Nevertheless, if you are unwilling to put up with monthly bleeding, the continuous method may be for you.

CAUTION! If bleeding is heavy or continuous, or if you have no bleeding for several months and it resumes, call your doctor.

Some doctors have started using the continuous regimen on a Monday-through-Friday schedule. This seems to lessen the problem of initial breakthrough bleeding. The total estrogen dose is reduced by about 30 percent with this weekend-off method; so CVD and osteoporosis protection may be compromised. Your blood lipoprotein levels should be monitored, and you should have a yearly bone density scan, if you use this method long term.

Summary

Two decades ago, this would have been a very short chapter; but the past twenty years have brought many changes to hormone replacement therapy. Scientific advance is often fraught with controversy, and HRT has certainly been no exception. Your primary responsibility to yourself regarding HRT it to become as fully informed as you can before you make a decision about using this therapy. You have a choice to use it or not to use it, but your choice is one of the most important health-care decisions you will make in your lifetime. If you are in the early stages of perimenopause, the information in this chapter may not apply to your immediate needs, but it should help make your future choices easier. The decision you make about using HRT should be the result of considering the benefits of symptom relief, CVD protection, osteoporosis prevention, reduced risk of colon cancer, and protection of brain deterioration with aging and weighing them against the risks of uterine or breast cancer and potential side effects. Your final decision should, then, be based on a composite of your knowledge, your trust in your health advisor, your intellectual perceptions, and your own body wisdom.

○ ○ ○

9

Alternative Medical Disciplines: Are They a Good Choice for You?

If you are experiencing the symptoms of diminishing hormone production that come with perimenopause, you will tend to seek out a health care provider who can give you relief. Your choices sort themselves out to traditional and alternative medical care. We've already looked at the benefits, along with the risks, of HRT, and explained the preventive benefits of that form of therapy. If you choose not to take hormones, there are alternatives for managing the symptoms of estrogen decline. Practitioners of both Western and alternative medicine tend to condemn each other's discipline. The loser in this case is you. Both traditional and alternative medical practices have benefits. If you make a choice to exclude one at the expense of the other, you may be throwing out the baby with the bathwater.

This chapter takes a look at a variety of alternative medical disciplines. All of the practitioners we discuss must be licensed in their particular field because the law requires it. The remedies offered vary from prescription medicine from licensed physicians, to a huge variety of naturally occurring plant and animal derivatives available without prescription. There are many options, and we've chosen to include the ones we think are representative—the ones hormone-deficient women tend to seek most frequently. They include Chinese and other herbal medicine, homeopathy, acupuncture, and holistic medicine. (Other alternatives, although we haven't included them in our discussion, include naturopaths, chiropractors, psychologists, hypnotherapists, and religious healers.)

Chinese Medicine

If it is prudent for us to take note of the experience of others, Chinese herbal medicine should get our attention. It has been practiced for five thousand years. When Western medicine was having its beginnings, Chinese herbal medicine was already ancient, and Chinese medicine has been successful in treating many areas of illness over the centuries. However, Western medicine has surpassed it in some well-known areas, such as control of infection, vaccine prevention of disease, treatment of acute illness such as heart attacks, and surgical emergencies.

A basic tenet of Chinese medicine is that good health requires that you remain in harmony with the world around you at all stages of life. The further belief is that your body is divided into five energy centers, controlled by five organs: kidneys, lungs, liver, heart, and spleen. Energy, called *Qi* (pronounced "chee"), flows from one control center to the next, in twelve channels. The channels are like meridians that intersect to form a grid or mesh-like pattern all over your body. Each channel has its own distinct pulse, which can be monitored to assess health status. If the flow of Qi is too much or too little in any channel, an imbalance is created in the network, which in turn increases your risk of disease. A finite amount of Qi exists in your body. It can be depleted by various problems in life, but Qi can also be restored by the use of herbs, diet, acupuncture, and relaxation techniques.

The *yin* and *yang* relationship is another Chinese concept fundamental to understanding energy balance. Yin and yang are opposite but balancing energies that are present in your body, and for that matter, throughout the universe. If one is at a low level, the other fills in the void and reestablishes the balance by becoming high. Yin is feminine, considered as representing things that are cold, dark, still, and heavy. Yang is masculine, and it is associated with things that are hot, light, mobile, and lightweight. A fever is yang, and a chill is yin. Low energy is yin, and hyperactivity is yang.

Your uterus and ovaries are in the energy sphere of your kidneys. Hormone deficiency problems are considered a kidney deficiency in yin energy. Since Qi flows from your kidneys to your liver, you also get a liver-yin deficiency. Now you have a yang excess in both energy centers as opposing balance is restored. A yang excess makes hot things—like hot flashes—happen. Yin deficiency causes insomnia and poor sleep. The liver Qi is associated with anger, so a yang excess here causes rising emotions and irritability. Anger and irritability in turn cause stagnation of liver Qi, which results in distention and bloating (Bienfield and Korngold 1991). Are any of these symptoms starting to sound familiar?

Chinese Herbs

Once your energy imbalance has been diagnosed, treatment may take a variety of forms. Chinese herbal treatments are usually a mixture of herbs from which a tea is brewed or a liquid extract is prepared as an oral tonic. The preparations are usually directed at a specific deficiency that is producing specific symptoms. The herb Rehmannia glutinosa is the main yin tonic. Other herbs are added to it to increase its potency or decrease side effects (Bienfield and Korngold 1991). With a variety of formulations, hot flashes with night sweats, irritability, and headaches may all be treated. If a yang deficiency is perceived to be the problem, dodder is added to Rehmannia to treat a diminished libido. Insomnia, heart palpitations, and nervousness are thought to be from altered flow of Qi between the heart and kidneys, so a Rehmannia preparation called Emperor Tea is used to treat it. As you can imagine, there are many, many more combinations of herbs for other specific situations. If you decide to use herbs, do it on the advice and under the supervision of an experienced herbalist (Bienfield and Korngold 1991).

Acupuncture and Acupressure

The intersections of the twelve energy channels near your skin surface form the basis for *acupuncture* treatment. Acupuncture involves the insertion of tiny needles into specific exterior body locations for therapeutic purposes. At the sites where these meridians cross one another, the flow of Qi can be enhanced, diminished, or redirected by the insertion of tiny needles at known locations. Acupuncture points have been shown to have differing electrical resistance. The needles stimulate electrical impulses causing release of neurotransmitters, which in turn raise the endorphin levels in your brain, as well as peripherally, in your tissues. Endorphins are your own internal pain relievers. They are opium-like chemicals that can produce sedation and a sense of well-being. (The "high" you feel after vigorous exercise results from endorphins.) Changing the flow of Qi can aid a faltering organ system. *Acupressure* is a means of using massage at known locations to accomplish the same results as acupuncture. Some practitioners also use electrical stimulation at acupuncture points.

These treatment regimes are primarily directed at symptoms. Relief from symptoms is widely reported by both patients and practitioners. There are no data available, however, as to whether you will have less cardiovascular disease or osteoporosis as a result using these techniques (Bienfield and Korngold 1991).

Homeopathy

The alternative medical discipline called homeopathy was founded in the late 1700s by Samuel Hahnemann, a German physician and chemist. Homeopathy involves administration of minute doses of drugs which in a healthy person are capable of producing symptoms like those of the condition to be treated. Its premise is that the mind and body are inseparable and mutually dependent. Symptoms displayed by your body are regarded as a signal that something has changed and that the mind/body is trying to heal itself. For example, hot flashes are a symptom of hormone depletion, fever is a symptom of infection, and a mood change is a response to an external or internal stress. The basic tenet of treatment is that like is cured by like (Ullman 1991). If you are having adverse symptoms produced by a toxic substance, the cure results from using an extreme dilution of that same offending substance. The theory is that these minuscule doses will stimulate your body to marshal its defense mechanisms and attack the source of your symptoms. Homeopathic remedies typically cause an initial exaggeration of symptoms. With continued use in progressively increasing doses, however, your body eventually overcomes the toxic effect, and health is restored. Allergists use this same principle in desensitizing you to things like pollens and bee stings. Because of the extremely small amounts used, the substance prescribed is not regarded as having cured you. Rather, your improvement is believed to have come from your mind/body being stimulated to heal itself.

Homeopathic practitioners are interested in all aspects of your life: age, occupation, general health, diet, moods, lifestyle habits, relationships, and other external and internal factors. The homeopathist integrates this information with your original complaint and selects a remedy. All the substances used occur naturally in plants or animals. Sometimes, two or three attempts are needed before the right remedy is found. Many months (up to two years) may be required to accomplish the goal of restoring your normal health on physical, mental, and emotional levels. Homeopathists emphasize that you must be committed to this mode of treatment to achieve success; homeopathic healing is a process, as opposed to traditional medical practice, which often consists only of an office visit and a prescription. No specific training is required to prescribe homeopathic remedies, but most practitioners are licensed health providers such as nurses, physicians, and acupuncturists.

As with Chinese herbal medicine, your hormone deficiency symptoms may be relieved with homeopathy, but there is as yet no body of scientific evidence that homeopathic remedies will protect you against cardiovascular disease or osteoporosis.

Holistic Medicine

Holistic practitioners sometimes use the term *complementary alternative medicine* to describe their field. *Holistic* refers to a system of preventive medicine that takes into account the whole individual, the individual's responsibility for personal well-being, and the total influences (social, psychological, environmental) that affect health, including nutrition, exercise, and mental relaxation. The basic premise is that all medical disciplines can be integrated and used to complement each other. These include homeopathy, herbal therapy, acupuncture, nutritional therapy, stress management techniques, and traditional medical practices such as X-ray, surgery, laboratory testing, and prescription medicines. Complementary medicine is practiced by licensed physicians whose orientation is patient centered, as opposed to disease centered. Conventional medical practices and techniques are regarded as secondary alternatives and used only if necessary.

Many of the nontraditional treatments of complementary medicine, such as megadoses of vitamins, especially C and E, are so widespread now that they are finding their way into mainstream thinking and practice. Some medical schools are researching the use of nutrition for the treatment and prevention of disease, an idea long held by complementary medicine practitioners.

Herbal Treatments for Hormone Deficiency Symptoms

A number of herbs are available to treat the symptoms of hormone deficiency, including:

- **Ginseng:** Ginseng is a widely advertised herb with estrogenic properties (not widely advertised). Herbalists combine it with dong quai (see the next item) and use them for menstrual disorders, depressed sexual desire, depression, insomnia, nervousness, hot flashes, chronic fatigue, and general old age (Wolfe 1990).

CAUTION! Used in large amounts, ginseng can cause abnormal uterine bleeding and ovarian cysts (Reichman 1996). Use ginseng with great caution if you have had breast cancer or have high risk factors for endometrial cancer. Large doses over a prolonged period of time provide a significant amount of unopposed estrogen, which carries risks for endometrial cancer (see Chapter 8).

- **Dong quai:** Dong quai is a phytoestrogen, meaning, as we explained in Chapter 8, that it is derived from a plant with estrogenic activity. The estrogenic potency of dong quai is far less than that used in hormone replacement therapy or birth control pills; if an estrogenic effect is desired, large doses are used. It is used to treat menstrual cramps, menstrual irregularities, and hot flashes. A recent double-blind and placebo-controlled study of dong quai used for hot flashes found that it was not more effective than a placebo (Ettinger 1997). The precautions regarding the use of unopposed estrogen apply to treatment with dong quai (Reichman 1996).

- **Black cohosh:** Black cohosh is an herb Native Americans have used traditionally for menstrual cramps. It is thought to have substances that relieve pain and act as sedatives. There is sufficient estrogenic activity to improve hot flashes and diminish vaginal atrophy. The estrogenic activity is even strong enough to lower FSH (follicle stimulating hormone) levels, just as birth control pills do. Black cohosh is also a vasoconstrictor, which accounts in part for the relief from hot flashes it provides. In a double-blind study of hot flash control at Purdue University School of Pharmacy, black cohosh was compared with Premarin (conjugated estrogen) and with a placebo. Black cohosh was found superior to both Premarin and the placebo for control of hot flashes and other estrogen deficiency symptoms. Because no studies exist on the risk for endometrial cancer with this herb, it is recommended that it be used not longer than three to six months (Tyler 1997). Remember from Chapter 7 that as little as six months of treatment with unopposed estrogen increases the risk of endometrial cancer fourfold, and the increased risk lingers for several years.

- **Red sage:** This is another phytoestrogen used for hot flashes (Wolfe 1990).

- **Chasteberry:** Chasteberry affects pituitary function sufficiently to lower FSH and LH (leuteinising hormone). This implies that it has a strong estrogenic component, which may be why it helps hot flashes. Some Mediterranean cultures have even used it to suppress the libidos of young women (Reichman 1996).

Homeopathic Remedies for Perimenopausal Symptoms

Earlier in this chapter we described the principles of homeopathy. Let's take a look at what's available for treating the undesirable symptoms of perimenopause.

- **Sepia:** Sepia is derived from the inky secretions of the cuttlefish. It is one of the most commonly used homeopathic remedies for fatigue, irritability, low sex drive, and vaginal dryness (Ullman 1991).

- **Evening primrose oil:** It is also found in seed oils of corn, wheat germ, sesame, sunflower, and safflower plants. The fatty acids develop a more effective cell membrane for diffusion of metabolic products, and this is said to improve function of the brain, adrenal glands, eyes, and reproductive organs (Ullman 1991). Evening primrose oil is also used to treat menstrual cramps and PMS symptoms. However, several placebo-controlled studies have shown that it has no beneficial effect on PMS (Khoo et al. 1990, Kleijmen 1994). It does not help hot flashes, but because of its weak estrogenic qualities, it may delay the age at which they first appear. Unopposed estrogen precautions are advisable.

- **Lachesis:** This substance is derived, believe it or not, from the poisonous venom of the American bushmaster snake. The venom is highly diluted and has no toxic effects. It is used for hot flashes, palpitations, and headaches. Candidates for treatment with lachesis are characterized as women who are overbearing, demanding, have fits of rage, and strong libidos (Ullman 1991).

- **Pulsatilla:** Pulsatilla comes from the windflower. The "pulsatilla type" is said to be women who are shy and nonassertive, weep easily, have low energy and low sexual desire, and feel chilled (Ullman 1991).

- **Nux vomica:** Made from something called the poison nut, nux vomica helps nausea, backache, disrupted sleep, perfectionistic tendencies, and chronic anger (Ullman 1991).

- **Bioflavinoids:** There are over 400 types of bioflavinoids. They are derived from soybeans, oriental spices, green tea, citrus fruits, and citrus rinds. They are mildly estrogenic, with a chemical structure that resembles estradiol. Women who have a high bioflavinoid intake in their diet have few symptoms of estrogen decline. Japanese women, for example, average about 5000 mg of bioflavinoids daily, compared to the American diet of 800 to 1000 mg (Ojeda 1995).

As you can see from the remedies we've described, homeopathic preparations can be directed at your specific symptoms or at your overall general characteristics. There are a great many homeopathic remedies available. Homeopathists urge that you not undertake self-treatment with these substances, because a broad knowledge of their indications is necessary for a successful outcome (Ullman 1991). If you are being treated for estrogen deficiency symptoms, ask the practitioner if the remedy has estrogenic qualities. You and your homeopathist must both have a clear understanding of the adverse effects of treatment with unopposed estrogen if unintended results are to be avoided.

Dietary Alternatives for Diminishing Hot Flashes

Some foods aggravate hot flashes and others diminish them. Consumption of hot foods and drinks, alcohol, and spicy foods should all be minimized to avoid food-related hot flashes. To lessen hot flashes, you can add more phytoestrogens to your diet. Japanese women have few complaints of hot flashes (only 1 percent), and their diet was studied by Finnish researchers in 1988. The typical Japanese diet is high in soybean products, such as miso, tofu, and soybeans, all of which contain phytoestrogen. Because of their dietary habits, the women studied had 1000 times more phytoestrogens in their urine than women on a Western diet (Aldercreutz et al. 1991).

The phytoestrogen in soybeans is a protein called *genistein.* The Finnish study of soy protein have showed that taking 25 to 50 grams daily (instead of animal protein) lowers cholesterol, raises HDL ("good" lipoproteins), and lowers LDL ("bad" lipoproteins) in both women and men. There is speculation that genistein may also have a positive influence on a woman's risk for breast cancer. The Japanese diet includes about 20 grams of soy foods per day (Aldercreutz et al. 1991). There are many ways to get more soy products into your diet:

- **Soy milk:** Substitute soy milk for cow's milk in flavored drinks and desserts.

- **Soy flour:** For pancakes, waffles, bread, cake, and thickeners, soy flour works well.

- **Tofu:** Tofu is a cheese-like curd made by adding calcium and magnesium to soy milk. It is a good substitute for animal protein in soups, sauces, and casseroles.

- **Soy nut snacks:** These beat high-fat cashews!

Of course, no soybean product can impersonate a two-inch filet mignon. Keep in mind, though, that the benefit of using more of the genistein in soybeans is a reduction in hormone deficiency symptoms. The more you consume this protein instead of animal protein, the more help you're getting in combating heart disease, obesity, and perhaps breast cancer.

Many other food plants also contain phytoestrogens, although none have quite the estrogen benefit you can get from soybeans. Table 9-1 lists a few of them.

Mind/Body Medicine

The thread running through most of the alternative treatment disciplines we've discussed is what is often called *mind/body medicine.* Dr. Deepak Chopra, in his book *Quantum Healing: Exploring the Frontiers of Mind/Body Medicine,* describes a new, non orthodox, and non Western approach to healing. The

Table 9.1. Plants Containing Phytoestrogens	
Type of Plant	**Example**
Grains	Wheat, barley, oats, rice, alfalfa
Fruits	Apples, cherries, pomegranates
Vegetables	Red and green beans, peas, potatoes, yams, sprouts
Odds and ends	Garlic, fennel, sesame seeds, parsley

Adapted from: Aldercreutz et al. 1991

premise of quantum healing is that in each of us is a package of intelligence, which happens to be contained in a body. All cells of the body use neuro-transmitters to stay in constant communication with each other. (Hormones are a good example of this.) Everything is under the control of the intelligence pool, the mind. In this sense, *mind* means more than just the brain and the nervous system. It includes the intelligence that resides in each of the trillions of cells of the entire body. If something goes wrong, such as a certain cell turning into a rogue cancer cell, the intelligence network is immediately aware of it, and healing is set in motion. According to Dr. Chopra, we may cure ourselves of cancer hundreds of times during a lifetime this way. Sometimes, though, the internal healing commands become overwhelmed by certain ill-nesses, such as cancer or infection, and the battle is lost. The challenge is to learn how to tap into this intelligence deliberately and consciously, rather than leaving it to work at the subconscious level, where it normally operates. The mind could turn out to be a *very* efficient healer, given its huge database of information and its capacity to fashion defenses to disease. This approach to medicine may, in time, make traditional and current alternative medical strategies seem crude.

Chopra indicates that mind/body medicine is being seriously explored by many talented people who have achieved remarkable success in improving a broad variety of ailments. Examples of currently used mind/body tech-niques are transcendental meditation, biofeedback, visualization/guided im-agery, hypnotherapy, and behavior modification. (We take a look at these in Chapter 12.) As for quantum healing, Dr. Chopra does not hesitate to point out that results to date are hard to interpret. As with most medical regimens, universal success is difficult to achieve. Nevertheless, mind/body medicine is now a field rather than a concept. As application of these techniques im-proves, future successes may be stunning.

Summary

Traditional versus alternative, orthodox versus nonorthodox, mainstream versus fringe, Western versus Eastern. These are all terms tossed about by the proponents of each of these schools of thought. Rather than choosing one of these categories of medicine over the other, it makes sense to seek the middle ground. All of these approaches to treatment have much to offer toward the goal of wellness, and also to each other.

It also makes sense to seek a total approach to your health care, integrating techniques of traditional Western medicine with those of Eastern traditions and other ancient healing approaches.

Your body is an exquisitely sensitive machine that demands balance to function properly and maintain wellness. The balance can be achieved in different ways and with different tools that traditional and alternative medicine can each supply.

○ ○ ○

10

Wellness for a Change: Good Nutrition and Exercise

Wellness is much more than the absence of disease. Wellness also means feeling vigorous, alert, robust, fresh as a daisy, and having the sense that you are in control of your body and your life. If you want to achieve and maintain wellness, you must assume the helm, guiding your lifestyle in ways that will ensure your goal. Wellness is also more than being conscientious about seeking care when you get sick. Contemporary health care is generally thought of as a problem-solving system: You go along day to day until you get sick, and then you rely upon your doctor to make it all better. You may get well from your disease this way, but your lifestyle may have been the *cause* of your illness. Antibiotics and a cough medicine will clear up your bronchitis, for example, but smoking may be the underlying reason you are susceptible to it. Physical therapy and an anti-inflammatory agent may help your backache; but a sedentary lifestyle and being overweight may be causing it.

Maintaining wellness involves becoming focused not just on the symptom that distresses you, but also on the larger issues that influence your overall health. These issues include adequate nutrition, a balanced diet, and exercise. These are the topics of this chapter. Weight control, limitation of destructive lifestyle habits, and management of stress are also involved in wellness. They are the topics of Chapters 11 and 12. Our goal is to show you how you can utilize these elements, how they are interrelated, and why they are necessary to your achieving wellness. If you have been thinking about losing weight, getting in shape, quitting smoking, and eliminating some other destructive lifestyle habits, your perimenopausal years represent an excellent time to start making these changes. This chapter and the next two are not just about making you live longer, but about your living well while you do it.

Changing Something

Changing anything that has been a long-term part of your behavior is not easy to do. Knowing some of the principles of change, however, can help you. The principles we discuss are the result of psychological studies of behavioral and intellectual factors involved in how people change (Landau et al. 1994).

- **Develop a realistic and positive plan:** You may have several changes you wish to accomplish, such as losing thirty pounds, reducing fat in your diet, and increasing fiber intake. It would not be realistic to set your goal at losing ten pounds every week, never eating another hamburger, and consuming oat bran muffins at every meal. A failed plan is too hard on your body; the common result of the "unreachable star" type of goal is no permanent accomplishment. Cut yourself some slack.

- **Take small steps:** If you lead a sedentary existence and are planning to increase your exercise activity, don't start with two hours of intense, heart-pounding activity every day, beginning tomorrow morning. There's a high likelihood that tomorrow morning would put an end to your plan. It is much better to set a target of, say, thirty to forty-five minutes, three to five days per week, but start with something easily accomplished. Make it thirty minutes of brisk walking for three to four days, and work up to your goal.

- **Think positive:** Regard the change you wish to accomplish as a challenge. Think of it as "doable," and something you know you can control. Not being in control is a stressor for many women; but successfully quitting smoking, for example, will make you feel better. It will give you confidence to tackle other changes you wish to make.

- **Make a commitment:** We're not talking about a resolution, like on New Year's Eve. A commitment must be deeply felt, and for the long haul. Your commitment will be permanent if you keep in front of you not only each change you wish to make, but the benefit it will afford you. For example, you might think. "I'll be able to play with the kids more," or simply, "My clothes will fit better."

- **Restructure your environment to avoid temptation:** If cutting back on fat consumption is your target, don't have lunch at McDonalds, where a Big Mac, fries, and a vanilla shake amount to 49.8 grams of fat—your entire day's fat allowance. If you are quitting alcohol, stay out of bars and avoid friends who drink. The same holds for smoking.

- **Reward yourself for success:** Revel in your small successes as you go along, rather than planning a big hoopla at the end. If you are losing weight, give yourself incremental rewards, like a new book each week that you have had a net loss. You might enlist the positive reinforcement of others, such as a weekly weigh-in on the family bathroom scale or a support group.

- **Avoid the all-or-nothing mind-set:** With this attitude, you can see yourself only as either totally successful or a total failure. The reality is that you are human, and you are going to have setbacks. When they occur, just regard them as part of the process of change. For example, perhaps you had a burger, fries, and a vanilla shake for lunch today. Remind yourself that this was the first time in a month you've eaten like this, you've lost ten pounds in the past two months, and this little incident was only a glitch in an ongoing process. No big deal.

- **Enlist a health care professional who will help:** This can be your physician, who may recommend a specialist in preventive health care, a dietitian, a local self-help group, or a university-based behavioral program. Or your doctor may just act as your cheerleader as your successful change progresses.

As you work your way through this chapter, you may identify several items in your life or in your body that you would like to change. Many American women are not happy with their bodies or how they function in some fashion or another. Once you have identified what it is that you wish to change, consider carefully and honestly what behavior you need to alter to accomplish your goal. Changing your wardrobe to disguise your broadening hips may seem like a solution; but you know that changing your diet is probably the fundamental answer. Taking the elevator to the second floor may solve your problem of being out of breath from climbing the stairs, but perhaps your leg muscles are out of shape or your lung capacity is diminished and you need to improve it with exercise. We urge you to keep these principles for successful change in mind, and maybe review them, as you read this chapter.

Nutrition

Protein, carbohydrate, and fat are the three principal categories of food. Water can be considered a fourth ingredient. Each of these types of food contains varying amounts of vitamins and minerals, and each serves an important role in a balanced diet. Over the years, nutritionists and other food scientists have studied these ingredients and their various effects on our bodies. As a result, they have been able to make recommendations for the most healthful combination of protein, carbohydrate, and fat in the diet. In general, however, Americans consume far too much protein and fat, and far too little carbohydrate.

First, let's consider the individual nutritional value of proteins, carbohydrates, fats, minerals, and vitamins. Then we'll put them together in a nutritional plan.

Protein

Your body makes protein by assembling amino acids into chains. There are twenty-two known amino acids, and your body can make all but eight of them. These eight are known as essential amino acids, and they must be supplied by your food intake. A complete protein is one that supplies all eight essential amino acids. Meat and dairy products are complete proteins, but fruits and vegetables are not.

Protein is second only to water as the most abundant substance in your body. It forms the basic structure of all parts of your body, including your bones. Muscle is mostly protein. Hormones, enzymes, and antibodies are all made from protein. When you are growing tissue or repairing it, protein is the essential ingredient. Protein in your body is also an energy source; but your body doesn't use it for this purpose as much as it uses carbohydrate and fat, unless your body is deficient in them. (This is what happens during starvation.)

Nutritionists recommend that you eat 0.42 grams of protein per pound of ideal body weight each day (Ojeda 1995). That comes to 55 grams if you weigh 130 pounds, but most Americans consume much more than that. The risk of a high-protein diet for you as a perimenopausal woman is that it causes you to lose calcium in your urine, and guess where the calcium comes from—your bones. Not good for prevention of osteoporosis. Another risk posed by a high-protein intake is that the typical American diet derives most of its protein from meat and dairy products. These are high in fat, and you may remember from Chapters 5 and 7 the problems that fat can cause with respect to cardiovascular disease, obesity, and certain cancers. Too much protein (more than 50 percent above daily needs) causes a net daily loss of calcium (Notelovitz and Tonnessen 1993). So not enough protein is bad, too much is bad too, and just right is just right. To see where you stand in protein consumption, calculate how much protein you need each day, at 0.42 grams per pound of your body weight. Then look over Table 10-1 for a list of commonly consumed protein foods to get a rough estimate of whether you meet the recommended intake.

Table 10.1.
Daily Protein Needs for Women
Formula using weight in pounds: _____lbs x 0.42 = _____grams per day

Food Source	Serving	Protein in Grams
Chicken	4 oz	36
Beef	4 oz	32
Fish	4 oz	28
Wheat cereal with milk	1 cup	28
Beans with rice	1 cup	17
Eggs	2	14
Cottage cheese	½ cup	14
Milk	1 cup	9
Cheddar cheese	1 oz	7
Beans	½ cup	7
Pasta	1 cup	5
Potato	1 medium	5
Whole wheat bread	1 slice	3

Adapted from: Ojeda 1995.

Carbohydrates—Pure-Burning Fuel

Carbohydrates consist of sugars, starches, and fiber. They are your primary energy source, with assists as needed from fat and protein. From your brain cells to your muscle cells, carbohydrates are the first thing they go for when they want to get something done that requires energy. Carbohydrates circulate in your blood as glucose, and this is your body's first choice when it comes to energy needs. Blood glucose can get used up quickly, though, so your liver converts some of it into a substance called glycogen and stores it for stoking the fire when necessary. If you have been really "carbing out," however, carbohydrates are converted to fat and tucked away in places that are not always inconspicuous.

Your body can make carbohydrate from components of protein and fat, so there aren't any *essential* carbohydrates. The three types of carbohydrates are worth discussing, though, because they have differing effects on your body and your health: simple sugars and refined carbohydrates, complex carbohydrates, and fiber.

Simple Sugar and Refined Carbohydrate

Simple sugars appear naturally in honey, fruits, and unrefined sugar. They are absorbed directly into your bloodstream without any significant digestive alteration, which is why you get such a quick energy surge from them. Refined carbohydrate foods are those made from white flour, refined sugar, and white rice. They are low in vitamins and minerals, which is bad enough, but the biggest problem with these foods is that they don't contain fiber. (We'll talk more about fiber in a moment.) Sugar is a great source of instant energy; but it is also a source of quick fatigue. When you load up on sugar, your blood glucose rises rapidly. This causes your pancreas to pour out insulin to get the blood glucose situation under control. Insulin production often overshoots the mark in reducing your blood sugar, and you end up with too little. Now you feel tired and weak again, so another shot of the sugar source seems irresistible.

A problem with sugar consumption for some people, aside from its lack of nutritional value, is that the high blood glucose levels it causes may require higher than usual insulin levels to control it. This is called insulin resistance. With larger amounts of insulin circulating to stanch the glucose tide, more of the glucose becomes converted to fat and stored. Obesity results, which increases the risk of diabetes. Insulin resistance increases with aging, so moderation in the your use of sweets during perimenopause seems prudent.

Complex Carbohydrates and Their Fabulous Fiber

Carbohydrates that need to be digested to be absorbed are called complex, not simple, carbohydrates. Complex carbohydrates are chiefly starches, found in potatoes, rice, pasta, corn, grains, and beans (lima, navy, kidney), but also in fruits and vegetables. When you eat them in an unrefined or unprocessed state, they provide abundant vitamins, minerals, and, especially fiber. Complex carbohydrates should constitute 55 to 60 percent of your daily caloric intake (Nutrition and Your Health 1995), but in the typical American diet, this is far from the case.

Dietary fiber is the indigestible part of these foods. It is found in the plant cell walls, and it does not become absorbed into the bloodstream. There are two types (Ojeda 1995).

- **Water soluble fiber:** This type of fiber is found in whole grains, oat-bran cereals, beans, and barley, plus many fruits and vegetables. Soluble fiber aids in lowering cholesterol, triglycerides, and low-density lipoproteins (LDLs).

- **Insoluble fiber:** Insoluble fiber is predominantly found in whole wheat products, wheat bran, corn and rice bran, and the skins of fruits and vegetables. This is the fiber that softens stools and prevents constipation. Consumption of insoluble fiber bulk also results in a form of intestinal calisthenics, by keeping the muscles of your gastrointestinal tract toned.

Nutritionists recommend 30 to 35 grams of fiber each day, which is in stark contrast to the average fiber-depleted American diet of 10 to 15 grams. There are numerous benefits to an adequate fiber intake:

- **Decreasing the risk of coronary heart disease:** While it is still somewhat controversial, the recommended level of dietary fiber appears to decrease the risk of coronary heart disease by enhancing the cholesterol-lowering effect of a low fat diet. LDL cholesterol is lowered, and so are triglycerides.

- **Controlling Moods:** A high complex-carbohydrate diet may assist in controlling some of the negative moods associated with PMS. Carbohydrates raise the brain level of an amino acid called tryptophan, which is converted to a neurotransmitter called serotonin. (See Chapter 2 for more about this neurotransmitter.) Serotonin influences sleep patterns, pain perception, and hormone secretion and has an overall calming effect. Inadequate serotonin levels are associated with depression. So start your PMS day with a large bowl of a high carbohydrate cereal, even if you hate the cereal, hate the bowl, hate the spoon, and hate the skim milk you pour over it. Chances are good you'll feel better within an hour or so.

- **Decreasing the risk of diabetes:** Fiber takes longer to digest than other food components, so it slows the absorption of carbohydrate into your bloodstream. This aids in blood sugar control. It decreases your risk of developing diabetes and helps blood sugar regulation in those who are already diabetic.

- **Decreasing cancer risks:** As we pointed out in Chapter 7, a high-fiber diet is clearly associated with decreased incidence of colon cancer. It may lower the incidence of other cancers as well.

- **Controlling weight:** High-fiber foods are lower in calories and fat than low-fiber foods. In addition, digestion of fiber is slow, which contributes to your feeling fuller longer.

- **Controlling intestinal problems:** Fiber prevents constipation because it absorbs water, creating a softer stool. (Stool softeners like Metamucil are powdered fiber.) Soft stools from an adequate fiber diet prevent the formation of diverticuli, which are little outpouchings from the wall of the colon. These can become inflamed and painful, causing a condition called diverticulitis.

When you increase your fiber intake, do it gradually. A big jump can result in gas and bloating. Be sure to drink plenty of water (six to eight cups a day) with your increased fiber diet. (There will be more bulk in your intestine; without water accompanying it, you can become constipated.) Also be aware that fiber can prevent or decrease the absorption of calcium and iron. If you are using these supplements, do not take them at the same time as a high-fiber meal. Table 10-2 lists the fiber content of common foods. When you select breads and cereals, stick to whole-grain products. Refining of these grains removes 60 to 90 percent of the vitamins, minerals, and fiber (Willet 1994).

The Skinny on Fat

Your body needs fat, but there's a limit. Fat is a very concentrated source of energy since it contains nine calories per gram, as compared to four calories per gram in both proteins and carbohydrates. Fat stores represent a valuable portable warehouse for energy and water to which your body can turn when your metabolic machine is running a little short. Fat insulates your body from cold and cushions vital organs from injury. Dietary fat aids in the absorption of the fat-soluble vitamins A, D, E, and K. Fat makes your food taste good. Because it digests more slowly than other foods, fat also gives you that pleasant feeling of fullness after a meal. That was the good news. And now the *rest* of the story.

McDowell and co-workers reported in 1994 that Americans consume about 34 percent of daily calories from dietary fat. Others have estimated the level to be as high as 40 percent. According to McDowell, the number should actually be about 25 to 30 percent to meet your body's needs and remain healthy. The American fat epidemic makes the news often enough, and maybe you have already cut back on your use of butter, and started to trim the fat off your meat, and drink low-fat milk. If so, you are heading in the right direction; but remember that there are fats in many everyday foods. You probably already know about items like cheesecake, potato chips, and nuts, that they're high in calories as well. Also watch out for fast foods and TV dinners, cream soups, lunch meats, avocado, cheese, and desserts like doughnuts and chocolate. These foods are high in calories, too, which end up as reserve stores of fat if they exceed your body needs. Dietary fat is more readily converted to body fat than either carbohydrates or proteins. It is less readily used for energy than carbohydrates, so it becomes more of a permanent fixture. Fat gets distributed to places you don't want it, like your hips, thighs, and around your middle. As we described in Chapter 8, perimenopausal women tend to have pear-shaped bodies. Postmenopausal women accumulate fat about the abdomen, as men do (the apple shape). Not only does a high-fat diet contribute to obesity, it raises your risk of cardiovascular disease, high blood pressure, diabetes, and certain cancers.

What about Cholesterol?

Cholesterol isn't really a fat. It is a waxy substance, called a lipid, found in animal foods and dairy products. We talked about cholesterol in Chapter

Table 10.2.
Fiber Content of Various Foods

Type of Food	Serving	Fiber in Grams
Cereals		
All Bran with extra fiber	½ cup	14.0
All Bran	½ cup	12.9
100% Bran	½ cup	10.0
Raisin Bran	¾ cup	5.3
40% Bran Flakes	½ cup	4.3
Oat bran, cooked	¾ cup	4.0
Oat bran cereal, cold	¾ cup	2.9
Corn flakes	¾ cup	2.1
Special K	¾ cup	1.2
Cream of Wheat	¾ cup	0.5
Rice Krispies	¾ cup	0
Breads		
Pita bread, whole wheat	1.5″ pocket	4.4
Pumpernickel	1 slice	2.7
Whole wheat	1 slice	1.5
Bagel, plain	1	1.4
White bread, French, Italian	1 slice	0.6
Croissant	1	0
Legumes (Beans & Peas)		
Black-eyed peas, cooked	¾ cup	12.3
Kidney or pinto beans, cooked	¾ cup	14.0
Kidney beans, canned	¾ cup	4.7
Lima beans, cooked	½ cup	3.5
Lentils, cooked	½ cup	5.2
Split peas, cooked	½ cup	3.1
Peas, canned	½ cup	2.8
Fruits		
Apple, large, with skin	1	4.7
Apricots, dried	10	3.6
Orange	1 medium	3.0
Pear, with skin	1 small	2.9
Peach, with skin	1 medium	2.0
Prune, dried	3 medium	1.7

Continued on the following page.

Type of Food	Serving	Fiber in Grams
Rasberries, fresh	½ cup	1.7
Grapefruit, medium	½	1.4
Pineapple, canned	½ cup	1.2
Banana, medium	1	0.7
Raisins	2 tbsp	0.4
Grapes, green, fresh	½ cup	0.4
Vegetables		
Peas, green, cooked	½ cup	4.3
Potato, baked + skin	1 medium	4.2
Brussels sprouts, cooked	½ cup	3.8
Corn, whole, cooked	½ cup	3.0
Carrots, raw	1 medium	2.3
Broccoli, cooked	½ cup	1.5
Spinach, raw	1 cup	1.4
Tomato, cooked	½ cup	1.0
Lettuce, iceberg	1 cup	0.6

Adapted from: Ojeda 1995 and Cutler 1992.

5, and about the role it plays in cardiovascular disease. Cholesterol itself, however, is not harmful; indeed it is vital to your existence! Cholesterol helps build cell membranes (all three trillion of them). Cholesterol is also the basic building block for hormones. Your body uses it to make vitamin D. Cholesterol also forms a protective sheath around nerves, which facilitates transmission of impulses, and it serves many, many other important biologic functions. You body can manufacture all the cholesterol it needs, but you add to the supply from the foods you eat, and there's the rub: If your cholesterol intake is too high, your blood level of cholesterol rises. Then you start parking the excess amounts of this waxy substance along the walls of arteries, which leads to hardening of your arteries, high blood pressure, and coronary heart disease. In other words, cholesterol is a "good guy" who can do bad things. You probably know people like that.

Cholesterol performs its marvels in your body's cells by being carried to them in your bloodstream. The carrier substances, called lipoproteins, are manufactured in your liver by combining fat and protein, to which cholesterol is attached for a free ride. Well, not always free—you may pay a price in the form of cardiovascular disease if your lipoproteins get out of whack. Don't get discouraged, though; you can control your lipoproteins.

Table 10-3 lists the amount of cholesterol in many common foods.

Table 10.3.
Calories, Fat, and Cholesterol in Foods

Food	Serving	Calories	Fat (grams)	Choles-terol (mgs)
Candy				
Milk chocolate bar	1 oz	150	9.2	5
Cheese				
Cheddar	1 oz	112	9.1	30
Cottage, 2% fat	½ cup	100	2.2	9
Monterey jack	1 oz	105	8.5	30
Swiss, pasteurized	1 oz	95	7.1	26
Cheese Whiz spread	1 oz	80	6.0	15
Condiments				
Mayonaise	1 tbsp	100	11.0	5
Diet mayonaise	1 tbsp	45	5.0	5
Miracle Whip	1 tbsp	70	7.0	5
Dairy Products				
Whole milk	1 cup	150	8.1	34
Low-fat milk	1 cup	122	4.7	20
Skim milk	1 cup	89	0.4	5
Yogurt, nonfat	1 cup	127	0.4	4
Yogurt, whole milk	1 cup	141	7.7	30
Egg, whole	1 med	78	5.5	250
Egg yolk	1 med	59	5.2	250
Egg Beaters	¼ cup	25	0	0
Fats & Oils				
Butter	1 tbsp	108	12.2	36
Margarine	1 tbsp	108	12.0	0
Vegetable oil	1 tbsp	120	13.5	0
Butter Buds	1 oz	12	0	0
Molly McButter	1 tsp	5	0	0
Seafood				
Crab, king	3½ oz	93	1.9	60
Fish sticks, frozen	3½ oz	176	8.9	70
Lobster	3½ oz	91	1.9	100
Mackerel	3½ oz	191	12.2	95

Continued on the following page.

Oysters	3½ oz	66	1.8	50
Salmon	3½ oz	182	7.4	47
Sardines, canned in oil	3½ oz	311	24.4	120
Shrimp	3½ oz	91	0.8	100
Tuna, canned in oil	3½ oz	197	8.2	63
Tuna, canned in water	3½ oz	127	0.8	63
Breads				
English muffin	1	133	1.0	0
Pita, pocket	1	145	1.0	0
White	1 slice	68	0.8	0
Whole wheat	1 slice	61	0.8	0
Meats				
Beef, trimmed, cooked	3 oz	192	9.4	73
Ground beef, 27% fat	3 oz	251	16.9	86
Ground beef, 10% fat	3 oz	213	11.9	86
Lamb chop	3 oz	188	8.9	82
Pork chop	3 oz	219	12.7	80
Spareribs	3 oz	338	25.8	103
Bacon	1 slice	40	3.0	5
Ham, 3% fat	3 oz	120	6.0	45
Chicken, light, no skin	3 oz	153	4.2	66
Chicken, with skin	3 oz	210	12.6	75
Turkey, light, no skin	3 oz	153	4.2	66
Turkey, with skin	3 oz	210	12.6	75
Veal, lean only	3 oz	120	2.7	84
Beef liver	3½ oz	140	4.7	300
Beef brain	3½ oz	106	7.3	2100
Bologna	1 oz	88	8.1	15+
Canadian bacon	1 oz	45	2.0	13
Liverwurst	1 oz	139	9.1	35
Salami	1 oz	112	9.8	22
Hot dog	1.6 oz	142	13.5	23
Salad Dressing				
Blue Cheese	1 tbsp	71	7.3	4-10
Russian	1 tbsp	74	7.6	7-10
French	1 tbsp	66	6.2	0
Italian	1 tbsp	83	9.0	0

Adapted from: R.E. Kowalski. 1990. *The 8-Week Cholesterol Cure*. New York: Harper & Row, and W. Cutler and C. Garcia, 1992. *Menopause: A Guide for Women and the Men Who Love Them*. New york: Norton.

Which Fat Is Which

There are several types of dietary fat. Too much of any of them is not good for you, but some are worse than others. All fats are composed of *fatty acids*, which are chemicals that are put together in a variety of ways to make each type of fat. Saturated fats and hydrogenated fats are the main trouble-makers. Monounsaturated and polyunsaturated fats are less harmful. Triglycerides are another form of fat that your liver makes from the food you eat. We discuss each of them below.

Saturated Fat

Saturated fat is dietary enemy number one. You get it from animal foods and dairy products. See Table 10-4 for a listing of common foods and their saturated fat content. Cholesterol has gotten a bad name because of saturated fat. A diet high in cholesterol does not necessarily raise the blood cholesterol if saturated fat intake is low. On the other hand, a high saturated fat diet raises LDL cholesterol and significantly increases the risk of CVD.

Table 10.4.
Food Sources of Dietary Fat

Saturated	Monosaturated	Polyunsaturated
Meat (beef, pork, lamb, veal, poultry)	Margarine with hydrogenated oil	Margarine with polyunsaturated oil
Butter	Shortening, partially hydrogenated	Cottonseed oil
Cheese		Corn oil
Lard	Olive oil	Safflower oil
Chocolate	Peanut oil	Soybeans, soybean oil
Coconut oil	Canola oil	Sunflower seeds and oil
Palm oil	Nuts (almonds, pecans, filberts, Brazil, macadamia)	Wheat germ and oil
Hydrogenated vegetable oil	Avocado and oil	Walnuts and oil
	Rice-bran oil	Mayonaise
		Salad dressing made with polyunsaturated oil
		Fatty fish

Source: C.J.W. Suitor and M.F. Crowley. 1996. *Nutrition Principles and Application in Health Promotion,* 2nd ed. Philadelphia: Lippincott.

TIP! If you've forgotten what all these abbreviations mean, take a look back at Chapter 5.

Saturated fats are usually solid at room temperature. Examples include butter, cheese, lard, meat fat, and chocolate. Some are liquid, like coconut oil, palm oil, and cream. Your daily fat intake should be less than half in saturated fat (Dreon et al. 1990). Your body does *not* have a biologic need for saturated fat; it can derive all the essential fatty acids it needs from unsaturated fat, which we talk about shortly.

Hydrogenated Fat (Trans Fatty Acids)

Hydrogenation is a chemical process that converts naturally occurring oils like coconut and peanut oil to saturated fat. These are the oils used in many processed products, such as corn chips, baked goods, potato chips, and french fries. Margarine and shortenings use hydrogenated fat. A tablespoon of margarine has two grams of saturated fat plus about two grams of hydrogenated fat, for a grand total of four grams of "bad" fat. (That still compares favorably with butter, at seven grams of saturated fat per tablespoon.)

Trans fatty acids are just as bad as saturated fat in raising your LDL, but they *also* lower your good HDL, which saturated fat does not do. A 1993 report from Harvard revealed a 66 percent higher risk of heart disease in women who used margarine four or more times daily compared to women who used it almost not at all (Willet and Stampfer 1993).

TIP! Manufacturers are not currently required to list the amounts of hydrogenated fat in their products. If the label say "partially hydrogenated vegetable oils," leave it on the shelf.

Polyunsaturated Fats

Polyunsaturated fats are generally liquid at room temperature. They include vegetable derivatives of cottonseed, corn, safflower, sunflower, soybeans, and wheat germ. Polyunsaturated fats lower blood levels of cholesterol, but they lower HDL *and* LDL, so it's a mixed blessing. Monounsaturated oils are considered safer.

Monounsaturated Fats

Monounsaturated fats have no undesirable effects on cholesterol. As a matter of fact, they make LDL cholesterol more resistant to oxidation, which reduces the tendency of cholesterol to be deposited as plaque on artery walls. This is a definite plus. Monounsaturated fats are vegetable products contained in olive oil, peanut oil, and canola oil. Mediterranean cultures consistently follow a diet that derives 30 to 40 percent of its calories from fat, yet their heart attack rate is half that of the United States (Notelovitz and Tonnessen 1993). It is believed that this is, in part, at least, due to their fondness for olive oil. Other genetic and cultural factors may also be involved, of course;

if you are choosing between olive oil and butter, go for the olive oil. But don't make olive oil a net addition to your fat intake. If you are going to emphasize olive oil in your diet, cut back on something else, like meats and fish. Too much fat is too much fat, no matter what form it takes.

Triglycerides

Triglycerides are another form of fatty acid that your body gets primarily from food. You store it in fat cells for energy use as needed. Most foods that contain fat have triglycerides. The significance of this fat to you as a woman is that high levels in your blood pose much more of a risk for coronary heart disease than the same levels in men (Lapidus 1986).

Fish Oils

There's been a lot of hoopla in recent years about omega-3 fatty acids, a polyunsaturated fat found in a large variety of fish. Studies of Eskimos and Japanese showed their traditionally high-fish diets resulted in less than half the heart attack rate of that experienced in the continental 48 states (Kromhaut et al. 1985). Eskimos have about the same cholesterol levels in their blood as we do in the continental U.S. but they have lower triglycerides than we do. This benefit was traced to the omega-3 fatty acids in fish oil. These fatty acids lower triglyceride levels quite effectively. They also have a beneficial influence on clotting factors, which is thought to be part of the reason for the lowered heart attack rate in the study.

Does this mean you should eat a lot of fish? Sort of. A Harvard study of middle-aged male professionals (women were not studied, unfortunately) demonstrated that eating as little as one or two servings of fish a week conferred as much protection as a high-fish diet (Von Schaky 1987). It makes sense to have fish as part of your weekly diet, but you don't have to get carried away with it. Fish oil is available in capsules, several of which must be taken each day. The experts who have studied fish oil capsules have sounded a different note on this issue. They found that concentrated fish oil use will lower your triglycerides, but it may actually raise your undesirable LDL. The current recommendation is not to use fish oil capsules, and to rely on fish consumption for the known benefits (Notelovitz and Tonnessen 1993). Sardines are very high in omega-3 fatty acids; other excellent sources with lesser amounts are sockeye salmon and Atlantic mackerel, albacore tuna, herring, and halibut (Bellerson 1993).

Vitamins and Minerals

Vitamins are essential in small amounts for regulation of your metabolism and for normal tissue growth and function. There are thirteen known vitamins, and they sort themselves into two categories: fat soluble and water soluble. The fat-soluble vitamins—A, D, E, and K—are dissolved by fat in the intestine and stored in your body, sometimes for surprising lengths of time. Vitamin A, for example, can remain in your liver for up to two years. Because these vitamins are stored, it is easily possible through the use of supplements to accumulate much more than you need and suffer serious toxic side effects. Water-soluble vitamins, such as the B vitamins and C, do not pose this risk because they are not stored, and any excess is passed in the urine.

With aging, your metabolic rate slowly falls. Caloric needs may decline while vitamin needs increase. Adjusting your daily diet to make up for the shortfall of vitamins can become a complex operation, so it probably makes sense to take a daily multiple vitamin supplement that provides a balanced regimen without providing mega-doses. As you will see in a moment, however, the Recommended Dietary Allowance (RDA) for several of the vitamins and minerals in a standard multivitamin preparation may be inadequate for you.

Antioxidants

Nutritional research has shown that oxygen, although it is necessary for survival, can actually cause you harm. At the cellular level, oxygen is used in the chemical reactions that produce energy and a host of useful metabolic products. A by-product of this molecular activity with oxygen is the release of particles called *oxygen-free radicals*. The problem free radicals have is that they are one electron shy of what they need to remain stable. They go whizzing around in their molecular soup looking for that missing electron. In the process, they smash into the cell wall and other molecules, causing damage. This damage at the cellular level speeds up the aging process in all cells of your body. Free radical attacks on LDL change it into plaque, which attaches to artery walls and clogs them. They may even damage the cellular genes, causing a mutation and setting up the cell for future cancerous activity. (Notelovitz and Tonnessen 1993)

Don't think you have to cut back on your oxygen consumption, though. Antioxidants can help solve the problem. The antioxidant vitamins are A, C, and E. Selenium is an antioxidant mineral. Their beneficial function is to gather up the cavorting free radicals and bind them into harmless, stable molecules that cause no cellular damage. The question, though, is whether your diet can supply you with enough antioxidant vitamins, or whether you need to take supplements. Let's look at each of these vitamins.

Vitamin E

Vitamin E occurs naturally in foods such as bran, wheat, nuts, seeds, sweet potatoes, fish, crab, and cold-pressed vegetable oils. It has been shown in a variety of studies to have the benefits in these areas (Stampfer and Willett 1993; Jandak and Richardson 1989; Kardinaal 1994).

- **LDL cholesterol:** Vitamin E prevents oxidation of LDL and subsequent plaque deposits on artery walls. This reduces hardening of the arteries, high blood pressure, heart attacks, and strokes.
- **Platelets:** Decreases the stickiness of platelets and thus reduces the risk of blood clots forming in plaque-damaged vessels. This also means fewer heart attacks and strokes.
- **Cell membranes:** Neutralizes free radicals inside the cell so they cannot attack the fatty acid components of the cell wall. This reduces cellular aging and, among other things, the brown marks on the skin known as "liver spots."
- **Vitamins A, C, and B complex:** Protects them from oxidation and inactivation.
- **Immune system:** Enhances this system's ability to resist genetic mutations and cancer formation.
- **Chromosome damage:** Together with vitamin C, reduces damage to chromosomes from carcinogens and radiation.
- **Muscles:** Improves muscular efficiency in using oxygen.
- **Cancer prevention:** An Iowa study showed a 70 percent reduction in colon cancer for women on high-dose vitamin E supplements (Reichman 1996).

Part of the Nurses' Health Study at Harvard was an eight-year follow-up of 87,000 women, ages 34 through 59, who took at least 100 IU (international units) of vitamin E daily. Those who used it for two years or more had a 40 percent reduction in risk factors for coronary disease. Those who took 30 IU or less also benefited, but with slightly less than a 25 percent reduction in risk factors. (Willet 1994)

So should you take a vitamin E supplement? The answer is maybe, maybe not. More research needs to be done for a solid recommendation, but there are no data suggesting that it's bad for you. Toxic levels are reached at about 3000 IU a day, and the recommended dose is only 100 to 400 IU a day. Reaching that level requires a supplement; because you just can't get that much from eating foods rich in vitamin E, such as sunflower seeds, filberts, and cucumbers, for example.

Vitamin A and Beta-Carotene

Vitamin A is a fat-soluble antioxidant derived from *carotenoids* in plant and animal sources. Carotenoids are contained in vegetable pigments, notably carrots, and their most noteworthy member is beta-carotene, from which vitamin A is made. About one quarter of dietary beta-carotenes are converted to vitamin A, and the rest are stored in fat tissues in your liver for later use, or passed out of your body through the intestine. Animal Vitamin A sources are fish, beef liver, and fish liver oil.

Vitamin A is essential in bone and tooth formation, growth and repair of tissues, maintenance of healthy skin, and normal night vision. When researchers found that vitamin A could halt the growth of breast cancer cells in laboratory cell cultures, studies got under way to see if this was true in real life. The Nurses' Health Study data showed a 25 percent higher risk for breast cancer in diets low in vitamin A or beta-carotene. Supplements of vitamin A did not affect the breast cancer risk in women whose diets were adequate in beta-carotene, suggesting that dietary beta-carotene sources are all that is needed for this benefit (Hunter 1993). In lung cancer and heart disease studies, a different story unfolded. They found either no protection or an increase in these diseases with vitamin A supplements. Some studies have shown a reduction in heart disease with vitamin A use, but not in mega-doses (Reichman 1996). Another study (Krasinski et al. 1989), reported that vitamin A supplements in mega-doses caused liver damage, and the higher the dose, the worse the damage. Obviously, more study is needed.

CAUTION! If you are planning to become pregnant, note this: A large study of 22,000 pregnant women found that supplemental vitamin A (not beta-carotene) in doses over 10,000 IU daily was associated with fetal malformations (Reichman 1996).

The bottom line is that you probably do not need vitamin A supplements. You can get what you need from dietary fruits and vegetables, and your body can store vitamin A for as long as two years. Good sources of vitamin A include beef liver, carrots, sweet potatoes, spinach, and cantaloupe.

Vitamin C (Ascorbic Acid)

Vitamin C is an antioxidant found in most fruits and vegetables. It is far and away the most widely researched of the vitamins. The RDA for vitamin C is 60 mg, but doses up to10,000 mg have been recommended in conditions of stress (Levine 1987). Since it is water-soluble, vitamin C is not stored in your body. Indeed, most of it is excreted in urine within three to four hours after you take it. Foods rich in vitamin C include orange juice, kiwi fruit, broccoli, and raw tomatoes. They must be consumed soon after they are cooked or otherwise prepared (sliced, pureed, juiced) because the vitamin quickly evaporates. Cooked foods that are stored quickly lose their vitamin C.

Vitamin C's health credentials are impressive:

- **Cardiovascular disease:** As an antioxidant, vitamin C prevents oxidation of LDL cholesterol and reduces the risk of plaque formation on artery walls. RDA levels are not sufficient for this protection. (Hallfrisch et al. 1994)
- **Collagen protection:** Collagen is the connective tissue that is responsible for smooth, wrinkle-free skin. It is also part of bone and many

other tissues. Vitamin C prevents free radicals from attacking collagen. Duke University has developed a skin product utilizing a form of vitamin C (L ascorbic acid) that appears to dramatically increase collagen formation and may play a role in preventing the effects of skin aging from ultraviolet light (Colvin and Pinnell 1996). As yet, the Duke studies have not been reproduced by other researchers.

- **Bones:** Vitamin C facilitates absorption of calcium from the intestine and therefore assists in bone formation.

- **Toxic effects of alcohol:** If you have red wine with a red meat dish, the tannin in the wine will prevent the iron in the meat from being absorbed. As little as 250 mg of vitamin C during such a meal appears to prevent this. A tomato salad does nicely. Vitamin C also seems to help avoid hangovers. (Zannoni 1987)

- **Nitrosamines:** Vitamin C inhibits formation of nitrosamines, cancer-promoting free radicals that result from the oxidation of nitrites in cooked meats, especially hot dogs, bacon, and other processed meat products (Ojeda, 1995).

- **Cancer:** According to Lohman (1987), vitamin C reduces the risk of death from all cancers by 14 percent. It has been shown to favorably influence the immune system in responding to several cancers, such as leukemia, advanced breast cancer, and colon cancer, as well as pre-cancers, such as high-grade abnormalities in cervical cells.

Studies have also shown that vitamin C helps prevent cataracts, promotes wound healing and iron absorption from the intestine, and plays a role in the formation of adrenaline, your stress-reaction hormone.

Vitamin C is depleted in your body if you have a wound, a fever, are under high stress, or are taking aspirin, antibiotics, or steroids. Smoking also depletes vitamin C. In these situations, you need more vitamin C than the RDA of 60 mg. Up to 10,000 mg a day in divided doses may be taken, usually without ill effect but this varies from person to person, as well as with the severity of the situation producing the vitamin C depletion. If your body needs vitamin C, it will absorb it; but if not, the excess is eliminated through bowel movements. The signal that you are taking more than you need is loose stools (Pauling 1986). So if diet alone doesn't supply the amount of vitamin C you need in a specific situation, take a supplement.

B Vitamins

The B vitamins are water soluble like vitamin C, but they are not antioxidants. The seven B vitamins are B-1(thiamin), B-2 (riboflavin), B-3 (niacin), B-5 (pantothenic acid), B-6 (pyridoxine), B-12 (cobalamin), and folic acid. Food sources include green vegetables, whole grain cereals, liver, and brewer's yeast. Your body also makes its own B vitamins, in your intestines. You can't store B vitamins, so your body needs a daily supply. They play a different role than the antioxidants, but they are no less important:

- **Energy:** B vitamins convert carbohydrates from food you eat into glucose for direct and immediate energy. They also provide your backup energy source by converting glycogen stores in your liver and muscles into glucose.

- **Fat and protein:** B vitamins are essential for metabolizing both fat and protein.

- **Vascular disease:** B6, B12, and folic acid are necessary to prevent the conversion of one amino acid, called methionine, to another amino acid, called homocysteine. Evidence exists that elevated homocysteine levels are an independent risk factor for vascular disease. As estrogen levels fall in women, homocysteine levels rise, so transitional women must maintain an adequate daily intake of vitamin C (Stampfer 1993).

- **PMS symptoms:** Vitamin B6 is instrumental in the formation of serotonin, which we described in Chapter 2. Many PMS sufferers are helped by taking 20 to 40 mg of B6 a day during the second half of the menstrual cycle. Large doses (over 200 mg) should be avoided because some women develop abnormal neurological symptoms (Reichman 1996, Ojeda 1995).

- **Central nervous system:** Folic acid is concentrated in your spinal fluid and is necessary for proper brain functioning. It is also necessary for proper brain development to prevent neural tube defects in a growing fetus. If you are planning to become pregnant, your baby's best protection comes from being on a folic acid supplement at the time of conception (Medical Research Council 1991, ACOG 1992).

- **Red blood cells:** Folic acid is needed to form the protein that, combined with iron, is used in your red blood cells as hemoglobin.

Vitamin D

Vitamin D is the last of the fat-soluble vitamins. Dietary sources are fatty animal products, such as fish liver oils, beef liver, tuna, salmon, butter, and milk. Most milk, the most common dietary source, is now artificially fortified with vitamin D in the U.S. Sunlight exposure of about 15 minutes per day allows ultraviolet rays to convert cholesterol molecules in your skin to vitamin D. It is also made synthetically and included in multiple vitamins and as a separate product. For ingested vitamin D to be absorbed from your intestine, fat, bile, and vitamin A are necessary. Once aboard, vitamin D can be stored in your liver and other organs.

As discussed in the osteoporosis section of Chapter 5, vitamin D is needed to absorb calcium from the intestines for incorporation into your bones. If your diet has sufficient vitamin D (400 IU) from foods such as canned tuna and salmon, whole milk, beef liver, and egg yolk and you get daily sun exposure, you, like most people in our culture, are probably not deficient in this vitamin.

Vitamin D is also associated with reduced risk for colon cancer. Additional evidence suggests that vitamin D may be involved in breast cancer prevention. Researchers have found the frequency of breast cancer is less in women who live in sunnier areas like San Diego and the American southwest (Notelovitz and Tonnessen 1993).

Calcium

Chapter 5 took a thorough look at the various roles calcium plays in your body's functioning. The bottom line is that you need about 1,000 mg of this mineral daily during your perimenopausal years and 1,500 mg after menopause.

Several foods and drugs can reduce your calcium absorption and utilization (Notelovitz and Tonnessen 1993):

- Excessive protein intake (50 percent above daily needs) increases calcium excretion. This is not an unusual amount of protein consumption in the U.S., so be alert to your dietary intake.
- Caffeine, nicotine, and alcohol all increase calcium loss in your urine.
- Phosphorus found in processed foods (especially soft drinks) causes the parathyroid gland to remove calcium from your bones and excrete it in your urine.
- High fiber intake binds calcium in your intestine and diminishes absorption. Stool softeners such as Metamucil cause this problem, so don't take them with your calcium supplement.
- Tetracycline antibiotics and cholesterol-lowering drugs (lovastatin, niacin, colestipol) interfere with calcium absorption and should be taken separately from your calcium supplement.
- Foods high in oxalates (spinach, chard, collards, turnip greens, parsley, rhubarb, peanuts, tea, cocoa, legumes) contain substantial calcium, but it is bound by the oxalates and therefore unavailable for absorption. The oxalates can also bind other calcium sources you consume at the same time. It's okay to eat these foods for other nutrient value, but it is best to avoid taking a calcium supplement for several hours afterward.

Iron

Remember when "they" used to tell you to take an iron supplement on a regular basis because you lose iron every month with your menstrual period? Turns out "they" were wrong. Ionized iron is actually an oxidant, and oxidants, as we've been discussing, do bad things to you. A Finnish study in 1992 (Notelowitz and Tonnessen 1993) correlated high iron levels with an increased rate of heart attacks in the 1931 men they studied. They postulated that part of the reason for women having few heart attacks before menopause is their relatively low iron stores during the menstrual years. When menstrual periods stop, iron levels rise in postmenopausal women, and so does the risk for heart attacks. You are probably getting all the iron you need in your diet, so don't use iron pills (aside from a multivitamin) unless you are proven to be iron deficient.

Magnesium

Magnesium is a trace mineral, and about 70 percent of it is located in your bones. It has functions similar to those of calcium in your body, with involvement in muscle contraction, nerve-impulse transmission, and heart muscle contraction. Magnesium is necessary for activation of enzymes that metabolize carbohydrates and amino acids. It is also part of tooth enamel.

You need magnesium to absorb calcium. These two minerals work together. Too much magnesium inhibits calcium absorption, and too much calcium does the same for magnesium. The current nutritional recommendation is that they stay in a constant ratio of 2 to 1, calcium to magnesium (Ojeda 1995). For you as a transitional woman, your daily calcium intake of 1,000 mg should be balanced with 500 mg of magnesium. After menopause, if your calcium needs increase to 1,500 mg, your magnesium should go up to 750 mg.

Like calcium, magnesium absorption is decreased by an excess of protein, oxalic acid foods (dark green leafy veggies), and alcohol. Use of diuretics also depletes magnesium. The Food and Drug Administration has set the Required Daily Allowance for magnesium at 280 mg, but this fails to take into account the increased calcium needs of mid-life women and the 2-to-1 ratio needed with magnesium. If your diet is low in fish, milk, grains, and green vegetables, it makes sense to use a magnesium supplement at half the level of your calcium intake.

Let's Plan a Diet

This section is about using nutritionally healthful principles to fashion a diet that you can stay with for the rest of your life. It is not a plan of deprivation and denial that will leave you hungry all the time; we know that won't work.

In 1995, the U.S. Departments of Agriculture and Health and Human Services published the *Dietary Guidelines for Americans,* which made these recommendations.

- Eat a variety of foods.
- Balance the food you eat with physical activity to maintain or improve your weight.
- Include plenty of grain products, vegetables, and fruits in your diet.
- Choose foods low in fat, saturated fat, and cholesterol.
- Choose foods moderate in sugar content.
- Choose foods moderate in salt and sodium content.
- If you drink alcoholic beverages, do so in moderation.

Since you want the second half of your life to be vibrant and enjoyable, following these recommendations is important.

According to the Senate Select Committee on Nutrition (1990), up to 80 percent of food consumed by the majority of Americans has minimal or no nutritional value. They issued a report that the average American's diet is high in fat, sugar, and calories and low in fiber and nutrients. Eating in America is a risk factor in itself for promotion of disease. Our diet has now been linked to high blood pressure, heart attacks, obesity, diabetes, cancer, gastrointestinal diseases, skin problems and accelerated aging.

According to a 1990 U.S. Department of Agriculture food consumption survey, only 3 percent of the population eats a balanced diet. Seventy-five percent of women over 35 fail to consume the Required Daily Allowance of calcium (Block 1991). The dietary lifestyle you establish is as important as anything you can do in determining your future health. Not only that, eating for wellness influences how you feel and appear right now. Physical fitness is an equal partner in this effort, and we'll get to that in the next section.

Before you plan your new diet, it makes sense to take a look at your current diet to see where you may need to change. According to Dr. Linda Ojeda (1995), you should avoid consuming any of the following more than four times each week:

- Fried or deep-fried foods
- Canned foods
- Frozen, prepackaged, or instant foods
- White bread, white rice
- Processed meats
- Fast foods
- Chips and dips
- Desserts, candy, ice cream
- Mayonnaise, sour cream, syrup

As for beverages, avoid more than two cups of coffee a day, more than four alcoholic drinks a week, or soft drinks, tea, or diet drinks more than five times weekly. You should also examine your general eating and exercise habits. Do you often skip one or more meals? Are you on a diet of fewer than 1000 calories per day? Are you sedentary (no regular exercise program)? Is there continuous stress in your life? Do you smoke? If you tend to go overboard in any of these areas, you owe yourself a major reevaluation of your habits, an overhaul of your diet, and probably some nutritional supplementation.

As the years pass, your metabolic rate slows, which means that if you continue to eat the same way as you did in your younger years, you will probably gain weight—the infamous "middle-age-spread." You need fewer calories to maintain your weight now. You still require the same amount of nutrients; but to avoid weight gain, they need to be contained in foods that add up to fewer calories.

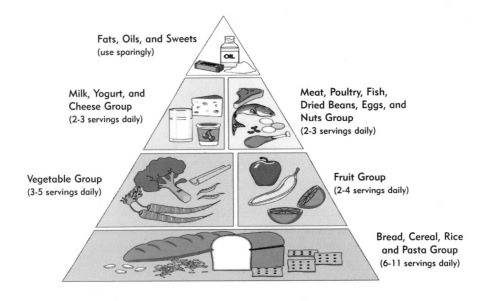

Figure 10.1.   The Food Guide Pyramid

Proportions of Food Types

In 1956, the U.S. Department of Agriculture (USDA) issued it's "basic four" food groups, with which you probably grew up. The recommendation was for more or less equally balanced portions of meat, dairy products, grains, fruits, and vegetables. Nutritional scientists began having another look at the basic four when it became apparent that as a nation, we were becoming too fat. In 1992, the USDA came out with "The Food Guide Pyramid," (figure 1-1) which represents current scientific thought about the proportions of the basic foods we should eat. The new focus of *Dietary Guidelines for Americans* is on foods rather than nutrients, and the food pyramid reflects this. It defines six food groups instead of four, with emphasis on complex carbohydrates, fruits, and vegetables as the staples. Meat and dairy products have been relegated to a far smaller role. A "balanced diet" now means a balance that reflects the proportions in the food pyramid. Don't try to eat the total recommended daily servings of all those foods—an astonishing twenty-six. You could start *resembling* a pyramid if you do that. The pyramid should be regarded as a guideline for deciding what proportions of each type of food you should incorporate in your diet.

Amount of Calories You Need

How many calories should you consume each day? There are a ton of charts that give you this crucial information, but they all vary quite a bit. Dr. Ojeda describes a formula for doing this, which is summarized in Table 10-5. The calculation is based on your knowing your ideal weight. (See Table 5-3 in Chapter 5.) Why don't you run those numbers right now and see where you stand?

Table 10.5. Daily Caloric Needs for Women	
General Activity Level	**Daily Calorie Intake**
Sedentary	Ideal weight x 11
Moderately active	Ideal weight x 14
Active	Ideal weight x 18
Adapted from: Ojeda 1995.	

Basic Rules for a Healthy Diet

It's important to educate yourself about food. Read all you can about healthful foods—including both how to select them and how to prepare them. The bookshelves and magazine racks are awash in excellent literature. See Appendix B for suggested reading. Also, read food labels. The front of the package may shout "No cholesterol," but the nutritional facts label may reveal that it is loaded with fat, or the recommended serving size may only fill a thimble.

Here are four principles for creating a healthy diet, along with some specific suggestions:

- **Select foods of high nutritional value that are not highly processed:** These include fresh fruits and vegetables that are harvested when they are ripe. Processing of foods, such as milling of grains, removes up to 90 percent of fiber.

- **Reduce fat in your diet:** Red meat is a great source for protein, but it's laden with fat. Try chicken breast instead. Think of meat as an additive rather than a main course—for example, use it in soups, stews, casseroles, and salads. Use low-fat or nonfat dairy products. (Try mixing whole milk and skim milk products until you get used to the new tastes.) Try low- or nonfat substitutes, such as evaporated skim milk instead of cream where possible, and eat low-fat snacks (fresh veggies in ice water, fresh fruit, low-fat baked crackers, whole grain crackers, pretzels, and plain popcorn).

- **Increase your fiber intake:** To increase your fiber intake, start with raw or lightly cooked fruits and vegetables. When your digestive system is able to tolerate them (not much gas), add more high-fiber cereals and breads to the mix. Then add beans, most of which are both high in fiber and a good protein source. Beans are a good foundation for a meatless dinner, but be sure to drink about eight cups of water each day when you are eating a higher-fiber diet to avoid constipation.

- **Increase antioxidants by eating more fruits and vegetables:** This includes green and yellow vegetables, citrus fruits, and wheat. As already discussed, vitamin C supplements may be needed from time to time, but the need for vitamin E supplements has not yet been proven. Recent studies reviewed by Harvard researchers show that dietary intake of E provides good cardiovascular disease protection without supplements (Rexrode and Manson 1996).

So have at it. Give some honest evaluation and thought as to whether or not your diet measures up to healthful standards. If it doesn't, take steps now to change it, and you will be protecting your future health.

Exercise

Among many other benefits, exercise helps hot flashes. It works its magic by increasing the endorphins in your brain. A decrease of this brain opioid is associated with inactivity and more hot flashes, so the more you exercise and raise your endorphins, the fewer hot flashes you will have. Women who exercise aerobically three hours each week have far fewer hot flashes than women who are sedentary (Reichman 1996). (Why not consider organizing a "Walking for Hot Flashes" march? You'd probably have so many participants, you'd need a parade permit.)

Exercise should share equal billing with nutrition in your program for achieving wellness. It's no longer necessary to carry water from the well or hunt for or grow your own food. Simple, ordinary walking has been replaced with automobiles, elevators, escalators, and "people movers" like those in airports. We can access the whole world with our fingers on telephones, computers, and television. Even our TVs have remote control. Strong muscles are no longer necessary for much of what you encounter in the average day.

The price of these work savers is what has been called "diseases of civilization." It is estimated that 25 percent of all deaths from chronic disease can be laid at the feet of physical inactivity (Reichman 1996). An osteoporotic hip fracture sentences a woman to a sedentary existence, and three to six months later she may be dead from pneumonia because of inactivity. Chronic heart disease may be so disabling that exercise is difficult or impossible, and that can bring on an earlier death from the disease. In other words, don't wait until exercise must be an element of your rehabilitation from a health problem. Work at avoiding the development of such problems by including regular and systematic exercise in your plan for wellness.

Do You Really Need to Exercise?

Let's look at the benefits of exercise so you can make an informed decision. It is common knowledge that exercise plays a major role in weight control. You probably know that it also contributes to strong muscles and sturdy bones. There's more to this story, though. Exercise benefits every part of your body—every organ, tissue, and cell. Further, your mind and your spirit become more agile and energized by the upbeat feeling that exercise brings with it. Exercise can help save your life; without it, your body deteriorates.

Weight Control

The short answer to the question of exercise and weight control is that exercise burns calories. It builds muscle, which is the most biologically active tissue in your body. The more muscle tissue you have, the more calories you burn; but you don't need to become a muscle-bound behemoth to benefit. You just probably need more than you have at the moment and exercise will accomplish this for you. Exercise speeds up your metabolic rate, which burns calories. Exercise also decreases your appetite and therefore the number of calories you take aboard to be burned in the first place (Ojeda 1995).

You can lose weight with a diet-only program; but if exercise is combined with it, you do not need to limit yourself to constant dieting. As a matter of fact, if you are exercising, it is not a good idea to severely restrict your diet; you need adequate calories for the energy your exercise consumes. Include nutritious foods; just avoid eating them with both hands.

Stress Control

Vigorous exercise brings oxygen to every cell in your body by stepping up circulation. This creates energy and improves your capacity for handling stress. Beta endorphins, your body's "feel good" drugs, are released during vigorous exercise, leaving you feeling relaxed and at ease after exercise. Also, exercise helps you to sleep more soundly, because your body is more tired. Researchers at Harvard have found that regular exercise reduces depression and is a practical means of handling the emotional stress of everyday living (Benson 1993).

CAUTION! Avoid exercising just before bedtime. The stimulation may actually prevent your getting to sleep.

Longevity

Regular exercise can prolong life. A large 1989 study by Steven Blair at the Institute for Aerobics Research in Dallas found that the death rates from all causes was reduced by 44 percent in women (and men) who exercise regularly. This list includes heart disease, cancer, and even accidents. The reduction in heart attack deaths was 50 percent.

Cardiovascular Disease

The dramatic reduction in heart attack deaths with exercise results from improving several parameters of cardiovascular disease (CVD) risk factors:

- It lowers your total cholesterol level, lowers LDL, lowers triglycerides (an independent risk factor for women), and raises HDL. All winners.
- It lowers blood pressure.
- It reduces the risk of blood clots by decreasing the stickiness of platelets and by increasing components of your blood that dissolve small but dangerous blood clots.
- It lowers the insulin level in your bloodstream by burning glucose, which diminishes the necessity for insulin. Too much insulin in your blood for too long a time promotes the formation of plaque on artery walls. This leads to hardening of the arteries and high blood pressure.
- It improves the strength of your heart muscle and its pumping efficiency; your heart pumps more blood per heart beat. If your exercise plan provides cardiac fitness, you can save up to 36,000 beats a day over an unfit heart (Reichman 1996). That works out to nearly 200 million saved heartbeats during your transition years alone!

Bone Strength

We made the case for preventing osteoporosis in Chapter 5. Weight-bearing exercise not only prevents bone loss, it has been shown to stimulate the formation of new bone in women who have low bone density. If you have risk factors for osteoporosis, get your bone density checked. Exercise is crucial for you if your bone density is below normal. If it turns out to be normal, however, just thank your lucky stars, and get (or keep) going with an exercise program to keep it that way. Exercise has a more beneficial effect for you as a perimenopausal woman in building bone than after you reach menopause. After menopause, exercise works mainly to keep the bone you already have. The point is this: Don't wait until menopause to start exercising; you want to arrive at menopause with a sturdy skeleton.

Estrogen Deficiency Symptoms

Exercise has been shown to be one of the best methods of relieving hot flashes. A study (Wallace 1982) showed that a moderate-intensity exercise program actually increased estrogen levels. Some researchers feel that low levels of endorphins in sedentary women are in part responsible for hot flashes. As you now know, exercise increases your level of this brain hormone.

Intestinal Function

Less constipation results from regular exercise because, along with the rest of your body, your intestinal tract is stimulated. Physical activity stimulates digestion and a more complete absorption of nutrients.

Cancer Risks

The Harvard School of Public Health found that former women athletes who continue to exercise have a 50 percent decreased incidence of breast cancer and a 60 percent decrease in reproductive organ cancers (in the cervix, ovaries, uterus, and vagina) (Frisch et al. 1989). That's impressive.

Brain Changes

Physically fit people are protected from several central nervous system changes that have traditionally been thought to be due to aging. Exercise increases blood flow to your brain and increases the release of brain chemicals called *neurotrophins*. These chemicals act like a fertilizer in your brain; they increase the number of connections between brain cells. This improves your ability to process and retain new information. In addition, your physical reaction time is improved (Brink 1995). These abilities are best protected with complex physical activities such as aerobic dancing, racquet sports, and swimming. Aerobic walking works also, but not quite as well. The ideal aerobic activity for brain improvement is one that also involves some decision making during the exercise, such as tennis and dancing. "Brain fade" and slowed physical reaction time may not be an inevitable consequence of time; fitness has a role in preventing these changes.

From all of the above, a fair minded person would have to conclude that exercise is an utter necessity to remaining well. A vibrant life can be yours if you exercise because you can look better, feel better, think better, and have a biological age that can be significantly less than your chronological age. From all of the above, any fair minded person would have to conclude that exercise is an utter necessity to remaining well.

Coming Up with a Fitness Plan

Now that we've listed all the reasons exercise is good for you, it's time to make some decisions. There are many forms of exercise, so you have choices. Which you choose should be based on the goals you set, your age, and current level of fitness. Goal-setting is probably one of the most important preliminaries to starting an exercise program. If you decide what you want out of it first, there is a greater likelihood that you will achieve it. These are the goals you might consider.

- Cardiovascular fitness
- Weight control
- Muscular strength
- Improved flexibility
- Coordination and balance
- Osteoporosis prevention
- Better brain functioning
- All of the above

Please don't regard these goals as just another wish list. Give sober and serious thought to them. What you decide for yourself should be something you really want to pursue. Cardiovascular fitness and weight control tend to be the most common choices. Don't regard your exercise plan as a temporary inconvenience, like a fad diet. This is going to become a new part of the rest of your life, so make it something you can realistically incorporate into your life and enjoy.

The Formula

Since the 1980s, the recommendation of most fitness experts has been to exercise three to four times weekly at a level that keeps your heart rate within a specified target zone continuously for 30 to 60 minutes at a time. The formula calls for aerobic conditioning, muscle strengthening, and flexibility exercises (Pollack and Froelicher 1990). This works quite well; but it takes a lot of planning to incorporate it into a busy life. In spite of the proliferation of health clubs, new athletic shoe and clothing designs, and exercise gadgetry, not enough Americans do anything about putting regular exercise into their lives.

A slightly different approach from the traditional one has been recommended by the Centers for Disease Control and Prevention and the American College of Sports Medicine (Reichman 1996). They found that acceptable physical fitness could be accomplished by moderate-intensity physical activity if it was carried out for half an hour a day. In addition, they found that the activity does not need to be continuous. If you accumulate thirty minutes of exercise in eight-to-ten-minute minute segments every day (or most days), you can become moderately fit. You just need to incorporate activities that burns 200 calories per day for a total of thirty minutes. How can you figure out how many calories you're burning? Some examples may help. Brisk walking on level ground, cycling under ten miles an hour, using a power lawn mower, general housecleaning, and playing golf all burn four to seven calories each minute. More strenuous activities, such as walking uphill, moving furniture, cycling over ten miles an hour, and using a hand mower (but not playing golf) burn over seven calories a minute. In other words, you may not need to bear the expense of a health club or buy a lot of special equipment to arrive at moderate physical fitness. Try cycling to work, walking briskly to lunch, and using the stairs instead of the elevator. Three ten-minute events performed at about the same pace as brisk walking can get it done for you. It's clear then that you can achieve fitness by many means, great and small. Without too much disruption of your average daily schedule, you can easily weave these things into your life. Just remember that moderate physical fitness will significantly decrease your chances of future illness and premature death! If you want to be more than moderately fit, then go for it. More effort is required, of course, but the payoff in better health and wellness is worth it. (Ainsworth 1989, Pollack and Wilmore 1990)

Exercises for Perimenopausal Women

The three basic forms of exercise are aerobic conditioning, muscle strengthening, and stretching exercises. Each category includes a wide variety of activities from which to choose, so you will not be required to get wired into a set routine.

Aerobic Conditioning

Aerobic exercise means systematic physical activity designed to increase oxygen consumption. The main objective is to increase the amount of oxygen your body can process in a given amount of time. This is called *aerobic capacity*. By improving your ability to utilize oxygen in aerobic exercise, you improve the functioning of your respiratory and cardiovascular systems, as well as muscle tone. This type of activity involves your body's large muscles, which speeds up your metabolic rate, increases your heart rate, and delivers more blood and oxygen to every cell in your body. Calories are burned in the process, too. Aerobic capacity reflects not only the condition of your muscles, but also the condition of your vital organs, so in that regard it is the best measure of your body's physical fitness.

Aerobic activity can be anything from running to dancing to climbing stairs or raking leaves. Your choice of activity should be based on your current level of fitness, how it will fit into your lifestyle, and the fitness goals you have set for yourself.

CAUTION! High-impact aerobic exercise is widely known to result in damage to tendons, muscles, and joint surfaces. This means any activity in which you are off both feet at the same time (jogging, jumping, aerobic dancing). Low-impact exercise does not provide as much cardiovascular conditioning, but it is still sufficient in this regard and is less likely to result in injury. (Garrick et al. 1988)

Your built-in speedometer for aerobic conditioning is your heart rate. The recommended *training rate* for any aerobic exercise is 60 to 80 percent of the maximum recommended heart rate for your age. (The simple formula for determining your personal training rate is to subtract your age from 220 and multiply by 0.6 to 0.8.) Do whatever level of exercise it takes to keep your heart rate in this range while you are exercising. As your fitness progresses, you will find that you can tolerate more exercise. As a matter of fact, once your physical reserves have increased, you will notice that it takes more aerobic activity to keep your heart rate in the 60 to 80 percent target range. This is a convenient way to track your progress, and it provides a potent motivation to keep you interested and involved.

To check your heart rate during aerobic exercise, slow down enough to feel your carotid artery pulse. (You can feel your carotid pulse by pressing your finger tips into the soft neck tissue just below the angle of your jaw bone.) Count this pulse for six seconds, and add a zero to whatever number you get to determine your beats per minute.

If you are a beginner, start in the lower part of your target range and work up gradually to the 80 percent level, but do not exceed the upper limit. Excessive exercise levels that put you beyond your target training heart rate only subject you to needless injuries, and result in sore muscles. For your exercise to be aerobic, it must be continuous for the duration of your specific program. This can be a mere ten minutes if you are you are making three short aerobic efforts each day, or thirty to sixty minutes three to five times weekly.

Muscle Strengthening

The value of stronger muscles to you as a perimenopausal woman is that they will protect you from joint and tendon injuries, which become increasingly common with disuse of your muscles. Strengthening your muscles and increasing their size dramatically increases your ability to burn calories and control your weight. A by-product of the effort this takes is the improvement in bone density that results from weight-bearing exercise. Stronger muscles translate to more competence in the way you use your body. You will be more agile, more graceful, and have better posture and a confident gait. This leads to fewer of the clutzy, clumsy accidents that we all hate.

For a muscle to be strengthened, it must be contracted against resistance. Most aerobic exercise involves some form of weight-bearing muscular activity.

The majority of aerobic exercises (walking, jogging, dancing, step-climbing, and so on) stress using lower body muscles; it might be a good idea to use hand-held weights during these activities to acquire upper-body muscle strengthening. You can target more specific muscle groups with free weight training and weight training machines like the Nautilus. Isometric exercise (active contraction of muscles against steady resistance), elastic resistance, and body weight resistance (push-ups, pull-ups) are also effective for muscle strengthening. Swimming is great for upper body training, and it is fantastic aerobic work.

TIP! Don't worry that muscle-strengthening exercises will turn you into a middle linebacker. You don't have enough male testosterone to get that kind of muscle bulk. As a woman, all you need is light weights and a higher repetition rate with each weight exercise.

Stretching Exercises

Stretching exercises promote flexibility. As the years pass, inactivity results in loss of elasticity in muscles, tendons and joints. We stiffen up. A program of stretching exercises, though, can keep you flexible. Stretching also will improve your posture and help relieve back pain.

There is risk of injury in stretching exercises, so be sure to get expert advice before venturing into a program on your own. Learn how to stretch properly—not herky-jerky and bouncy, but slow and sustained. A stretch should be sustained for about 20 seconds to be effective. Your muscles must be "warmed up" before your stretch them if you are to avoid injury. This means that you must not start a workout with stretching. If you are an exercise walker, for example, do some slow walking first to warm up your muscles, and then stretch them before you set out on the vigorous part of your exercise program. Stretching your muscles again at the conclusion of your routine, while they are still warm, will contribute to your being supple and prevent post-exercise soreness. Yoga is an excellent method for improving and maintaining flexibility. Hatha (pronounced ha-ta) yoga is the more vigorous of the various branches of yoga. In recent years, hatha yoga has enjoyed an incarnation in our country as more people interested in fitness recognize that it is not merely a cultural fad. From glitzy gyms and spas to local YW-CAs, yoga is starting to shape new trends in exercise and diet. (Davis 1996)

Components of Your Ideal Workout

There are four components to the ideal workout:
- **Warm up and stretching:** This is an important part of the exercise routine for every age; but it is especially important for you at mid-life. If you have been sedentary, your chances of injury are much increased if you don't spend a few minutes on mild activity to increase the

blood flow to your muscles. This can be as simple as a few minutes on the rowing machine or some slow walking. Once your heart rate has increased somewhat or you have broken into a slight sweat, do your stretching exercises to get your muscles ready for increased range of motion and stepped-up activity.

- **Aerobic workout:** As we said, your choice of aerobic exercise can be any type of activity that gets your heart rate into the desirable range for your age and level of physical fitness. You can vary it depending on your personal schedule of work and family obligations. Working out with a friend or your partner or in a class can add variety and interest.

- **Muscle strengthening:** These are good exercises to add after your aerobic workout, when your muscles are warm and supple. Ideally, they should include all major muscle groups. An alternative is to do these exercises on one or two days when you are not doing aerobic work. This can add some variety to your program and prevent the boredom of doing the same thing every time you exercise.

- **Cool down and stretching:** This is the opposite number of the warm-up; but it is of equal importance. A gradual slowdown of your heart rate allows the increased blood flow to your muscles and skin to subside. The cool-down can be as simple as slowly walking around until your heart rate is back to normal. This is an ideal time to do some more stretching exercises to prevent muscle stiffness.

CAUTION! After exercising, avoid a cold shower until your heart rate has slowed. Cold water on blood-engorged skin can force massive amounts of blood back into your central circulation by constricting the blood vessels in your skin. This puts a huge strain on your heart. Also, wait to cool down before using a saunas or hot tub; additional heat on blood-engorged skin can draw even more blood out of your central circulation into your skin, which may result in fainting.

Summary

Wellness involves conducting your life in a fashion that decreases your chances of disease and enhances your verve for living. This chapter has shown you the principles of good nutrition, how to plan a healthful diet, and the value of exercise. The next chapter puts all these elements together in considering of another aspect of wellness that has a profound influence on your second half of life: weight control.

◯ ◯ ◯

11

Wellness from Lifestyle Changes: Weight Control, and Detoxifying Your Body and Mind

"If I knew I was going to live this long, I would have taken better care of myself." This famous lament of the elderly does not need to be yours. What you do to your body now, while you are young, will have a major impact on your future health. We know that destructive behaviors are responsible for many illnesses, and we're talking major diseases like high blood pressure, heart disease, diabetes, stroke, emphysema, osteoporosis, and cancer. Habits that seem innocent and apparently harmless in the beginning can cause monstrous problems a few years down the road. It's better to have never started overeating, smoking, or using alcohol or recreational drugs, but what if you did? You still have time to protect your health. Changing a long-ingrained behavior is not easy, but the physical and psychological benefits are powerful. This chapter will give you the reasons to try, and some of the ways to get it done.

Weight Control

Are you sure you have a weight problem? If you think so, it is probably based on what your bathroom scale tells you, or on a standard weight chart that uses your height and frame size to determine your "ideal" weight. Table 5-3 in Chapter 5 is such a chart. The problem with this method is that it only tells you your weight. It fails to distinguish between overweight and overfat. There's a difference. Too much body fat is the real culprit when it comes to increased health risks for high blood pressure, heart disease, diabetes, and certain cancers, such as colorectal cancer. It is possible to weigh more than the standard tables prescribe, yet not be overfat. For example, a trim-looking aerobics class instructor may appear to weigh twenty pounds less than her actual weight simply because she has good musculature and less body fat than usual. On the other hand, a woman of normal weight may be considerably overfat if she has a small muscle mass, and she has the least healthy body composition.

Determining your percentage of body fat is the most accurate way to assess your body composition of fat versus lean body weight (in other words, your total weight minus body fat). This can be done in a variety of ways. One way is to use skin calipers on your upper arm. Another is to take girth measurements of waist and hips, and another is to have your body weighed underwater. Conversion tables are then used to interpret the measurements. Ultrasound, dual-energy X-ray absorptiometry (DEXA), and CT scans are also being used to make these determinations. A newer method, using bioelectric impedance shows promise (Roubenoff 1995). These are all rather complicated methods that require third-party help in dealing with the numbers.

Body-Mass Index

There's a simpler way to do an estimate of your proportion of body fat. You calculate your body-mass index (BMI) using the following formula:

(Weight in lbs. x 702.95) ÷ (height x height).

If you weigh 130 pounds and are 5 feet 5 inches tall (65 inches), your calculation would be

(130 x 702.95) ÷ (65 x 65) = 21.6

A BMI less than 19.8 is underweight, 19.8 to 26.0 is normal weight, 26.0-29.0 is overweight, over 29.0 is obese, and over 32.3 is severe obesity. These BMI determinations are all about 20 percent higher than the 1990 USDA suggested weights for adults (Table 5-3). BMI is being used increasingly for reference levels of body weight for women and men rather than guidelines like Table 5-3. The drawback is that it is based on averages and fails to take into account differing frame sizes. Still, it is a reasonable guide to determining whether you may be carrying too much fat (Notelovitz and Tonnessen 1993). If you don't want to do the calculations, refer to Table 11-1, which does it for you.

Table 11.1.
Body Mass Index

Weight in Pounds	Height in inches																
	58	59	60	61	62	63	64	65	66	67	68	69	70	71	72	73	74
110	23.0	22.2	21.5	20.8	20.1	19.5	18.9	18.3	17.8	17.2	16.7	16.2	15.8	15.3	14.9	14.5	14.1
115	24.0	23.2	22.5	21.7	21.0	20.4	19.7	19.1	18.6	18.0	17.5	17.0	16.5	16.0	15.6	15.2	14.8
120	25.1	24.2	23.4	22.7	21.9	21.3	20.6	20.0	19.4	18.8	18.2	17.7	17.2	16.7	16.3	15.8	15.4
125	26.1	25.2	23.4	23.6	22.9	22.1	21.5	20.8	20.2	19.6	19.0	18.5	17.9	17.4	17.0	16.5	16.0
130	27.2	26.3	25.4	24.6	23.8	23.0	22.3	21.6	21.0	20.4	19.8	19.2	18.7	18.1	17.6	17.2	16.7
135	28.2	27.3	26.4	25.5	24.7	23.9	23.2	22.5	21.8	21.1	20.5	19.9	19.4	18.8	18.3	17.8	17.3
140	29.3	28.3	27.3	26.5	25.6	24.8	24.0	23.3	22.6	21.9	21.3	20.7	20.1	19.5	19.0	18.5	18.0
145	30.3	29.3	28.3	27.4	26.5	25.7	24.9	24.1	23.4	22.7	22.0	21.4	20.8	20.2	19.7	19.1	18.6
150	31.4	30.3	29.3	28.3	27.4	26.6	25.7	25.0	24.2	23.5	22.8	22.2	21.5	20.9	20.3	19.8	19.3
155	32.4	31.3	30.3	29.3	28.4	27.5	26.6	25.8	25.0	24.3	23.6	22.9	22.2	21.6	21.1	20.4	19.9
160	33.4	32.3	31.2	30.2	29.3	28.3	27.5	26.6	25.8	25.1	24.3	23.6	23.0	22.3	21.7	21.1	20.5
165	34.5	33.3	32.2	31.2	30.2	29.2	28.3	27.5	26.6	25.8	25.1	24.4	23.7	23.0	22.4	21.8	21.2
170	35.5	34.3	33.2	32.1	31.1	30.1	29.2	28.3	27.4	26.6	25.8	25.1	24.4	23.7	23.1	22.4	21.8
175	36.6	35.3	34.2	33.1	32.0	31.0	30.0	29.1	28.2	27.4	26.6	25.8	25.1	24.4	23.7	23.1	22.5
180	37.6	36.4	25.2	34.0	32.9	31.9	30.9	30.0	29.1	28.2	27.4	26.6	25.8	25.1	24.4	23.7	23.1
185	38.7	37.4	36.1	35.0	33.8	32.8	31.8	30.8	29.9	29.0	28.1	27.3	26.5	25.8	25.1	24.4	23.8
190	39.7	38.4	37.1	35.9	34.8	33.7	32.6	31.6	30.7	29.8	28.9	28.1	27.3	26.5	25.8	25.1	24.4
195	40.8	39.4	38.1	36.8	35.7	34.5	33.5	32.4	31.5	30.5	29.6	28.8	28.0	27.2	26.4	25.7	25.0
200	41.8	40.4	39.1	37.8	36.6	35.4	34.3	33.3	32.3	31.3	30.4	29.5	28.7	27.9	27.1	26.4	25.7
205	42.8	41.4	40.0	38.7	37.5	36.3	35.2	34.1	33.1	32.1	31.2	30.3	29.4	28.6	27.8	27.0	26.3
210	43.9	42.4	41.0	39.7	38.4	37.2	36.0	34.9	33.9	32.9	31.9	31.0	30.1	29.3	28.5	27.7	27.0
215	44.9	43.4	42.0	40.6	39.3	38.1	36.9	35.8	34.7	33.7	32.7	31.8	30.8	30.0	29.2	28.4	27.6
220	46.0	44.4	43.0	41.6	40.2	39.0	37.8	36.6	35.5	34.5	33.5	32.5	31.6	30.7	29.8	29.0	28.2
225	47.0	45.4	43.9	42.5	41.2	39.9	38.6	37.4	36.3	35.2	34.2	33.2	32.3	31.4	30.5	29.7	28.9
230	48.1	46.5	44.9	43.5	42.1	40.7	39.5	38.3	37.1	36.0	35.0	34.0	33.0	32.1	31.2	30.3	29.5
235	49.1	47.5	45.9	44.4	43.0	41.6	40.3	39.1	37.9	36.8	35.7	34.7	33.7	32.8	31.9	31.0	30.2
240	50.2	48.5	46.9	45.3	43.9	42.5	41.2	39.9	38.7	37.6	36.5	35.4	34.4	33.5	32.6	31.7	30.8
245	51.2	49.5	47.8	46.3	44.8	43.4	42.1	40.8	39.5	38.4	37.3	36.2	35.2	34.2	33.2	32.3	31.5
250	52.3	50.5	48.8	47.2	45.7	44.3	42.9	41.6	40.4	39.2	38.0	36.9	35.9	34.9	33.9	33.0	32.1

Interpretation:

Underweight: less than 19.8

Normal Weight: 19.8–26.0

Overweight: 26.0–29.0

Obese: greater than 29.0

Source: National Academy of Science 1992

Fat Distribution

The way your body fat is distributed is another consideration that influences your health. Total weight is important, but the distribution of fat is an added factor. The greatest distribution risk is if your fat is concentrated around your waist as opposed to around your hips (the apple shape versus the pear). A simple method of determining this is to measure your waist and hips with a nonstretch tape. Here's how to do it:

1. Measure the circumference of your abdomen at a point on your side just above where you feel your pelvic bones flair out (the iliac crest). This is just below the point where your waist measurement is the smallest.
2. Measure your hips around the largest part of your buttocks at the level of the iliac crest.
3. Divide your waist measurement by your hip measurement.

If the value is 1 or more, your fat is distributed too much in your abdomen. In addition to the known risk of weighing too much, your distribution of body fat adds to it. As discussed in Chapter 10, the "apple" shape is associated with greater risk for cardiovascular disease.

If a determination of your body-fat composition is available to you through your doctor or your health club, compare it to the norms for your age in Table 11-2. Your percentage of body fat slowly rises as you grow older. This is important. If you are now forty-five, you don't need to return your body composition to what it was twenty years ago!

Table 11.2. Female Body Composition (Percent Body Fat) By Age					
	Age				
	26–35	36–45	46–55	56–65	Over 65
Good	18–20	20–23	23–25	24–26	22–26
Average	21–23	24–26	26–28	27–29	27–29
Poor	31–33	33–36	35–38	36–38	35–37

Adapted from: Goldring et al. 1989.

Most women gain weight during the transition years, and weight gain is greater after menopause. We are talking here about over-gaining; not the gradual increase referred to in Table 11-2. Using body mass index standards, Kuczmarski and co-workers published a study in 1994 showing that 38 percent of women between the ages of forty to forty-nine are overweight, and the numbers rose to 52 percent between 50 and 59. Although men tend to reach their peak weight gains between thirty-five and sixty-four; women continue their gain even beyond their middle years. See Table 11-3 for the data collected by the National Health and Nutrition Examinations Survey. This table shows that during the five decades between ages thirty and eighty, an average of 40 percent of American women are overweight. Are you thinking that you are doomed to this weight gain? That it is inevitable? Maybe not, if you know what causes it.

Table 11.3. Percentage of Overweight Women by Age	
Age	**Percent of Women Overweight**
30–39	34.3
40–49	37.6
50–59	52.0
60–69	42.5
70–79	37.2
80 +	26.2
Source: National Health and Nutrition Examination Surveys 1992.	

What Causes Overweight?

Fat storage is the fundamental cause of becoming overweight, but things are more complex than that. Several factors are involved in fat accumulation (Notelovitz and Tonnessen 1993):

- **Aging:** Aging results in a gradual slowing of your metabolism. It seems related to the fact that after age thirty, women start losing about 1 percent of their muscle mass each year as a result of lessened physical activity. By age thirty-five, this amounts to about one pound a year. With each lost pound of muscle, you burn fifty fewer calories per day. If your caloric intake remains unchanged as time passes, you end up taking aboard more calories than you burn, and the excess becomes stored as fat. By the time you have lost as much as five pounds of muscle mass, your body is storing 250 calories a day. If your daily dietary intake remains the same, you can gain up to twenty pounds in a year.

- **Appetite:** The neurotransmitter norepinephrine stimulates hunger; serotonin suppresses it. Overweight results when these regulators of appetite become short circuited and the wrong signals are sent. This is not specifically a perimenopausal event; it can happen at any age. The only evidence that it has happened in you is a large appetite that you can't attribute to other causes, such as hyperthyroidism. Why does it happen? We don't know. This is one of the confounding perplexities of obesity.

- **Genes:** Genetics may play a role. We seem to have a genetic mechanism that controls how much body fat we accumulate. It operates much like a thermostat, in that there is a "fat setting" in the brain that programs and regulates the amount of body fat you maintain. An "obesity" gene has been located in humans (Baron 1997). Not surprisingly, it has been named "the OB gene." The gene controls production of a protein called leptin, which sends messages to your brain on the status of your overall body fat content. If the gene is defective or missing, leptin is not produced in adequate amounts. If your brain is insensitive to leptin, the fat setting may be too high, and obesity results. Research is continuing to develop products that will increase the brain's sensitivity to leptin.

- **Gender:** The fact that you're a woman is a factor. Women of normal weight have an average of 25 percent body fat, as compared to 15 percent in men. Women who have only 6 to 12 percent body fat (as a result of excessive athleticism or starvation) are at risk for suppression of ovarian function and resulting osteoporosis (Somer 1993). Because a woman's body accepts fat more readily than men, you can gain weight more easily, and it may be more difficult to lose it. Not fair perhaps, but that's a gender-fact.

- **Metabolism:** Your metabolism plays a definite role. One factor is the muscle tissue story we discussed in the last chapter. The more muscle you have, the greater your metabolic rate and the more calories you burn. Another metabolic factor is an enzyme in fat cells called lipoprotein lipase. This enzyme is active in removing triglycerides from your bloodstream and tucking them into fat cells for energy storage. This enzyme increases after dieting—your body is trying to get the weight back. (This supports the genetic theory that we are all preprogrammed to have a certain amount of body fat.)

- **Hormones:** Hormones can influence your weight, but contrary to popular thought, glandular obesity is rare. Thyroid, insulin, and female sex hormones can all play a role.

The Part Hormones Play in Weight Changes

Let's take a closer look at the role of hormones in influencing weight. Thyroid hormone levels are influenced by what you eat. Levels of T4, the metabolically active thyroid hormone, are lower during fasting. This is one reason your metabolic rate is lower during a weight loss diet. Your body is trying to conserve its energy resources and resist losing tissue, whether it be fat or muscle. Some diet programs use thyroid supplements to counteract this normal effect, but this is at the risk of increasing calcium excretion and the risk of developing osteoporosis. Overeating increases T4, which raises your metabolic rate in an effort to burn some of the excess calories. However, this weak regulatory effort by your thyroid gland does not work well enough.

Insulin may play a role in keeping obesity in check. It is known to stimulate heat production and increase the metabolism of fat—but at the expense of causing more insulin to circulate in your bloodstream. This puts you at risk for plaque formation on artery walls and hardening of the arteries. Overeating challenges this protective mechanism.

Estrogen and progesterone production during the childbearing years also influence your weight. Estrogen causes fat deposits to accumulate in your breasts, hips, and thighs, which contributes to your body's feminine contours. Progesterone stimulates your appetite (which you can probably confirm—you may tend to eat more in the second half of your cycle, when progesterone levels are highest). However, this doesn't mean that HRT with estrogen and progesterone causes weight gain, because the doses used are very low. The gain is from the other factors we have been discussing. Concern over weight gain does not need to be part of the equation when you are considering whether to use HRT.

It may sound as though what you weigh is beyond your control, so why worry. It's a bit late, of course, to choose your gender or rechoose your parents, who gave you their genes, but there is still plenty you can do. Obesity is hereditary 50 percent of the time (Baron 1997), but the other 50 percent is under your control—over your diet and over how much you exercise. These things, along with your genetic makeup and psychological and sociological factors, are the ultimate determiners of your weight.

Weight-Loss Diets

We've already talked about your "fat thermostat," or internal fat-setting mechanism. The question is, can your thermostat be reset if it is currently too high and you are overweight? It isn't easy, but it's doable. It involves fundamental changes in how you eat, how you exercise, and in how you think. Let's take them one at a time, starting with diet.

Horm and Anderson reported in 1993 that at any one time, approximately 40 percent of American women are on a diet, even if their weight is normal. The problem is, diets don't work in the long run. The implication of the word diet is that it has a beginning and an end. You set out to lose some predetermined amount of weight, lose it on a specific diet plan, and then you're done with the diet. A 1995 study report by the Institute of Medicine on this type of weight loss in both women and men showed that a high percentage will regain most of the lost weight within a year, and all of it within three to five years! Women often end up weighing more than they originally did. In other words, a temporary diet won't succeed in resetting your fat regulator. When you resume your normal eating habits, your lipoprotein lipase enzyme, discussed earlier in this chapter, is still programmed to take as much of the triglycerides as possible from the food you eat, refilling those fat cells you so recently emptied. This often leads to another go at dieting, and another cycle of loss and regain—the infamous yo-yo pattern of weight fluctuation.

Part of the reason for this pattern of weight gain is that losing weight does not eliminate fat cells. Your body contains about 30 billion fat cells, which hold about 135,000 calories, and serve a vital energy storage function (Notelovitz and Tonnessen 1993). Your fat cells can sustain your body's energy needs for about six to seven weeks, even without any food. When a fat cell is full, it can store up to 95 percent of its volume in pure triglyceride. When all 30 billion of them are full, your body makes more fat cells to accommodate whatever additional storage requirements your diet imposes, and those cells are permanent as well; they're there for life.

The take-home message for you as a transitional woman is to avoid excess weight to begin with. (Your children will benefit from your guidance in this regard; you can help them by carefully managing their food intake and training them in habits of healthful nutrition.)

Another reason for regaining weight after a weight-loss diet is that calorie deprivation reduces your muscle mass. Weight loss from a diet is 75 percent fat (which is good), but 25 percent lean muscle mass (which is bad) (Kayman et al. 1990). Since muscle mass helps burn calories, losing some of it lowers your metabolic rate, and your post-diet return to normal eating habits makes it less likely you will burn the increased calories and much more likely that you will store them as fat. An important point is that yo-yo dieting is dangerous to your health. The thirty-plus–year Framingham Heart Study of 3000 women and men in this Massachusetts town found that those who had frequent and dramatic fluctuations in weight had a twofold increased risk for heart disease and premature death (Brody 1991). This was even true for those who were not seriously overweight. By contrast, the Nurses' Health Study, which has been going since 1976, concluded that a ten- to twenty-pound weight gain or loss over a ten-year period did not correlate with an increase in mortality (Willet 1994). This study found that it took a fluctuation of more than forty pounds to show a slight increase in premature death from heart disease. Their "Shakespearean" conclusion was that it is better to lose weight and try to keep if off, even if you fail, then never to have tried at all.

For all these reasons, chronic or repeated dieting cannot be relied upon to control your weight. This does not mean you should not reduce your caloric intake to lose excess pounds. Calorie cutting is a powerful tool in weight loss. The point, though, is that success hinges on your adopting a weight control program that incorporates foods you will keep in your diet for the rest of your life. This is not a "diet" in the usual sense of the word, because it is not temporary. It is a new way of life. Such an eating program will not shed weight as quickly as crash dieting; but it is a reliable method to lose weight permanently—especially if it is combined with exercise. A continuing and consistent change in your eating habits is your best shot at resetting your body's internal fat-regulating mechanism.

A Weight-Loss Plan

The key to a weight-losing plan is to reduce the amount of fat you consume. The opposite is also true: Increased fat intake is the primary cause of increasing weight. Carbohydrates and protein have calories too, but fat is the main culprit, because it has a higher concentration of calories. Fat has nine calories per gram, while protein and carbohydrate each have only four. When you cut back on fat consumption, you then reduce your calorie intake substantially more than an equivalent reduction in either protein or carbohydrates. In addition, your body metabolizes fat differently than it does carbohydrates or protein. Dietary fat is very similar to body fat, so converting dietary fat to body fat requires only 3 percent of the dietary fat's calories. In contrast, converting dietary carbohydrates or protein to body fat uses up 25 percent of their calories. The net result is that you can eat more carbohydrate and protein and not pay the price of stored fat, as long as you don't go overboard (Insull et al. 1990). Just remember that if you eat more calories than your body needs, the excess will be stored as fat, no matter what type of food it is.

On average, American women consume 80 to 100 grams of fat daily (Ojeda 1995); that's 720 to 900 calories. If you are not seriously overweight, you will lose about one or two pounds a week on a 1,000 to 1,200-calorie regimen. That 720 to 900 calories from fat must obviously be cut back significantly if you are going to squeeze any protein and carbohydrate into those 1,000 to 1,200 daily calories. The American Diabetes Association (ADA) recommended in 1994 that 20 percent of the calories in a weight-losing diet should come from fat, 20 percent from protein, and 60 percent from complex carbohydrates, which contain 25 grams of fiber. For women with diabetes, the ADA has guidelines that individualize the recommendation for each person. It is based on such things as BMI, blood sugar levels, lipid levels, physical activity, and personal preferences of weight level.

CAUTION! Do not attempt a diet with fewer than 1,000 calories on your own; it can be very dangerous. Deaths have been reported as a result of severe caloric restriction (Baron 1997). Such diets have been used for extreme obesity; but they must be under the strict supervision of a physician who understands the potential hazards and can recognize serious problems if they arise.

For a 1,200 calorie diet, 20 percent of fat works out to 26 grams of fat per day. The good news is that when you start eating low-fat foods, you can eat more—they have fewer total calories. But remember this: To lose weight, you must eat fewer calories. Changing your calories from fat to carbohydrates may help, but it doesn't fool your body if your total calories are not reduced.

Stick with the following general principles for reliable and safe dietary weight control (Notelovitz and Tonnessen 1993):

- **Go slow:** Don't cut calories to fewer than 1,000 to 1,200 per day. Losing one pound a week, or two pounds, is about the right pace.
- **Emphasize foods high in nutrients and low in fat and calories:** The best choices are raw vegetables and fruits, plus complex carbohydrates, such as whole-grain breads and cereals, pasta, legumes, and rice. (Refer to Chapter 10 for more information on nutrition.)
- **Avoid quick-fix diet programs:** If they promise weight losses of more than the recommended one to two pounds a week, they are usually counting on your losing water, not fat. It won't last.
- **Eat most of your calories early in the day:** This increases the likelihood that they will be used for energy during the day. Meals just before bedtime result in more fat storage.
- **Take a multivitamin supplement:** It is unlikely you can get enough nutrients in a weight-losing diet to supply the vitamins you need.
- **Regard your new diet and the accompanying exercise program as a permanent part of your life.** We can't emphasize this enough.

There are many books on the market to help you make up your individual diet. Weight Watchers International produces a new cookbook almost annually with recipes that are low in calories, low in fat, high in fiber, and well balanced. Sonja and William Connor's The New American Diet System details their cholesterol-saturated fat index (CSI) to selecting healthful foods. Jane Brody's Good Food Gourmet provides a wide array of recipes. Cooking Light magazine is a another good source of low-fat menus.

Very Low-Calorie Liquid Diets and Diet Pills— Are They Any Good?

The very low-calorie liquid diet concept for seriously obese people (100 percent overweight, for example) has been around for twenty years. It got a very bad name in the seventies because its use caused some significant medical problems, and even some deaths. For these reasons, these regimens have been largely abandoned. The newer products in very low-calorie diets don't carry the same risks as those of twenty years ago and do get the weight off you very fast (40 to 50 pounds in four to five months), so some doctors do recommend them. Remember, though, that only 20 percent of dieters keep the weight off, no matter what type of diet they use. The rest gain it all back, and more, in the first year and a half after completing the diet. Success has to do with behavior modification. Those who learn to permanently modify their eating habits keep it off, and those who don't are back where they started, and then some (Baron 1997).

What about Diet Pills?

A number of diet pills on the market successfully suppress appetite, but none of them keep the weight off unless you take them permanently. They do not change your internal fat-regulating mechanism, even with long-term use. What they can do is give you a reasonable jump-start on losing weight. If you are significantly overweight (more than 30 percent over your ideal weight), diet pills can produce a weight loss in a few weeks that may motivate you to continue on a long-term plan of dietary control. And if you combine such a regimen with exercise, your chances of permanent change are even more enhanced.

Two diet pill regimens that were in common use until withdrawn from the market in 1997 were "fen-phen," the combination of fenfluramine (Pondimin) and phentermine (Fastin, Adipez, Banobese, Zantryl), and dexfenfluramine (Redux). Over 30 million people had used one or the other of these regimens until it was discovered they could cause heart valve abnormalities (leaky valves) and pulmonary hypertension, a rare but potentially fatal abnormality in half of those who developed it (Langreth 1997; Abenheim et al. 1996). These drugs enhanced serotonin production in the brain which dampens appetite.

Other anti-obesity drugs are in the research pipeline. A drug being used in Europe, Xenical, inhibits fat absorption from the intestines. Unfortunately Xenical results in severe fatty diarrhea with multiple bowel movements every day. Another serotonin-targeting drug that mimics the effect of fenfluramine and dexfenfluramine, *sibutramine,* is being considered but is not on the market.

Five genes have been discovered that influence fat storage. They produce a hormone called *leptin* that attaches to specific brain receptor sites and regulates how much fat your body stores. Obesity results if the receptor sites are insensitive to leptin or if not enough leptin is produced. Leptin (by injection only, unfortunately) is being used in research projects.

Another approach to obesity control involves *neuropeptide Y* (nicknamed NPY), a brain chemical that has been shown to be a potent stimulus to feed in laboratory animals. Researchers are trying to develop a drug that will prevent NPY from attaching to brain receptor sites and dampen the desire to eat.

In the absence of fenfluramine and dexfenfluramine, a serious promotion of what is called "herbal fen-phen" has begun. This is a mixture of St. John's Wort, a plant derivative, and ephedra, an ancient chinese herb. St. John's Wort elevates serotonin levels resembling the effect of fenfluramine and ephedra is a stimulant which mimics phentermine. As yet there are no studies supporting the safety or effectiveness of these plant derivatives. Ephedra has been reported to cause states of severe agitation (Langreth 1997).

The bottom line for using drugs to combat obesity is that they are unlikely to result in more than a 5-10 percent reduction in body weight. Starting a weight reduction program with such drugs may be initially helpful, but long-term success still depends on permanent changes in your dietary lifestyle.

Exercise—A Must for Weight Control

If you cut back on calories and fat, you will reliably lose weight. Eventually, however, your body will start resisting this self-imposed tissue destruction and start slowing the metabolic rate. You burn fewer calories, and weight loss slows. A major cause of this metabolic change is the loss of muscle that results from food deprivation. If you lose twenty pounds from dieting alone, a quarter of it will have been muscle mass. You already know that a pound of muscle will burn about fifty calories each day, so losing five pounds of muscle cuts your calorie furnace by two hundred fifty calories every day. This looks good on the bathroom scale, but your body composition has been compromised. The answer to this problem is to combine exercise with your new diet. No weight loss program is complete without it.

There are several reasons why exercise plays such a vital role in weight control:

- Exercise burns calories and fat.

- It keeps your muscles from deteriorating (very important!).

- A workout sharply raises your metabolic rate, and the increased rate may persist for several hours afterward. The studies on this residual effect are conflicting. Nevertheless, it is known that dieters who also exercise do not experience the slowdown in their metabolic rate that diet-only weight losers do (Notelovitz and Tonnessen 1993).

- Exercise suppresses appetite. Total food consumption is less in people who exercise regularly. If exercise is combined with your new way of eating, you can make fewer cuts in your food intake. As a matter of fact, it is important to allow yourself a few more calories to compensate for the energy expended by exercise. Not a bunch more—just more than you would allow yourself on a weight-loss diet. This, in turn, may make it easier to stick with your new dietary program.

- Exercise helps to diminish the risks of being overweight, including high blood pressure, abnormal lipid profile (high cholesterol, high triglycerides), diabetes, heart disease, and certain cancers.

- When exercise is combined with a weight-losing diet, it becomes the most efficient way to lose weight. It has long been known that neither exercise nor diet alone is as effective as they are in combination (Johannessen 1986).

- Strenuous exercise releases endorphins in your brain, which generates a feeling of well-being and relieves depression. This helps create a feeling of equanimity that can help you accept your new weight control program and stay enthusiastic about sticking with it. When you have reached your target weight, continuing exercise has been shown to increase the likelihood that you will maintain it. Nonexercisers more consistently regain weight. The Harvard studies (mentioned in Chapter 10) of athletes showed that once you have become physically fit, you continue to benefit: You have a higher level of fat-burning enzymes, so keeping your weight under control becomes easier.

What Kind of Exercise?

The decision as to which type of exercise you choose is an important one. Muscle-strengthening exercise will keep you from losing vital muscle mass, so it is an important part of the mix (Butts 1994). On the other hand, while the use of free weights and the machines at the health club make for better muscles, they do little to burn fat. You need aerobic activity to accomplish that. (We described some aerobic activities in Chapter 10.) With weight control as the goal, you need a type of aerobic exercise that differs from what you need for cardiovascular fitness. It revolves around your need to burn fat. In the first half hour of aerobic exercise, the energy you expend is provided by glycogen, which is stored sugar in muscle tissue. It isn't until your glycogen stores are exhausted that your body turns to fat for energy (Notelovitz and Tonnessen 1993). This means that a longer workout, of about forty-five minutes, is necessary. For this reason, select a form of exercise that you can sustain for that length of time, such as cycling or walking. As discussed in Chapter 10, you will need to gradually build up to that level if you are unfit or a beginning exerciser. It should be low impact, to protect your tendons and joint surfaces; this is especially important if you are overweight. Ideal exercises might be brisk walking, whether around the neighborhood or on a treadmill, and cycling around town or on a stationary unit. Platform step-aerobics and aerobic dance are also excellent as long as they remain low impact. Swimming is good aerobic exercise and great for muscle strengthening, but it is hard to sustain it long enough to get to the fat-burning stage. Watch out for jogging, running, and some forms of aerobic dance; they are high impact and therefore risk injury to your knees, hips, and ankles.

Be sure to alternate aerobic exercise with weight training to maintain your muscle mass. Exercising three to four days a week may be sufficient for cardiovascular health, but weight loss needs a seven-days-a-week commitment (Kayman et al. 1990). Never go to bed without a plan for exercise the next day. If you planned to walk three miles but you wake up at seven instead of six and it's raining cats and dogs, have a backup plan. Never go to bed without planning what you will eat the next day, either. By having your diet and exercise plan firmly in mind, you are more likely to succeed with both endeavors.

A suitable exercise program can be designed for almost anyone. If you are a beginner, get some advice from your physician. You need to be as sure as you can that the exercise program you are undertaking will not be harmful to you. If you are over forty-five, many experts suggest a treadmill electrocardiogram (ECG) to determine whether your heart can sustain the increased workload. A treadmill ECG hooks you up to a machine that monitors your heart while you undergo an increasing workload of walking. It may also be helpful to have your exercise program set up by a professional fitness expert who can steer you around situations that may injure you. This is especially true for stretching exercises. (Many health clubs employ certified training experts.)

The guidelines for weight control exercise are essentially the same as for anybody else, with some added precautions if you are overweight (Notelovitz and Tonnessen 1993):

- **The warmup phase:** The warmup phase of exercise is especially important because being overweight tends to make you less flexible. Your muscles and tendons are more easily injured. For these reasons, do some slow walking, cycling, or rowing until your heart rate has increased or you have begun to sweat. Then do your stretching exercises. Don't do any exercise that hurts; wait until you have lost some weight and try again.

- **Underdo it at the beginning:** If your goal is to walk three miles in forty-five minutes, start with something like three blocks in ten minutes, and work up to it in later sessions. Your tolerance for exercise is considerably less if you are overweight, and you need to sneak up on it. Remember, this is a new lifestyle for you, and there is plenty of time to ease into your new role.

- **The cool down:** Cooling down after exercise is more important for you because there is a greater tendency for blood to pool in your legs if you stop suddenly. This can make you feel faint or actually faint. Gradually diminish your level of activity over five to ten minutes, and let your heart rate return to normal before you become inactive.

- **Temperature awareness:** If you are overweight, you will overheat more readily, especially in the early stages of becoming an exerciser. Avoid hot rooms and, if you exercise outside, the hottest hours of the day. Be sure to drink plenty of fluids before and during your workout. Wear loose-fitting, lightweight clothing. Cottons and linens are best because they wick moisture away from your body for evaporation and its cooling effect.

The Head Trip—Think More to Weigh Less

Eating isn't just a means of staying alive. It's also a behavior. You may eat because you are hungry, or you may be trying to fulfill a secondary need. It may be anything from a political statement to a plea for acceptance. It might be that eating relieves boredom, quiets anxiety, calms anger, and vents frustration. One of the important aspects of weight control is to sort out which of these needs is operative when you are eating. Being conscious of why you are eating can go a long way toward modifying eating habits.

Behavior modification techniques can make an important contribution to your being successful in losing weight. You must first identify your personal eating patterns. This involves keeping a written record of how you eat for a period of two to three weeks. Estimates of what you eat usually do not work because most women underestimate their daily food intake by anywhere from 500 to 900 calories. The record should include when you ate, what it was, where you ate it (home, restaurant, snack stand, and so on), and how you felt at the time (angry, guilty, frustrated, lonely). Long-term success in changing a pattern of overeating depends on graphically demonstrating how, what, when, and why you really do eat (Ojeda 1995). Once you have an understanding of your eating patterns and what foods are packing on the weight for you, you can begin to make some positive changes.

For example, if you find that you frequently eat high-calorie snacks while watching TV, try a low-fat substitution—such as low-fat yogurt instead of ice cream. When you feel hungry, it may be that you are only thirsty. Try drinking a glass of water. You may be surprised at how many times your "hunger" is sated when you slake your thirst. Here's another suggestion: Go for a brisk walk instead of walking to the refrigerator after a disagreeable confrontation. You can probably think of other substitutes.

You can gain help in modifying destructive eating habits from successful diet programs such as Weight Watchers International, Jenny Craig, and TOPS (Take Off Pounds Sensibly). These organizations specialize in helping dieters identify the eating habits contributing to being overweight and in establishing new habits to reverse these trends. They will teach you every aspect of formulating a new diet, how to shop for healthful foods, and how to prepare your meals. Support groups like these abound in most communities. You might even want to start your own.

You can probably also improve your exercise program by keeping a record of your daily activities for a week or so. The record may show you where you can squeeze in some exercise without a lot of fuss. Maybe you can get off the commuter train a mile from work and walk the rest of the way, or park your car somewhere that provides a comfortable walk to your destination. Riding a stationary bicycle while you watch the evening news is healthier than consuming a cocktail and snacks during that time.

Weight control may be a challenge for you in your transition years, but it is a major component of wellness and deserves a prominent position on your agenda of things to do to stay healthy.

Smoking

There has probably been more said and written about the destructive effects of smoking than about any other human habit. Americans must be listening, because the number of Americans who smoke has been declining over the last two decades.

If you are still smoking, you probably would like to quit. Earlier in this book you learned about the relationship of smoking to cardiovascular disease, osteoporosis, lung cancer (the number one cause of cancer death for women), the aging process, skin wrinkles, and earlier menopause. The number of deaths attributable to smoking for all Americans between ages 35 and 64 is nearly one in five. This exceeds the combined total from suicide, murders, fire, auto accidents, AIDS, alcohol, cocaine and heroin (Warner 1991). When used as directed, setting fire to tobacco leaves and inhaling the products of combustion is a waste of a perfectly good body. Thirty-five percent of smokers die from a smoking-related disease. As a woman, you currently can expect to outlive your male contemporaries by seven years. If you are a smoking woman, however, this advantage may be lost entirely.

Then there is the issue of passive smoking. Secondhand smoke is estimated to be responsible for 30,000 to 60,000 cardiac deaths each year, as well as for 100,000 to 200,000 nonfatal heart attacks and strokes. Dr. Fontham reported in 1994 that overall, nonsmoking women exposed to tobacco smoke are 30 percent more likely to develop lung cancer than those who aren't. (Note: Childhood exposure was not shown to increase the cancer risk in women unless it was combined with adult exposure, but infants and children being raised in a smoking household have a much higher incidence of asthma, bronchitis, pneumonia, and middle-ear infections.)

Why You May Still Be Smoking

One of the keys to quitting smoking is to be aware of the reasons that you do smoke. A 1992 report indicated a variety of reasons women continue to smoke (Rigotti 1992):

- **Addiction to nicotine:** It's official: Nicotine is addictive. This is a very difficult problem to conquer. Nicotine gum and skin patches may help you.

- **Weight control:** A 1990 Surgeon General's report indicated that three quarters of women gained an average of five to seven pounds after quitting smoking. The American Cancer Society disagrees. They found only about one third gained weight, and if exercise is combined with an effort to cease smoking, one third actually lost weight. It may be that you gain weight after quitting because your metabolic rate drops, or it may be simply that you end up using eating as a substitute for the strong oral stimulus of smoking. You may well gain some weight, but estimates are that you would need to gain at least 75 pounds before the risks of obesity began to outweigh the risks of smoking (Reichman 1996)!

- **Pleasant associations with smoking:** After-dinner conversation, coffee breaks, and smoking after sex are three examples.

- **Psychological dependence:** Like overeating, smoking may represent a coping mechanism for dealing with anger, boredom, stress, frustration, and pressure.

- **Coping with stress:** You may use smoking to handle stress; when you stop, you experience more stress, which causes you to light up again.

There are many books and programs available to assist you in your effort to quit smoking. Check Appendix A for the addresses and phone numbers of the American Cancer Society, National Cancer Institute, American Heart Association, and American Lung Association.

Alcohol

As you sip your evening cocktail after another harrowing day of just being you, you are consuming a very unusual substance. Alcohol is a tiny molecule with no nutrient value, but it is readily absorbed into your bloodstream. Because it is so small and is soluble in water, it is carried to every cell in your body. Other drugs with larger molecules are not as widely distributed, but alcohol, once consumed, is presented with near-endless opportunities to do harm. The array of effects on your body and your life from alcohol abuse is astonishing. It is a potent, and sometimes deadly, force in aging. Alcohol can destroy your liver, raise your blood pressure, lower your bone mass, enlarge your heart, cause gastrointestinal bleeding, impair your brain function, shatter your sex life, hasten your menopause, decrease your fertility, suppress your immune system, worsen diabetes, increase your cancer risk, sap your energy, increase your stress level, trigger depression, and create social problems, including marital and occupational difficulties.

The Gender Difference

It takes less alcohol over a shorter time span for women to sustain the serious and sometimes fatal outcomes of alcohol consumption (Landau et al. 1994). Part of the reason is that women are generally smaller than men, so they have a smaller volume of blood and other body fluids. If you consume the same amount of alcohol as a man, it will probably not be diluted as much in your body. The effect on your tissues is therefore more intense.

Another important difference is that as a woman, you have less of a stomach enzyme called gastric alcohol dehydrogenase than men do (Frezza 1990). This enzyme's job is to partially break down alcohol in your stomach and reduce the amount of alcohol's active ingredient, called ethanol, that you absorb into your bloodstream. With less enzyme breakdown, your blood alcohol level rises much faster than in men. Your organs and tissues are once again subjected to a more concentrated solution of alcohol.

Alcoholism

Most people who drink overdo it occasionally. The morning after reminds you of it. This doesn't mean you have an alcohol problem. You do have a problem, though, if you fall into either of these two categories:

- **Alcohol abuse:** When drinking impairs your normal life functions, such as your marriage, job, and other relationships.
- **Alcohol dependence:** When, in spite of these impairments, you have an unrelenting compulsion to continue drinking.

Your genetic background can influence your chances for alcohol dependence. If you have a first-degree relative (parent or sibling) who is an alcoholic, your risk is fourfold. (Just having this information can serve as a potent preventive force for you.) Approximately 5 million American women have serious drinking problems. This may even be an underestimate, since women are more introspective about their drinking problems than men and may seek to disguise their overuse of alcohol. Many more women drink alone than men. Although more than twice as many men as women are reported to be serious problem drinkers, this may be the result of underreporting of alcohol use by women (Gold 1991).

Health Consequences

For women, heavy drinking is considered to be more than two drinks a day (Gold 1991). By now, you are probably already aware that alcohol affects your brain (and therefore your behavior, coordination, and reflexes) and that it can cause cirrhosis of the liver. It is also a significant factor in fatal accidents and in heart disease. How else does alcohol abuse affect you?

- **Skin damage:** Overuse of alcohol can severely damage skin (Ojeda 1995). It has to do with free radicals, which we described in Chapter 10. Collagen and elastin are damaged, which leads to decreased skin tone, sagging, blotching, puffiness, and brown spots. Long-term use may even give you rhynophyma—in other words, a red "W. C. Fields" nose. Severe alcoholics in their forties commonly appear to be in their sixties.

- **Effects on sex:** With lowered inhibitions, you are more likely to engage in risky sexual behaviors. These can range from socially risky flirtations to health risks of sexually transmitted diseases from new or multiple partners. Heavy alcohol use can also suppress orgasms and diminish your sexual desire.

- **Breast cancer:** In the 1980s, alcohol and breast cancer were linked, but more than a dozen studies since then have shown either no association or a slightly increased risk. Two studies showed that perimenopausal women who drink are at greater risk for breast cancer than those who are postmenopausal (van Veer et al. 1989, Young 1989). One large review study of about three dozen other studies found that the increase in risk was 11 percent at one drink per day, 24 percent at two drinks, and 38 percent for three (Longnecker 1988). No one knows the reason for the alcohol-breast cancer association, but speculation is that alcohol causes decreased estrogen levels, abnormal liver function, immune system suppression, and free radical damage to DNA in breast cells. If you have risk factors for breast cancer (you have first-degree relatives with breast cancer, are overweight, have never been pregnant, or had your first term pregnancy after age thirty), abstinence from alcohol is your safest course.

- **Obesity:** Alcohol contains seven calories per gram, compared to four calories per gram for carbohydrate and protein and nine calories per gram for fat. There is no nutritional value in alcohol, so any of those calories you do not burn are stored as fat. Since your metabolic rate slowly declines during perimenopause, your need is for fewer calories containing more nutrients. You may not gain weight, but you sure won't become better nourished.

- **Fetal damage:** If you are planning a pregnancy, drinking alcohol is a very bad idea. This is true both while you are trying to get pregnant and once you've succeeded. Heavy drinking can cause fetal alcohol syndrome, which causes low birth weight with deformities of the heart, limbs, and face, as well as mental retardation (Autti-Ramo et al. 1992). The specific safe minimum for alcohol in pregnancy is still unknown, so abstinence is safest for your baby. Heart disease: Heavy drinking can cause high blood pressure, which in turn is linked to an increased workload for your heart and to damaged heart muscle. Alcohol also raises serum triglycerides, which represents a specific risk for heart disease in women. But there's some good news. The Harvard Nurses' Health Study found that moderate alcohol intake (two or fewer drinks a day) can reduce your risk for heart disease (Stampfer and Willett 1988)! As if that weren't enough, moderate alcohol use also raises your good high-density lipoproteins (HDL). Moderate alcohol intake has a positive effect on blood-clotting mechanisms, which decrease your risk for strokes and heart attacks.

- **Osteoporosis:** Low bone mass is common in heavy drinkers, including women who have not reached menopause. The reason is that alcohol interferes with calcium absorption. It also impairs activation of vitamin D by your liver, and this further lowers calcium absorption. In addition, if your diet is nutritionally poor (common for heavy drinkers), your intake of calcium and vitamin D may be deficient. If you have personal risk factors for osteoporosis, limit your consumption of alcohol to fewer than two drinks daily.

- **Immune suppression:** Not much has been published on this subject, but alcohol apparently lowers or alters your immune response to foreign intruders and cancer formation (Reichman 1996). When oncogenes trigger the formation of a cancer cell, your immune system normally resists this abnormal cell and tries to destroy it, but this effect is lessened in heavy drinkers. If your immune system is suppressed, you are more susceptible to infections—everything from the common cold to HIV (the AIDS virus).

There is not much disagreement that drinking alcohol in moderation can do a little good, but it can do a lot of harm if consumption gets out of control. The transition from a moderate "social" drinker to alcohol abuse and dependence is often a subtle one. The profile of the transitional woman who develops a drinking problem is that of a divorced or separated woman, a woman who lives with an alcoholic partner, a married woman who does not have an outside job, and a woman whose children no longer live at home. A very common trait of the alcoholic woman is that she is a solitary drinker, and often a secret one (Gold 1991). The good news is that, like quitting smoking, healing begins immediately when you stop drinking.

As we mentioned earlier in this chapter, drinking problems are categorized as either alcohol dependence or alcohol abuse. If your problem is alcohol dependence, and alcohol is literally controlling your life, your best choice for treatment is to enter a detoxification program, either as an inpatient or an outpatient. Inpatient therapy usually requires about a month of treatment. Most communities have such facilities.

If alcohol abuse more accurately describes your situation, a detox program may still be the best plan, but for some, a lesser level of treatment may also work. Alcoholics Anonymous and Women for Sobriety are two effective 12-step support groups that can help you. Here are some additional tips:

- **Acknowledge your drinking problem:** The longer you put it off, the more likely you are to suffer permanent damage to your body and to your life.

- **Go public:** Make an announcement of your intention to stop drinking. It's easier for you to quit this way. Tell people important to you (your partner, friends, co-workers) that you are quitting alcohol. The value is twofold. First, you are more likely to stick with your commitment because you have announced it to them. Second, your peers may avoid putting pressure on you to drink when they realize your genuine intention to quit alcohol.

- **Ask your partner to help:** Ask your partner not to drink in your presence. Also, invite your partner to attend counseling and group sessions with you. It may turn out that your partner is enabling (unwittingly encouraging) you to be a drinker and does not realize it. If your partner refuses to participate, you may have to choose between ending your relationship and jeopardizing your recovery.

- **Decline the offer of a drink:** At a party, simply say, "I don't drink." If your hosts insist, leave the party.

- **Avoid drinkers:** Seek out friends who don't drink. One source of new friends is the people you meet in a support group. In the early stages of recovery, when you are most vulnerable to backsliding, it is reasonable to ask friends who do drink not to do so around you. You can't impose that limitation forever, of course, but they may be willing to help you during the early stages. If not, avoid them.

- **Refuse alcohol substitutes:** Avoid nonalcoholic beer and wine. The tastes are similar enough to their alcoholic cousins that they may conjure up the old cravings.

- **Keep busy:** Now may be a good time to invest yourself in volunteer community work, join a theater group, or go back to school. Just make sure it's fun. You may soon realize that being sober is really more rewarding than drinking.

- **Exercise:** Join a health club if you can. Regular exercise relieves stress, improves your body's condition, and puts you in the company of people who enjoy good health.

The overall mortality rate for alcoholic women is four and a half times that of nondrinkers. Your life expectancy is shortened fifteen years by heavy drinking (Reichman 1996). Foreshortened also are relationships with your partner, children, and friends. Time and human closeness are too precious to throw away on a tiny but deadly molecule like alcohol.

Drug Dependency

Just as you are not immune to alcohol dependence, neither are you immune to dependence on addictive drugs. You may not know a single person who set out to become addicted, but you probably know some addicts. Much has been said and written about inner-city abuse of illegal drugs. As a perimenopausal woman, however, you are more likely to become dependent upon legal than illicit drugs. Drug dependency cuts across all social, cultural, and economic boundaries. One in twenty American women abuse or are dependent on drugs of some type (Gold 1991).

The effects on you of drug dependency can be widespread and devastating. It can turn your body into a toxic waste dump and rapidly age you. You may lose your money, your partner, your children, your job, your friends, and your dignity. You can become malnourished. Neglect of exercise and personal grooming habits contribute to further deterioration. Your intellectual capabilities will become blunted. And the bottom line is that you can die from drug dependence.

How Drug Dependence Can Happen

People take drugs because they make them feel good. If you sprain your ankle, a prescription painkiller makes you feel better. For sinus congestion, an over-the-counter decongestant helps. A line of cocaine may make your brutal daily schedule more tolerable. A tranquilizer gets you some much needed sleep. That's the start of it. These drugs fill a need in your life. For most people, however, relief is short-lived. Long-term use causes decreased production of endorphins, your own internal opium-like drug, which, as you know from Chapter 5, you rely upon for relief of pain and other stresses. This encourages greater use of your drug of choice and may eventually result in dependence—you need it just to get by.

What Drugs?

While marijuana, cocaine, and heroin are the usual suspects, there are many, many more prescription and over-the-counter drugs upon which you may become dependent:

- **Psychotropic drugs:** Medications such as tranquilizers and sleeping pills are common sources of drug abuse in women. Diazepam (Valium), chlorazepate (Tranxene), chlordiazepoxide (Librium) and similar drugs are commonly prescribed for short-term stress control, but these drugs are well known for their addicting capabilities.
- **Amphetamines and other appetite suppressants:** Amphetamines and a whole panoply of similar appetite suppressants, such as phentermine (Fastin) and mazindol (Sanorex) may give you a diminished urge to

eat; but the stimulant effect of these "uppers" makes you want to stay with them indefinitely.

- **Painkillers:** These are intended for relief of acute pain, but some pain is chronic and poses the threat of addiction if these drugs are continued for an extended time. They include oxycodone with aspirin (Percodan), propoxyphene (Darvon), codeine-containing drugs, and other analgesics, such as pentazocine (Talwin), hydrocodone (Lortab, Vicodin), and levorphanol (Levo-Dromoran), may become avenues to addiction.

- **Over-the-counter medicines:** These, too, can become addictive. Phenylpropranolamine is the active ingredient in diet pills such as Dexatrim, Acutrim, and Dex-a-Diet. This drug is also found in many other medications, including nasal decongestants (Entex, Ornade), cough medications (Dimetane, Hycomine, Triaminic), and drugs for treating PMS. Phenylpropranolamine has a stimulant effect, and therein lies the trouble—it's another feel-good drug.

- **Alcohol abuse:** A National Institute of Mental Health survey found that women who abuse alcohol are six times more likely to abuse other drugs as well (Gold 1991).

Are You at Risk?

As a woman, you are at greater risk than men for abuse of tranquilizers, stimulants, sedatives, and other prescription drugs (Prochaska et al. 1992). This stems from the fact that women are generally more health conscious than men and seek care more frequently. Women tend to be more open about their concerns and in touch with their feelings about common disorders such as anxiety, insomnia, weight control, and chronically painful conditions. The drugs warranted for these problems often have a high potential for addiction. Adding to your risk is the fact that women are less likely to come forth with a dependency problem, which results in a more advanced stage of addiction when care is finally sought. The exception to this is in women who work outside the home; if drug abuse is causing trouble at work, help is usually sought earlier.

If you suffer from a mental disorder, such as depression or anxiety states, your risk of drug dependency is raised. Depression quadruples your risk of abuse or dependency. For panic disorder and obsessive-compulsive states, the increase is doubled (Gold 1991). (See Chapter 12 for more information about these disorders.)

Another gender-related risk is that women generally have more body fat than men. Sedatives and tranquilizers are deposited in body fat, and they are cleared from your body more slowly than in men who have less fat. This means that the desired effect lasts longer, and you can get to like it. In addition, the smaller your body, the greater the concentration of the drug, resulting in a more intense response. If the response is a positive one, you may be reluctant to give it up.

Heredity also has a role to play. In his book *The Good News about Drugs and Alcohol*, Dr. Mark Gold writes that drug dependence, like alcoholism, can run in families. His estimate is that one in ten people is genetically predisposed to drug dependency. There is no genetic test for this, so if your family history includes drug or alcohol dependency, be extremely cautious. Avoidance is a whole lot easier to deal with than dependence.

Prevention

There is no question that never getting started on drugs beats trying to stop. Experimentation with illegal drugs, even briefly, can quickly lead to dependency. Addiction is certainly not what you had in mind when, just for a lark, you snorted your first cocaine. But it can be a pretty slippery slope after that. And it's a long way down. Dependency on legal drugs, although it starts with legitimate treatment, can follow the same downward path. Consider these suggestions for steering around a drug problem:

- **Know what you are taking:** When a new medication is prescribed, ask your doctor or the pharmacist about its potential for addiction. This is especially important if you have risk factors that make you prone to dependency—prior drug abuse or mental illness, or a family history of addiction.

- **Use as directed:** Your interests are best served by following the prescription label precisely. Take the medication as frequently and for as long as directed, and then stop. Avoid saving what is left over unless your doctor advises you to do so. Prescription drugs may be even more dangerous than illegal drugs because they are made available to you for a legitimate purpose, and you might worry less about misusing a legal drug than a street drug.

- **Resolve conflicts in your life:** Attempts at using drugs to relieve the stress created by a conflict is only avoidance; it's a temporary measure. Seek out the cause of your frustration, boredom, anxiety, work pressure, or poor relationship and deal with it. Change partners, get a new job, compromise with an adversary, or do whatever is appropriate to get it off your back. Don't risk having drug dependency on your back along with your conflict. Know your family history: If there is drug abuse, be cautious about drug use of any kind.

When to Get Help

There are some very clear signs that your drug use has overstepped normal bounds:

- You can't think of anything except the drugs you are using. Without them you can't start the day, go to work, be happy, be relaxed, go to a party, have sex, get to sleep, or do anything normal.
- You are neglecting your family and friends to obtain and use drugs.
- You are lying to get prescriptions refilled.
- You are missing work because of drug use or drug hangovers.
- You are neglecting your nutritional needs and personal grooming habits.
- You are depleting your savings or selling possessions to buy drugs.

How to Get Help

Drug dependency can happen to you. It doesn't mean that you are of low moral character or unworthy of compassion. For a variety of reasons, some of them not of your choosing or in your control, you may have drifted into dependency. Chronic illness, overwhelming stresses, ignorance of the risks, and many other factors may have played a part in bringing you to this point. You didn't intend to get addicted. You just are. If this is your situation or you think it is, the following suggestions can be helpful (Larson 1993):

- **Ask for help:** Your chances of getting out of this morass alone are not good. Tell someone—your partner, a friend, your doctor, a clergy member—about your problem. This alone will make you feel better. If someone knows about you and cares, you've acquired some support and taken the first step toward recovery.
- **Seriously consider a treatment program:** Drug recovery centers offer both inpatient and outpatient services. As an inpatient, you will be in a nonthreatening environment during which your body is detoxified. This setting also provides skilled people to help you address the underlying causes of your drug dependency. Both are necessary to full recovery. The costs are now covered by many insurance companies and even by some employers.
- **Join a support groups:** Support groups can be very helpful. Many twelve-step programs, for example, are conducted by people who have experienced drug dependency. The people you meet will greet your problem with understanding and empathy. Contact Narcotics Anonymous, Alcoholics Anonymous, or Cocaine Anonymous for a chapter near you (see Appendix A).
- **Get back on a healthy diet:** Very few drug-dependent women regard eating well as a priority item. The problem can arise from binge eating and obesity in marijuana users to severe undereating and malnutrition

in cocaine users. If you are starting a recovery program, a balanced diet will not only supply the needed calories, it can provide the sense of orderliness in your life that you may have lost.

- **Start exercising:** You have probably neglected your body during your drug dependency. If so, starting a regular program of moderate exercise, as we described earlier in this chapter, will make a big difference during your recovery. Your body will feel better, and your spirits will be raised. Depression is common during dependency, and exercise is an excellent mood elevator.

Summing Up

Destructive behaviors are common human frailties. For some of you, they result from an unfortunate shuffling of the genetic deck. For others, these behaviors arise from bad choices. Fortunately. the latter is the most common cause of destructive behavior (Prochaska et al. 1992). If you chose it to begin with, you can also "unchoose" it. It isn't easy to change long-standing habits and behaviors, but as a perimenopausal woman, you have years ahead of you in which to benefit from changing destructive behaviors that can endanger your wellness.

O O O

12

Relax for a Change: Management of Stress and Depression

As a perimenopausal woman, you have no doubt had your share of stress. It is not age related; nothing about your transitional years makes stress any different from what you have known in the past. You may encounter some new stressors (hot flashes, sleep disruption, mood shifts, short term memory changes), but your stress response will likely be similar to your past experiences with stress. However, like most people, you probably don't have a perfect handle on coping with stress. The first half of this chapter explains what stress is, how to recognize it, how it can affect your health, and how to cope with it. The second half of the chapter takes a look at the relationship of stress to the development of depression—both minor and major—and other psychological problems.

What Is Stress?

You might think a term as widely used as stress would be easy to define, but it isn't. Different people perceive stress differently, which makes a universal definition difficult. One description is that stress is the sum of your biological reactions to any adverse stimulus that tends to disrupt your homeostasis, or balanced state. (Homeostasis is a constantly changing balance in the physiological, psychological, and social spheres of your life.) Stress throws you off-kilter. The adverse stimulus can be physical, such as threat of an impending injury; it can be mental, as when you worry about paying your bills; or it can be an emotion, like anger. A stressor is any change arising internally or externally, whether real or imagined, that requires you to react or adapt to it. If your compensating reaction to stress is inadequate or inappropriate, it can lead to trouble.

Stress control is an important part of your wellness program. By understanding the relationship between stress and your health, you can control it.

What Link Does Stress Have to Other Disorders?

If someone tells you a particular complaint you have is "just" from stress, you may come away feeling belittled and humiliated. However, stress can play a large role in your health. Estimates are that 60 to 90 percent of office visit complaints are rooted in lifestyle habits and stress (Notelovitz and Tonnessen 1993). In addition, while infections of various sorts have always been the predominant cause of death and disease, stress-induced disease has now assumed this mantle in industrialized cultures. Stress is now linked to cardiovascular disease, respiratory disease, arthritis, insomnia, infertility, chronic pain, depression and even cancer. There is now solid evidence that stressors such as negative emotions, anxiety, loneliness, grief, and depression will suppress your immune system (Kiecolt-Glaser and Glaser 1991). This puts you at risk for a variety of illnesses, including common colds. In one study (Kiecolt-Glaser 1996), medical students who were studying for finals (an immensely stressful situation) were given hepatitis vaccine. This normally triggers the immune system to develop protective antibodies. A month later, when their booster shots were due, their antibody levels were much lower than expected. They were still at risk for hepatitis, and stress appeared to be the reason.

How Does Stress Do It to You?

Stress upsets your body's homeostasis. Even though events frequently disturb that balance, a series of ongoing minor adjustments will usually bring you back into balance. This fine tuning occurs at many levels: biochemical, cellular, organ-system, psychological, interpersonal, and social.

For example, let's say your stressor is that you are very cold. Your homeostatic responses might be

- **Biochemical:** Your stress hormones, epinephrine (adrenaline), norepinephrine, and cortisol, are increased. These prepare you to take whatever action might be necessary to combat the cold. This is your "fight-or-flight" capability.

- **Cellular:** Your declining body temperature causes certain cellular metabolic functions (like digestion) to slow, in an effort to conserve energy for more important tasks.

- **Organ-system:** The heat-regulating mechanism in your brain signals your skin capillaries to constrict and keep more blood located centrally in your body, where it is warmer. Your brain triggers shivering to generate heat from your muscles.

- **Psychological:** You worry that you might be freezing to death.

- **Interpersonal:** "May I borrow your coat?"

- **Social:** "Let's get off this frozen lake and go home."

Voila! Saved by homeostasis and appropriate responses to stress.

As we have described, a stressor is something that threatens your physical or psychological well-being. The magnitude of the threat (and therefore the stress) depends on whether you feel you can cope with it. The very cold person we described above coped very well and spent a pleasant evening in front of the fireplace. Each time you are confronted by a stressful or threatening situation, your brain instructs your sympathetic nervous system to rapidly release stress hormones into your bloodstream. Each time you are readied for fight or flight. This served our distant ancestors very well when they were being charged by a Woolly Mammoth perhaps, and it still works for us in emergencies. But most of the stresses we face don't require coping techniques like a primal scream with fists balled or taking off like a scalded cat. The fight-or-flight reaction is hard on your body and your health, which is why it's important to find ways to control your responses to stress.

This issue turns out to have more significance for you as a woman because stress hormones appear to stay in your bloodstream longer than in men. A study of 90 newlywed couples (Kiecolt-Glaser et al. 1987) found that, following a marital disagreement, the blood level of stress hormones in the wives rose suddenly and sharply. The husbands had increased levels too, but not as suddenly or as high. The next day, before the couples left the clinic where they had stayed overnight, the stress hormone levels in the men had returned to normal, but in the women they were still quite high. This suggests that women are more sensitive to negative behavior than men. As explained above, stress hormones suppress your immune system which, in turn, suggests that you are more at risk for infectious diseases and other illnesses if such episodes are frequent or chronic. Damage control for these responses centers around recognizing stress, and then coping with it.

Recognizing Stress

It is often easier to recognize the symptoms of stress than the source of it. The symptoms may be emotional, physical, behavioral or cognitive, and you may sometimes have symptoms in all of these categories. Take a look at Table 12-1 for a listing of some typical symptoms. The source of stress that shows up in these symptoms is sometimes obvious, such as loss of a family member, divorce, a job change, or moving to a new town. Some aren't so obvious. For example, biological changes that may occur during your transitional years can be sources of stress. The perimenopausal symptoms of estrogen decline represent a few of them.

Table 12.1.
Symptoms of Stress

Emotional	Physical	Behavioral	Cognitive
Anxiety	Rapid heart rate	Critical of others	Forgetfulness
Nervousness	Restlessness	Can't get things done	Can't make decisions
Anger, acute or chronic	Headaches	Bossy with others	Fuzzy thinking
Irritability	Stomach aches	Overeating	Diminished creativity
Loneliness	Insomnia	Excess smoking	Lost sense of humor
Boredom with life	Sweaty palms	Overuse of alcohol	Constant worrying
Feeling pressured	Fatigue	Neglect of personal habits	Trouble concentrating
Fearfulness	Breathlessness	Decreased sexual desire	
Crying	Tension, neck and shoulders		
Unexplained sadness			

Adapted from: Benson and Stuart 1993.

If you are also experiencing other biological changes (unrelated to hormones), such as graying of your hair, the need for glasses, and the appearance of wrinkles, you might not recognize any one of them as a stressor, but you may nevertheless feel stressed without other apparent causes. In this case, it could be that the aging process itself is unacceptable to you. In situations like this, finding the source can sometimes require some expert help from a psychological counselor.

Whatever the cause of your stress, once you recognize it, you are in a much better position to effectively deal with it.

Tolerating Stress

Some people adapt to stress more naturally than others. One investigator (Kobasa 1982) refers to people like this as having "stress-hardy" personalities. Such individuals are able to experience stress without undergoing the typical physical or mental stress responses. People with stress-hardiness are characterized by three important attitudes toward life's events: acceptance of challenge, a sense of control over life's vagaries, and a commitment to their families, their work, and in life in general. They tend to take control of their lives instead of passively accepting their lot. They are more likely to regard challenges as opportunities for personal growth than as threats to be avoided or escaped. When stressful situations confront a person with a stress-hardy personality, their response is to embrace it, explore the possibilities the conflict presents, and get involved in problem solving. According to the study, the opposite number of stress-hardiness is represented by people who react to stress more passively, with an attitude of helplessness. Most of us fall somewhere between these extremes.

According to *The Wellness Book* (Benson and Stuart 1993), closeness is a fourth characteristic of the stress-hardy personality. This refers to the ability to establish relationships in which a person can both provide and receive social support. This type of person appears to be much more stress resistant than someone who feels isolated from personal contact.

Are you getting the impression that stress doesn't need to have a negative impact on you, that it can be turned to your advantage? The larger view of stress is that it is not always bad for you.

Your reaction to stress is what governs its effect on your life and your health. It makes sense to reduce heavily stressful influences in your life as much as you can and to learn strategies for coping with stress. But adopting a strategy of avoiding or escaping from all stress may not make sense. Instead of regarding all stress in largely negative terms, you can try to perceive it as an exciting challenge—a stimulus to achievement. Actively coping with hardship (stress) challenges your intellect and engages your emotions. Indeed, you may obtain a more desirable result by changing your reaction to a stressful situation than by changing the situation itself.

In addition, many studies have demonstrated that up to a point, performance and efficiency increase as levels of anxiety and stress increase, but then, as stress continues to increase, performance and efficiency decline

(Yerkes and Dodson 1989). (Ever notice how a slightly messy office is the most productive one, or how happy seemingly disorganized families are?) The point is that total stress avoidance can be unhealthy. You do, however, need to know how to handle the heavy stuff.

Strategies for Coping with Stress

Effective coping is dependent on a number of factors, some of which we've already talked about in this book: a healthy diet, adequate exercise, relaxation techniques, and psychological adjustments that produce a positive attitude. Not all kinds of coping are equal, though. Eating a balanced diet is a good way of coping with stress; a food binge is not. Regular exercise is a good coping mechanism, but being a couch potato is a bad one.

Restoring homeostasis by psychological means involves what are called defense mechanisms. These are relatively automatic mental maneuvers that modulate the intensity of your emotional reaction to a stressful situation so that your behavior in dealing with it is appropriate. Good coping utilizes mature defenses, and poor coping uses immature defenses. The long-term problem of poor coping is that it can lead to a number of social maladjustments, such as chronic anger and estrangement. It also may become the lead-in to true psychological illnesses, such as depression and anxiety states.

Your built-in homeostatic mechanisms help you counteract the everyday stresses of life: when you've misplaced your car keys, your child's soccer team just lost, or you have incinerated the family dinner. You may handle these stresses without even noticing how you did it. When the stresses are extreme (as when a spouse dies) or long-lasting (you lose your job), they can overwhelm homeostasis, and their effects can become harmful to your health. There are several ways you can reduce the negative impact of stress.

Avoid the Quick Fix

Many health care professionals and their patients rely on the prescription drug route for managing stress. Our "instant relief" society has been conditioned to expect a "pill cure" from tranquilizers, and antidepressants. These drugs do indeed have usefulness in acutely stressful situations, but drug therapy tends to deal with symptoms only. It fails to address the underlying causes of severe stresses and the importance of taking responsibility for dealing with them. The same may be said for alcohol use during stress. In addition, the National Institute of Alcohol Abuse and Alcoholism has stated that if you consume alcohol during stress, you become more intoxicated and experience a worse hangover than when you use it during more relaxed periods. And lighting up a cigarette to relax is counter-productive because nicotine releases epinephrine, the very stress hormone you already have circulating in abundance. Use of street drugs also falls into the category of temporary avoidance (Notelovitz and Tonnessen 1993).

Prioritize the Tasks That Face You

Sometimes your stressor is not a major one, but an accumulation of little things that are annoying. They may have taken months or years to pile up on you, or maybe the list just started yesterday morning. Try ranking these tasks into categories according to their relative priority: (1) essential, (2) important, and (3) trivial. A good way to assign rank is to ask yourself: "What is the worst that could happen if I don't get this done?" You'll find that many things you first thought were crucial, just aren't. You can downgrade many items on your list of "things to do immediately" to "what the heck" when you have subjected them to the "what is the worst that could happen" test. Then concentrate on the essential items, delegate to others as many of the important tasks as possible, and ignore the trivial stuff altogether (Landau et al. 1994). When assigning priorities to your list, be sure to include "time for myself" near the top of your "essential" column. Even if it is for only a few minutes, plan something that pleases you and is just for you—perhaps luxuriating in a warm bath.

Eat a Healthful Diet

If you are under stress, you may be too distracted to focus on your nutritional needs. Nevertheless, good nutrition is more important than ever; stress raises your metabolic rate and increases your energy needs. As discussed in Chapter 10, a diet emphasizing complex carbohydrates and high in fiber is known to be beneficial during PMS because of the calming effect from increased serotonin availability. It works for stress control as well.

Get Regular Exercise

Aerobic exercise such as brisk walking, cycling, step-aerobics, and swimming are dependable methods to reduce stress. (Chapter 10 discusses the role of exercise more fully.) They provide a useful outlet for your fight-or-flight energy. As you know from Chapter 10, endorphins are released into your circulation during vigorous exercise. They elevate your mood, leaving you in a state of natural relaxation at the end of your workout. Your blood pressure declines, your pulse rate decreases, your muscles become relaxed, and tension is released. You will sleep better, and your mind will also participate in the general relaxation. Exercising for stress relief is most beneficial if you do it twice daily for about thirty minutes (Notelovitz and Tonnessen 1993). It doesn't need to be two trips to the health club every day. A brisk walk will do nicely, and it can also qualify as time for yourself. Remember this, though: If you exercise just before bedtime, you may become overstimulated, which can prevent sleep.

Get Plenty of Rest

Insomnia is a common accompaniment to stress. The problem this creates is chronic fatigue, which in itself can be an additional stressor. Prescription sleeping pills can provide relief in acute situations, but they are too addicting for long-term treatment. Even over-the-counter sleeping aids can result in your becoming dependent on them for sleep. Improving your sleeping habits is your best long-term option. Regular exercise can contribute to your sleeping well. In addition, consider the following recommendations for helping you sleep (Benson 1993; Notelovitz and Tonnessen 1993):

- **Spend less time in bed:** The belief that everyone needs eight hours sleep is a myth. The average adult needs only seven to seven and a half hours (Hauri and Linde 1990). This Mayo Clinic study showed that spending too much time in bed is the most common mistake you can make if you have problems with insomnia.

- **Eat a light carbohydrate snack an hour or two before bed:** A snack such as cookies or cereal may help to increase your production of serotonin, the brain chemical that promotes sleep.

- **Control your sleeping room:** It should be dark, quiet, and reasonably cool. Pull the shades, wear eye covers, and use ear plugs if necessary to manage your sleeping environment.

- **Maintain a sleeping schedule:** Try to establish a sleeping rhythm by going to bed at the same time every day and getting up at the same time. Your body will accommodate to your schedule.

- **Avoid caffeine late in the day:** Coffee, tea, and cola-like soft drinks are the chief suppliers of this sleep-robbing stimulant.

- **Use your bed exclusively for sleep:** Except for having sex, of course. Don't eat, watch TV, talk on the phone, or work in your bed.

Look for Social Support

The transitional years can be accompanied by some major life stresses: perhaps divorce, infidelity, work dislocation, children leaving home, financial problems, or single parenthood. You may find solace in joining a group of women who are facing similar problems. Talking about your stresses and sharing your feelings with others who are experiencing similar disruptions in their lives can reduce stress significantly. Support groups for various health concerns abound in most communities. You can make contact with them through newspaper listings, community hospitals, religious organizations, mental health clinics, and the ever reliable word of mouth.

Learn Some Relaxation Techniques

There are a number of relaxation techniques from which to choose. Deep breathing is one of the simplest, yet effective relaxation methods. Others include meditation, self-hypnosis, biofeedback, yoga, t'ai chi, massage, visualization and guided imagery, acupuncture, and acupressure. We'll describe these techniques in a moment. Find out what works for you. The goal of all of them is to elicit what Benson (1993) calls the relaxation response. This is a state of consciousness during which you have succeeded in diminishing oxygen consumption and lowering your breathing rate, heart rate, and blood pressure. This is the opposite of what happens during a fight-or-flight stress response.

Deep Breathing

Deep breathing is one of the most widely used methods to relax. (It is effective in relieving hot flashes too.) Deep breathing is often used as the starting point for other relaxation techniques, such as meditation, visualization, and yoga. To elicit the relaxation response, try this simple method:

- Seat yourself comfortably in a quiet room and close your eyes.
- Relax all of your muscle groups by consciously thinking of each of them one at a time. (See the next section.)
- Breathe in and out slowly through your nose, and concentrate on the air you are moving both into and out of your body.
- Repeat a word or phrase silently. Any neutral word—one that does not provoke anxious thoughts—will do. This repetition tends to keep extraneous thoughts out of your mind.
- Allow about ten to twenty minutes to complete this routine.
- At the end, sit quietly for another minute or two before slowly opening your eyes.

Progressive Muscle Relaxation

The technique of progressive muscle relaxation is a great way to relieve muscle tension when you feel it building up. You alternately tense and relax all muscle groups in your body, starting with your toes and feet and progressing through your calves, thighs, buttocks, back, hands, arms, neck, and face. It is most effective if you start with slow breathing. This routine takes ten or fifteen minutes to complete, so be sure to allow for enough solitude to do it. Try this technique a couple of times a day.

Transcendental Meditation

The value of meditation, often greatly underestimated in Western cultures, is a well-known alternative in relieving a wide variety of ailments, and stress relief is not the least of them. Meditation uses the same breathing techniques that we have already covered. In addition, it often involves repeating a mantra (word or phrase) and incorporates a variety of additional relaxation methods.

Meditation involves learning to have a quiet inner self and to live more actively in the moment. As you learn to meditate, you may become both more alert and energetic and more serene. There are a number of effective ways to meditate. You can do it sitting or lying down, while enjoying a peaceful walk, or even during other forms of exercise. It takes some training to get started, so look for a beginners class at your community center, church, or local mental health clinic. See Appendix B for a listing of books that can help you on your way.

If you decide to try meditation, make a commitment of several months. It can take this long before you appreciate the positive effects that meditation can have on your stresses and your life.

Visualization and Guided Imagery

Visualization is a way of filling your mind with a relaxing image. You close your eyes, doing the deep breathing exercise we've already described, and focusing on an image of utter serenity or profound joy. For example, you can focus on a past event in your life that made you feel that way. Think about every detail of the event: the time of day it happened, the surroundings, who was there, what was said, what you were wearing, how it felt, how it smelled, what you were feeling. If focusing on an actual event doesn't work for you, guided imagery can help you out. Guided imagery involves listening to a voice, either in person or on tape, that helps you create an image of serenity in your mind. Visualization and guided imagery can be both exquisitely relaxing and a lot of fun.

Hypnosis can also be used as a form of guided imagery. It is a safe and effective means of relaxing; but it requires the help of someone specifically trained. You can also learn to relax using self-hypnosis.

Laughter

Humor is a proven stress reliever, both psychologically and physiologically. Everybody knows there's nothing like a good laugh to break up a tense situation. It relaxes muscles, puts more oxygen into your system, and lowers blood pressure, not to mention laughter's unique ability to defuse a confrontation. Keep in mind Victor Borge's observation: "Humor is the shortest distance between two people." From everyday events like missing twelve consecutive traffic lights to serious events like a major illness, humor can help you cope. Look for the humor in seemingly sober moments; there usually is a thread of it somewhere. Start remembering jokes people tell you instead of immediately forgetting them; then retell them with your own embellishments. Keep a scrapbook of really great jokes or cartoons you see in newspapers and magazines. Reviewing it can turn a rainy afternoon into sort of a grin. Make a point of seeing funny movies; if possible, go to a theater instead of renting a video—the laughter of an audience is infectious. (Just listen to how different people laugh; that's funny in itself!)

A sense of humor is like a first-aid kit that you carry with you at all times. It is available at a moment's notice to improve your mood, defuse a confrontation, lower your blood pressure, and relieve your anxiety. Here is a five-point plan for improving your health and your life with laughter (Wilde 1997):

- **Laugh out loud:** Physically laughing, as opposed to just grinning or thinking about it, increases your oxygenation, improves your circulation, lowers your blood pressure, and even has a positive influence on your immune system. Laughter and longevity apparently go hand-in-hand. George Burns made it to 100, Lucille Ball to her late '70s, and Bob Hope, Milton Berle, and Red Skelton are all deep into advanced age.

- **Laugh at yourself:** At its roots, laughter is an expression of love. If you can laugh at your own shortcomings, you basically like yourself and you have a healthy self-esteem. Abraham Lincoln, never known as a handsome man, had this comment when he was accused by someone of being two-faced: "If I had two faces, would I be showing you this one?" Abe was comfortable with himself.

- **Maintain a lighthearted attitude:** Attitude is a choice you make in any situation, so why not make it upbeat? A joyful spirit makes you a more productive worker, helps control stress, defuses resentment, and improves loyalty in your employees. When things are tense, take a ten-minute humor break. Open a joke book or listen to a tape; and then see how smoothly things go afterward.

- **Find something funny every day:** Some days you may have to dig pretty deep to find something funny; life is like that. Maybe it will be only a cartoon in the newspaper; but find something.

- **Find the funny side of life even when you are up to your neck in alligators:** You might as well laugh instead of cry. When everything has seemingly turned against you, it is not inappropriate to resort to humor. A famous humorist wrote that just as life does not cease to be funny when we have a serious problem, life does not cease to be serious when we laugh.

Laughter is good for you. It doesn't cost a dime, is tax-free, fat-free, cholesterol-free, and nontoxic. Humorist Josh Billings said: "There ain't much fun in medicine, but there's a heck of a lot of medicine in fun."

Religion

Many people benefit from a commitment to a formal religion and a deeply felt set of values and beliefs. By this time in life, you may be starting to become aware of your own mortality. Perhaps you have already experienced a health threat, or you realize that your parents are nearing the end of life, or they are already gone. Religious traditions and beliefs can provide a sense of depth and meaning at a time in life when you have acquired the wisdom to appreciate them. A commitment to religion can help you in developing an awareness of a larger reality and promote an understanding that life has meaning and significance (Moyers 1993). The peace you derive from this kind of awareness is a good antidote for stress.

Yoga

Yoga is a system of physical exercises, postures, and stretching combined with deep breathing that requires you to focus on your body. As a transitional woman, you may discover that yoga is not just a wonderful way to relax, but hatha yoga (discussed in Chapter 10) is a way to improve flexibility in your body. Look for yoga classes at your local community college or on a videotape. (It is probably a good idea to start with a class to learn the basics.)

T'ai Chi

T'ai chi (pronounced "tie-chee") is a discipline of exercise and breathing that originated in China. It is a "Salute to the Sun" that is the exercise of choice for aging Orientals to greet the new day. It is well known that Orientals enjoy much better health as they age than Americans, and many claim that practicing t'ai chi is one of the reasons (Reichman 1996). T'ai chi emphasizes breathing, body alignment, and flexibility, which makes it similar to yoga. The difference is that the techniques of t'ai chi are designed to stimulate your body as well as to relax it, which is why it is an effective way to start your day. It is becoming increasingly popular in the U.S., so look for announcements and ads for local classes.

Acupuncture

Acupuncture is an ancient Chinese technique for treating many health problems, and it works for stress as well. We described the principles of this technique in Chapter 10. As you may recall, it involves insertion of tiny needles at specific locations to positively alter the flow of energy, called Qi (pronounced "chee"). It works for many people to advance healing, promote overall well-being, and induce relaxation. The benefit you receive is quite dependent upon the skill of the practitioner, so be sure you see a licensed acupuncturist. (Acupressure, a similar technique applies pressure, but not needles, to the appropriate locations.)

Massage

Massage can be an extremely pleasurable and relaxing experience. You can learn many of the various techniques yourself, but it is probably better to start with a professional. You can often find massage therapists at beauty salons and health clubs. Once you know that thumping, pounding, pinching, and jerking are not really part of therapeutic massage, you can get a video or a book on massage and try it yourself. Mutual massage is another good option; in addition to its relaxing benefits, it can provide an affectionate and romantic interlude for you and your partner. Many women find it relaxing to have a facial performed by an experienced and sensitive esthetician.

Hot Tubs and Saunas

Hot tubs and saunas feel great after a workout, or even if you just want to relax before going to bed. Usually, about fifteen minutes in water around a hundred degrees is all it takes.

CAUTION! After exercising, avoid water or a sauna that is too hot; it can divert too much blood from your central circulation into your skin and cause you to faint. If you have not cooled down after exercise or you have just consumed a large meal (which concentrates blood in your abdomen for digestion), plunging into a hot tub or entering a sauna can lower your blood pressure sufficiently to cause you to faint. So tubbing or taking a sauna alone is not always a good idea (or as much fun).

Biofeedback

Biofeedback is a method of inducing relaxation that uses various recording devices that monitor heart rate, blood pressure, and skin responses. When you are tense, the recordings are dramatically different from when you are relaxed. Biofeedback teaches you to identify tension in your body. Then, using visualization, guided imagery, and other relaxation techniques, you can monitor whether, and how much, your tension is being relieved. In this fashion you are taught how to do it for yourself.

Psychotherapy

Short-term therapy with a psychologist (rather than a psychiatrist, whose training is in mental illness) is yet another method of handling stress. This is less structured than most of the above techniques, and its advantage is that it is personalized. A major goal of stress management is to first identify the stressor. In many instances the underlying source of stress is obscure, and you may need some counseling to help identify it.

Beyond Stress—Psychological Illnesses

If a healthful diet, exercise, relaxation techniques, and other psychological adjustments are not successful in controlling your stress, it may be that you are suffering from a more serious mental illness, such as major depression, a variety of anxiety states, and panic attacks. If the causes of your stress have long passed but the symptoms of stress persist and are causing serious disruptions in your life—perhaps making it impossible for you to work or threatening the functioning of your family), you may have a significant problem that requires professional intervention. Let's examine several of these illnesses so you'll know what to look for—or better yet, what you probably don't have to worry about.

Major Depression

The word depression is one of the most overused words in our culture. We use it to describe everything from economic hard times, to satellite weather conditions, to a bad-hair day. Like most people, you probably have occasional bouts of the "blues." These short-lived episodes that result from "life junk" to produce moodiness, discouragement, sadness, or loneliness are a normal part of life, and they are referred to as minor depression. For the most part, minor depression is self-limiting and does not pose a health threat. Our homeostatic balancing act and psychological defenses are usually adequate to cope with minor depression.

Serious depression that just doesn't go away, or major depression, however, is a true psychiatric illness. Depressive disorders are characterized by a persisting disturbance of mood, a loss of sense of control, and intense mental, emotional, and physical anguish. Depression tends to disrupt relationships like family, job, and social functioning. (Depression Guideline Panel 1993). This is the kind of depression that requires psychotherapy and antidepressant medication. (The American Psychiatric Association categorizes severe depression in two ways: major depression, also known as unipolar depression, and manic-depressive illness, now known as bipolar depression. We'll look at bipolar depression in the next section.)

To put the importance of this disorder in perspective, it should be pointed out that the lifetime chances of your dying during a major depression are greater than your lifetime risk for dying from breast cancer. This of course is related to the 15 percent suicide rate (Gise 1996).

Diagnosis of Major Depression

The Diagnostic and Statistical Manual of Mental Disorders (1987) outlines some markers for major depression. Two factors are feeling depressed most of the day, nearly every day, and taking markedly diminished (or no) interest or pleasure in most or all activities of the day, most of the day, nearly every day. If you have either of these symptoms together with at least three of the following, you may have a major depression:

- Significant weight loss or gain (about 5 percent in a month) even when you are not dieting, or increased or decreased appetite nearly every day.
- Insomnia or hypersomnia (sleeping too much) nearly every day.
- Psychomotor (mental and physical) agitation or retardation nearly every day.
- Fatigue or loss of energy nearly every day.
- Feelings of worthlessness; excessive or inappropriate guilt nearly ever day.
- Diminished ability to think or concentrate, or indecisiveness nearly every day.
- Recurrent thoughts of death (not just fear of dying), recurrent suicidal thoughts without a specific plan, a suicide attempt, or a plan for suicide.

(Note: Hypothyroidism, unrecognized diabetes, adrenal disorders and other metabolic illnesses can mimic depression, and their consideration must be part of the evaluation when the diagnosis of depression is being considered.)

CAUTION! If the above describes you, or comes even close, you may be suffering from major depression. Since only 20 to 25 percent of those who meet the above criteria receive appropriate treatment (McGrath et al. 1990), we urge you to avoid inadequate treatment and seek immediate help from a physician experienced in diagnosing and treating depression.

Causes and Risk Factors

A number of factors may predispose you to depression (McGrath et al. 1990):

- A childhood loss such as death or prolonged illness of a parent, or divorced parents.
- Physical or sexual abuse by a parent, spouse, or partner. Twenty-five percent of depressed women have been sexually abused as children.
- Low self-esteem.
- Socioeconomic deprivation. Inadequate education plays a major role.
- Family history of depression. In some families it occurs generation after generation.
- Stress from multiple lifestyle roles, such as spouse, mother, homemaker, occupation outside the home, community responsibilities.

- Unhappy marriage or unhappy divorce.
- Young children at home.
- Recent childbirth. Up to 8 to 10 percent suffer major depressive symptoms (O'Hara 1991).
- Bodily disfigurement from trauma or surgery.

Depression was considered solely a psychiatric illness until abnormalities in serotonin were revealed in the last decade. Depression is now believed to be caused by a chemical imbalance in brain chemicals: Too many serotonin receptor sites on brain cells remain empty. In such women, the predisposing factors mentioned above influence the likelihood and severity of depression (ACOG 1993).

One factor that may influence major depression is hormonal changes. Perimenopausal symptoms do not generally cause major depression, but symptoms such as hot flashes, which disturb sleep, can contribute to it (Sherwin 1993). Do not confuse serious depressive symptoms with those of perimenopause; symptoms of major depression are much more pervasive, severe, and disruptive. Major depression and perimenopause do not go hand in hand, although there appears to be a slight increase of the rate of depression in transitional women. The stress induced by perimenopausal changes may trigger a major depression in a woman who is already teetering on the brink of it, but it is rare for perimenopausal symptoms to be a solitary cause.

Hypoglycemia, or low glucose levels in the blood, is a common cause of depression-like symptoms. Brain function is hampered by low serotonin levels, creating such symptoms as irritability, fatigue, anxiety, headaches, and depression. Once this source of symptoms is recognized, removal of refined carbohydrates from the diet is often enough to solve the problem (Notelovitz and Tonnessen 1993). Food allergies can play a major role for people suffering from depression (Ojeda 1995). It is thought to be a leading cause of undiagnosed depressive symptoms. (If your therapist can't get a handle on why you are depressed, this would be a reasonable avenue to explore.)

The Harvard Women's Health Study found that about five to ten percent of all women experience major depression at some time, regardless of age (McKinley et al. 1987). There was a slight increase in the rate of depression during the perimenopausal transition, but women over age forty-five were shown to have less depression than younger women. According to this study, the profile of a women at risk for depression is someone who has children under age five at home, is divorced or has a poor relationship, has less than a high school education, and is undergoing economic hardship—any of which might be true of any contemporary transitional women.

There appears to be a gender difference in the incidence of major depression. A study of major depression in North America, Europe, the Middle East, Asia, and the Pacific Rim (Weissman et al. 1996) found that women are more likely to experience major depression than men. In North America, the incidence in women is twice as high as in men. The gender difference for women begins at puberty and ends at menopause, when rates of depression become higher in men. The fact that depression is more common during the "high-hormone" years suggests that a hormonal factor may exist.

Another factor that may explain the gender difference is the differing ways that women and men define themselves. Psychologically, women tend to define themselves primarily through their relationships with other people: partners, children, family members, lovers, friends, co-workers (Kaplan 1986). Relationship issues take center stage for women, and problems in this area are common sources of depression. When women start feeling depressed, they may turn inward and examine their responsibility for a relationship gone awry (Nolen-Hoeksema 1987). This tendency to analyze relationships, if combined with little power to create a positive change, can lead to feelings of helplessness, despair, and depression. On the other hand, men define themselves on the basis of physical ability, sexual prowess, occupational success, and societal impact. When stressful problems arise in these areas, men tend to turn outward. They become involved with hobbies, sports, other women, more work, and other pursuits to distract themselves. This difference may in part explain why men have a lower rate of depression than women.

To summarize, there are multiple bio-psycho-sociological factors that put you at risk for major depression. You and your health care advisor must take all of them into account if you are experiencing major depression.

Treatment of Major Depression

People suffering from depression are often embarrassed by their perceived "weakness." In addition, far too many depression sufferers and their physicians erroneously believe that a "pep talk," a "stiff upper lip," and a "chin up" attitude are all you need. Unfortunately, failure to get proper treatment usually results in prolonged suffering, lost productivity, and a severely diminished quality of life. The good news is that major depression is treatable.

Treatment is successful for 70 percent who use antidepressant medications, and the success rate is higher still if psychotherapy is used in addition (Gise 1996). Major advances in the understanding of the neurobiology of depression have led to the development of newer and safer antidepressant medications. Treatment is no longer dependent upon "talk" therapy as the sole modality, although psychotherapists have a continuing major role to play. The serotonin-booster medications prescribed for major depression, such as Prozac, Zoloft, Paxil, and Serzone have been especially helpful for women whose depression has been aggravated by the serotonin-lowering effect of diminished estrogen. (Note: If you are seeing a psychiatrist, that person can prescribe antidepressants for you. If you are seeing a nonphysician therapist, your regular doctor may be able to prescribe them.)

When you are under care, make sure your physician or therapist knows of any relationship problems you are having. Remember that strong relationships are a core constituent of your psychological well-being. It is also important to disclose any history of depression in your biological family, and your use of alcohol, prescription drugs (including HRT and high-blood pressure medications, which can influence depression), and over-the-counter and street drugs.

What You Can Do to Diminish Your Symptoms

In addition to treatment by a **nonphysician** therapist or psychiatrist, there are steps you can take on your own to alleviate the symptoms of a major depression. Here are some suggestions:

- **Incorporate healthy habits:** As in treatment for stress, a healthy diet, regular exercise, relaxation techniques, and support groups are important parts of the mix in dealing with major depression.

- **Avoid isolation:** Don't cut yourself off from other people. A family member, your physician, a member of the clergy, or a trusted friend can all serve the need you have for a close and intimate human contact. A study in England (Brown et al. 1986) found that being able to confide in an intimate and trustworthy friend can actually avert major depression if it occurs early on in the disease.

- **Avoid self-treatment:** Persistent fatigue from lack of sleep may tempt you to power up during the day with caffeine or ride the crest of quick energy from sweets. Then at night a couple of cocktails or some wine may seem to be the way to relax. Maybe you have some tranquilizers or sleeping pills left over in your medicine cabinet that become your bedtime buddy, to help you get to sleep. These, though, are only avoidance techniques, and they do not help depression.

The bottom line is that major depression is a highly treatable, biologically based disorder. If you are aware of the warning symptoms and knowledgeable about the principles and availability of successful treatment, you can get help early if you need it.

Bipolar Depression (Manic-Depressive Illness)

Bipolar depression, which affects women and men equally, is characterized by cycles of alternating depression and elation. The lows are very low and the highs are very high. Changing from the trough to the peak is usually gradual; but occasionally it can be dramatic and rapid. Symptoms of the manic phase include hyperactivity, decreased sleep, decreased appetite, racing thoughts, and often psychotic behavior, as well as inordinate elation, grandiose notions, disconnected thoughts, racing thought streams, inappropriate or embarrassing social behavior, poor judgment, bursts of energy, non-stop talking, irritability, insomnia, and a startling increase in sexual desire. During the depressive cycle, you may experience all the symptoms of major depression.

Bipolar depression, like major depression, is believed to be related to chemical imbalances in the brain's neurotransmitters. There are also emotional and situational factors. It is therefore not surprising that treatment involves both medication (Luvox, Depakote, Eskalith) and psychotherapy.

Summary

Stress is an unavoidable fact of living. In some ways, stress plays a positive role in your life, requiring you to interact with events, adapt to them, and evolve with changing circumstances. However, when stressors start to threaten your equanimity (overwhelm your homeostasis), it is crucial to recognize and take steps to cope with them; your physical and emotional health may be on the line. You can use a variety of coping techniques to bolster your ability to handle stress positively.

Sometimes, though, in spite of all your efforts to resist the slings and arrows of life, you may be overwhelmed by events to the point where major depression or other mental illnesses result. Fortunately, a number of treatments are available if mental illness does strike.

○ ○ ○

Section III:

Making Change Easy

13

Sexuality: Good Sex Doesn't Need to Change

Sex can be one of the most pleasurable experiences that life has to offer at any age. However, in a youth-oriented, media-driven society like ours, it is easy to get the impression that sex is only for the young and firm-bodied. Sex, like your body, changes as you progress through life; but the desire to be sexual is never extinguished for most people. Young couples might feel that no one on the planet could possibly experience the pinnacles of sexual pleasure they enjoy. A few years later, the same ardent couple might remain intensely interested, but they might start to wonder whether their former ecstasies will ever be achieved again, what with children dashing through the house, the phone forever ringing, and appointments to be kept. In this couple's later years, the desire to be sexual persists, but conditions have probably changed a little. The feverish athleticism of youth has been replaced with sex at a more measured pace. The sexuality of youth, mid-life, and later years should not really be compared because each phase has its own unique perspective.

This chapter starts out by discussing the all-important role psychological factors such as attitude and self-image play in determining how full your sex life is. Then we take a look at certain biological factors that, in your perimenopausal years, may have a negative impact on your sexual pleasure. You will see how to deal with these changes in ways that protect your sexuality. Armed with this information, you can proceed with confidence toward (and beyond) menopause with your sexuality intact.

Psychological Influences on Sexual Desire

Your brain is the most important sexual organ throughout life (Landau et al. 1994). So it should not be surprising that lost or diminished sexual desire may have its roots in psychological influences. If you have this problem, you may be reticent to admit or discuss it. You may regard it as a personal shortcoming. This makes it difficult to confront the situation and effectively deal with it.

A variety of factors can combine to cause your libido to decline during perimenopause. Declining female hormone production is responsible for some anatomic and physiologic changes that can decrease your sexual desire (we look at these later in the chapter), but many psychiatrists and sex therapists believe, though, that the most influential factors, by far, are psychological. Attitude is the keystone of a healthy libido.

Let's talk about some things that influence your attitude toward sex.

Past Experience

If sex has been an enjoyable and integral part of your life, you and your partner have probably learned to communicate effectively with each other about your wishes and desires. Good sex leads to more good sex. Partners who are physically affectionate (frequent hugs, kisses, and pats) are usually well connected sexually. If this describes your relationship, you can reasonably expect that your sexual desire will persist in spite of the biological changes that perimenopause and menopause bring.

At the other end of the spectrum are mid-life women who no longer want sex. This may be related to such past experiences such as cultural and religious influences, trauma, and relationship problems. If your desire for sex has diminished for any of these reasons, or if sex has never been enjoyable or fulfilling for you, the biological changes of late perimenopause and menopause may provide a convenient reason to opt out of being sexually active.

CAUTION! Childhood sexual abuse has been a past experience for perhaps one quarter to one third of adult women (Lechner et al. 1993, Russell 1986). Many women who had such childhood experiences often do not remember them until they are over forty (Bolen 1993). If you are a victim, you may just now be finding out about or remembering it. If you believe you have a history of childhood sexual abuse, get professional help. The complicated problems arising from childhood sexual abuse often take years of therapy and hard work to resolve.

The complicated emotions, such as guilt and anger, that result from childhood sexual abuse and adult remembering can interfere with your sex life in some very specific ways. Survivors of childhood sexual abuse often have a difficult time trusting their sexual partners, even though they love them, because love was associated with pain when they were children (Russell 1986).

There may be physical symptoms as well. You may unexpectedly begin to have pain or have trouble lubricating your vagina when you try to have sex. You may experience vaginal muscle spasm called vaginismus; vaginal penetration during vaginismus is extremely painful or simply impossible.

In addition, more than 35 percent of women with abdominal and pelvic pain are really the victims of sexual abuse as children (Lechner et al. 1993). That is an astonishing datum. Nevertheless, the psychological and physical manifestations mentioned here can be from a variety of causes other than childhood abuse, so we urge caution in considering such sources.

Physical Vitality

You already know, from earlier chapters, many good reasons to remain physically active and in good physical health. Here is one more: If you feel good about yourself, concerns you may have about the aging process become less pervasive. The psychological lift from regular exercise may also be associated with increased sexual energy. Sexual desire can remain high if you feel good physically.

Routinized Sex

If you are in a long-term relationship, you and your partner may have spent years together making career decisions, raising kids, purchasing property, and negotiating family vacations. Your pattern of living as a couple is likely to have become routine. An element of tedium may now creep into the relationship as both of you become more predictable in your behavior and responses.

Sex is one area where these characteristics can arise. It may get boring. You know in advance what happens first, followed by what happens next, and concluding with what happens last. You may start thinking about your grocery shopping list during sex. If romance, sensuality, and intimacy are left out, sexual desire may wither. You may start blaming your slumping sexual desire on PMS or on perimenopause and diminishing hormone levels. You may blame your partner for your dampened desire. (You may be right if your partner is experiencing similar feelings about your humdrum sex life.)

To escape this situation, some women (and men) seek a new sex partner or turn more to self-stimulation. These methods of dealing with decreased sexual desire can lead to misgivings and feelings of guilt. (More on this topic later in the chapter.) To protect against this, another avenue is to try differing positions, lubricants, sexy lighting, music, and more verbalizing; allow your fantasies to lead you.

Self-Image

Another psychological challenge for women in the perimenopausal years is to resist the cultural stereotype of what constitutes a sexy woman. Worry about physical attractiveness quickly translates to worry about sexual attractiveness, and dampens desire. Your body is not like it was two decades ago. This is true of men, too, of course, but in many ways, they've been let off the hook: It is culturally more acceptable to be a man whose hair is thinning a bit on the top or graying around the sides and whose middle is growing than to be a woman with physical characteristics of mid-life. The media have finally begun to represent some women over forty as being romantic and having a sex life—although they usually don't have wrinkles, graying hair, reading glasses, or a few extra pounds. Your healthy sexual desire is intimately involved with your understanding that good sex is not dependent upon the superficial concept that a perfect body is required.

Your marital status may also affect your self-image. One study of late perimenopausal and early postmenopausal women showed a significant difference between married and single women (Cone 1993). Single women at mid-life reported less dismay with their body changes and regarded themselves as generally attractive. Married women reported a greater decline in sexual desire and interest. Frequency of sex was only slightly different for married versus single women: sixty-seven times yearly for marrieds, sixty-six for divorced, and fifty-five for never-married singles. These statistics appear to implicate committed relationships in promoting diminished desire.

Stress

If you are worried about a serious illness, a family crisis, or a financial problem, having sex may be very low on your agenda of important things to do. In situations like these, along with the other stress-related symptoms we described in Chapter 12, you may experience depressed sexual desire. Solving the problem usually restores your sexual desire.

Partner Availability

Dr. Gloria Bachman and co-workers (1991) found that many women without partners report that their sexual desire progressively recedes the longer they remain sexually inactive. The same appears to be true for women who have partners but have infrequent sex. You could say that partner availability is a problem for them too. There are some biological benefits related to sexual frequency, which we will discuss in a moment. Psychologically, the partner issue is an important one. Sexual desire, multifaceted though it may be, is dramatically influenced by your partner's interest in you sexually. For example, if your partner is having erection problems, he may be profoundly embarrassed by his diminished prowess and reluctant to display his incapacity. His interest in you sexually may actually be undiminished, but you may interpret this behavior as a symptom of disinterest. Your self-esteem may be damaged, causing sexual desire to plummet. (A number of other issues can be at the root of infrequent sex; good communication between you and your partner, which we discuss later in the chapter, is essential for dealing with them.)

Biological Influences on Sexual Desire

Along with the significant psychological factors we have described, a broad range of biological factors influence sexual desire. While these factors can have a potent effect on your desire, they are not nearly as influential as your sexual attitude.

What Is Sexual Response?

According to the landmark work of Masters and Johnson (1966) female response to sexual stimulation falls into four stages:

- **Sexual excitement:** Sexual excitement can begin in any number of ways—with fantasies, hugs, stroking, whispered endearments, X-rated movies, a full moon, a sunny day, a rainy day, a foggy day .... Your pelvic blood vessels dilate and congest the region with blood. Vaginal lubrication results, as very slick secretions pour out through your vaginal walls. Muscles throughout your body begin to tense.

- **Plateau:** In the plateau phase, your sexual arousal increases dramatically. Your clitoris, situated just below your pubic bone at the top of your outer genitalia, becomes enlarged from blood engorgement and exquisitely sensitive to being touched. The folds at the entrance of your vagina (labia) become swollen from blood engorgement. Your heart rate and rate of breathing have increased, and you may be perspiring. Your upper vagina becomes dilated and lengthened, while the muscles surrounding your lower vagina tense.

- **Orgasm:** This is the climactic moment, or moments, of sexual response. The physical and emotional excitement generated is maximized and you may feel compelled to relinquish your sense of control. Rhythmic contractions occur in your uterus and lower vagina. There may be multiple orgasmic peaks or a single intense one.

- **Resolution:** During resolution, pelvic vascular congestion promptly subsides. You are engulfed in a feeling of profound relaxation during which peace and warmth and closeness may be maximal. A few moments of hypersensitivity may occur occasionally in your vaginal lips, and particularly your clitoris, during which you are too sensitive to be further stimulated. Once this passes, repeat arousal and additional orgasms are possible.

This four-stage pattern of sexual response generally remains unchanged throughout life, although individual components may vary as time passes. What excited you sexually at twenty may be very different from what works a couple of decades later. Lubrication may take longer. Reaching an orgasm may also take longer, be less intense, and occur less reliably; and the intensity may change from rocket-like to Roman-candlesque. The number of orgasmic contractions may diminish. During your perimenopausal years, none of these may be an issue. If they are, as a result of the psychological factors and biological changes we have been talking about, there are many steps you can take to manage them. As for those postmenopausal years down the road, take comfort in knowing that women at any age can enjoy sex. Keep reading to learn more

Better Sex Through Chemistry

There's no question that hormone levels and sexual desire are linked. Women generally have a higher level of sexual interest at the midpoint of their cycle, when production of estrogen, progesterone, and testosterone is at its peak. (Of course, nonhormonal factors, such as low self-image, may interfere with this beneficial effect.) Chapter 8 was devoted to the topic of hormones. Here we look specifically at their links to sexuality.

The Role of Male Hormone

A 1985 study on sex hormones (Sherwin) reported on a group of women who had undergone menopause with surgical removal of their ovaries. The women were randomly divided into four groups, each to take one of four types of medication: estrogen, testosterone (both of which are normally produced in the ovaries), a combination of estrogen and testosterone, or a placebo. Each woman was asked to rate the intensity of her sexual desire before and after their surgery.

The groups on testosterone alone and estrogen plus testosterone reported an increased level of desire, arousal, and sexual fantasizing. The groups on estrogen and those taking a placebo did not. Testosterone, according to this study and others since, appears to be the driving hormonal force behind sexuality, influencing your sexual desire, motivation, and sexual fantasies. By contrast, estrogen's role is more closely connected to physical aspects of sexuality, such as vaginal lubrication, other arousal responses, and orgasm (Sarrel 1990). Estrogen mediates these responses through receptor sites on the nerves that supply your vagina, clitoris, and other pelvic structures. This study and others have resulted in the use of testosterone to boost female sexual interest and fantasizing (Cohen 1994).

As we mentioned earlier, sexual problems from lowered hormone levels are not common during perimenopause, but there are exceptions: If your ovaries have been removed or if you are taking low-dose birth pills during perimenopause, you may need a testosterone supplement to maintain normal levels of sexual desire.

The Role of Estrogen

If your sexual anatomy is normal, your physical response to sexual stimulation will generally be unimpaired. The primary anatomic problems, if there are any during perimenopause, come from declining estrogen availability. The functioning of your clitoris, vulva (outer visible genitalia), vagina, and uterus are dependent upon estrogen support. As you know from earlier chapters, when estrogen is withdrawn, these structures undergo atrophic changes. These changes can have an adverse impact on the effectiveness of sexual arousal and pleasure.

Your vagina may be the first to complain of estrogen decline. As estrogen diminishes, blood supply your pelvic anatomy does as well. This causes thinning of your vaginal lining and a reduction in mucus production. Long before your doctor can see any evidence of thinning, you may notice a reduction in moisture. Your vagina may produce less lubrication and feel dry. After menopause, if you take no preventive measures, these changes can become more extreme. Your vagina can eventually lose up to 90 percent of its thickness, as well as its elasticity (Sachs 1991). Attempting to have sex if you have a thin, inelastic, shortened vagina can be extremely painful.

Vulvar changes from estrogen deficiency are slow and subtle also, and mainly postmenopausal. The skin covering of both the outer and inner folds (labia) of the vulva become thin and inelastic. Fatty tissue under the vulva is lost, and the labia appear shrunken. There is less pubic hair. Vulvar dryness may cause a very itchy condition, called pruritis.

With estrogen depletion, your uterus, including your cervix, also shrinks over time. In rare cases, painful uterine contractions occur during orgasm. In addition, your clitoris will have fewer functioning nerve fibers because of a diminished blood supply and it will be less sensitive to stimulation.

Other estrogen-related changes can also interfere with your sex life. For example, if hot flashes are depriving you of sleep, you may be too tired to enjoy sex. Your sensory perceptions may also be altered; estrogen level is a factor in the sensitivity of skin nerves.

Don't panic over all this information. The changes we've described are slow to develop; they may not become bothersome until after menopause. And if you provide your genital anatomy with estrogen when appropriate, these atrophic changes may never be a problem. Don't just jump into a tub of estrogen, though. There are better ways to manage these changes, as you will see.

Other Drugs

Dopamine is a neurotransmitter that is instrumental in testosterone production for both genders. Commonly used to treat Parkinson's disease, dopamine has been noted to increase sexual arousal, although there hasn't been much study of this effect (Notelovitz and Tonnessen 1993). This suggests that in the future other nonhormonal drugs may be found to be effective for improving sexual arousal and desire.

Medical Illness and Your Sex Life

A major physical illness at any age can affect both your interest in having sex and your physical ability to do so. If the illness is temporary, desire usually returns when you start feeling better. However, some chronic diseases may have long-term effects:

- **Arthritis and orthopedic problems:** Joint pain and reduced range of motion from arthritis and other orthopedic problems can interfere with the mechanics of having sex. Experiment with different positions, strategic use of pillows, and sensuous hot baths to accommodate your disability. (That might be interesting even if there are no orthopedic problems.)

- **Chronic heart or lung disease:** If you have severe heart or lung disease, you may be fearful that having sex can be dangerous to your health. In fact, this concern can come up in terms of any disease that makes you physically unfit. It may be helpful to know that the energy required is about the same as climbing two flights of stairs. Sex, of course, is generally a lot more fun.

- **Diabetes:** If poorly controlled, diabetes causes loss of orgasmic ability in about one third of women within four to six years after diagnosis of the disease (Reichman 1996). It pays off sexually to take care of yourself if this disease is diagnosed. In addition, diabetes in a man can cause impotence, which can drastically reduce sexual encounters for you.

- **Hypothyroidism:** Because hypothyroidism (which we talked about in Chapter 6) can cause profound fatigue and depression, it can also seriously dampen sexual interest and your ability to reach an orgasm.

Sex after Surgery

The major problems in the area of sex posed by major surgery are generally not that you will lose sexual capability through surgery; that seldom happens. The problems lie in what that surgery may do to your self-esteem and body image. For example, some women feel, after a hysterectomy, that they are no longer whole because they can no longer reproduce, and their partners may feel the same way. In addition, you (or your partner's) negative assessment of your body after surgery can undermine your self-esteem and depress your sexual desire.

If you have a hysterectomy, it may temporarily dampen desire because of postsurgical tenderness in your vagina. If this surgery results in shortening of your vagina (unlikely unless it is radical surgery for cancer), this may make sex feel different for a few weeks, until stretching takes place. Some investigators feel that the cervix functions as a trigger for orgasm in about 10 percent of women and that uterine contractions are an integral part of orgasmic pleasure (Helstrom 1994). In spite of uterine loss, however, women who had good sex preoperatively still had it postoperatively. In addition, surgical removal of both ovaries (oophorectomy) cuts off your major source of estrogen and testosterone. Sexual desire may plummet if testosterone is not replaced.

Disfiguring surgery, such as a mastectomy or a colectomy followed by colostomy (removal of the colon and diversion of fecal material through the abdominal wall into a collecting receptacle) can have potent negative effects on self-image and desire. Surgical reconstruction of a new breast often helps in diminishing post-mastectomy emotional turmoil. Fortunately, more and more breast cancers are being treated by lumpectomy (removal of a cancerous lump with conservation of the breast) a less drastic measure.

Later in this chapter you'll find some suggestions for dealing with issues like these.

Medications and Alcohol

A variety of prescription and over-the-counter medicines, while helping one type of health problem may be detrimental to your sexual health. Antidepressants (Prozac, Nardil) and tranquilizers (Valium, Tranxene) can relieve your stress in some ways, but they may create another stressful problem by blunting your sexual responsiveness. Beta blockers (Lopressor, Timolide) are effective for lowering high blood pressure, but in up to 50 percent of women and men who use beta blockers in high doses, they lower sexual desire and the ability for arousal and orgasm (Drugs . . . Dysfunction 1992).

Antihistamines do a good job of drying up a drippy nose or congested sinuses, but they may also cause vaginal dryness and decreased sexual lubrication. Selective serotonin reuptake inhibitors (SSRIs—see Chapter 4) such as Prozac may cause a decreased sexual desire in 30 percent of users of either gender (Drugs . . . Dysfunction 1992).

Alcohol can also cause sexual problems. It is well known to lower inhibitions, which may make you feel like you are about to be a sexual Olympian. However, arousal levels are actually lowered in about 40 percent of intoxicated people of both genders in spite of their feeling sexually uninhibited (Reichman 1996).

Some Keys to Good Sex

The perimenopausal years, and the entire process of aging, do not preclude your need for intimacy and sexual pleasure; these are lifelong. But unless you make the effort to understand and cope with the changes in your body, your sex life may suffer. Let's look at some ways that can help you cope.

Communication

Communication is more than mere talking. Communication involves being understood and understanding in return, but communicating about sexual issues is often not easy. You may talk about it, read about it, see references to it on TV, and watch it on videotape. But that does not help your ability to communicate about the more important sexual issues, such as caring, sharing, intimacy, and personal preferences for sexual satisfaction. However, partners who do discuss sexual issues (what feels good, what doesn't, erection difficulties, lubrication) can do a great deal to resolve sexual problems.

In a recent lecture (1997), psychiatrist Jeanne Leventhal stated that all humans tend to think that other people think the way they do. If your own sexual desire decreases, for whatever reason, you may think your partner feels the same way. Instead of making assumptions like this one, communicate. That way, each of you knows how the other feels, which can help avoid damage to your relationship.

In *Making Sense of Menopause,* author Faye Kitchner Cone presented guidelines for improving your ability to communicate. She called this "getting your verbal juices flowing." To effectively communicate about a problem, you must be patient, caring, open, and avoid a self-centered approach. The principles involved are as follows:

- Enlist your partner as a fellow problem solver. Agree in advance that your goals are to improve mutual satisfaction and harmony. This gives you an agenda and a common goal. Cooperation in the pursuit of a common goal will promote a sense of intimacy.

- Find out more about your partner's sexual needs and preferences. It may be true that your unsatisfied needs and preferences are the reason you have convened this committee of two. Nevertheless, if you have shown an interest in your partner's needs, this unself-centered approach can result in your partner becoming more sensitive to, and inquisitive about, your needs. In addition, you may learn some things about your partner's preferences that vary considerably from your previous impressions.

- Don't be confrontational. The last thing you want is to turn this into an argument, so don't ambush your partner with your pet grievance: "I fake orgasm because you fake foreplay." Drawing a line in the sand does not serve your purposes. Instead, make your partner feel safe in talking to you. Be evenhanded and explain that you are interested in making your sex life satisfying for you both. Keep in mind that this needs to be a dialog, not a lecture.

- Regard this as a process, as opposed to an event. Your newly formed committee of two may need to be convened several times to accomplish your mutual goal. This attitude of a process is especially important if your first attempt at communication stumbles and bumbles a bit. You have too much riding on resolution of your differences to gamble on a single all-or-nothing conversation. If you need to table the discussion for a better time or a more appropriate setting, decide on a time to resume. In the meantime, both of you will have time to think. Total agreement may not be a realistic possibility; but compromise is a wonderful way to come together.

- Nonverbal communication works too. The primary goal of this communication process is not mere talking, valuable as it might be, but rather that you and your partner are meeting each other's needs. If either or both of you are aware that a positive change is needed, you may be able to communicate this by altering your approach to having sex. For example, buy a new teddy, burn scented candles, take a warm bath together, introduce lubricants, or try new verbal expressions during sex. Then depend upon positive or negative feedback for deciding whether or not to keep your innovations on the menu.

In communicating with your partner, the obligation you both have is to be receptive to new thinking and suggestions, be sensitive to personal preferences, and be nonjudgmental. Avoid canned speeches; communicate from your heart.

Maintaining Vaginal Moistness

As we've pointed out, after age forty, you may notice slightly less abundant secretions in your vagina. Penetration during sex may become uncomfortable. By your mid- to late forties, this may have progressed to a sense of dryness, with painful sex. After menopause, if your vaginal lining has atrophied, the dryness can be even more accentuated.

Regular Sexual Activity

Masters and Johnson (1970) noted an interesting exception to the scenario we just described. Their research showed that women who experience sexual stimulation on a regular basis, about twice weekly, do not lose their vaginal secretions or sexual lubrication. Self-stimulation appears to work just as well for this purpose as sex with a partner, and the study showed this was true for women well into their sixties. Masters and Johnson coined the phrase "Use it or lose it," which has since been used for advice on everything from athletic prowess to government funding.

Lubricants

Lubricants, even if you are on hormone supplements (see the next section), are often helpful. Some women are reluctant to use sexual lubricants because they feel somehow defeated by having to admit the need for them. They can make a big difference in your sexual enjoyment, and your partner's. Try introducing a lubricant as part of your sex play, and use it on your partner as well. There are many water-based commercial products available, including Astroglide, H-R Jelly, Today Personal Lubricant, K-Y Jelly, good old reliable saliva (not sold in stores) also works. One drawback of the above water-soluble lubricants is that they dry quickly; you may need more than one application. Vegetable oils (right out of your kitchen) last longer and work well as lubricants.

CAUTION! Avoid lubrication with petroleum-based products like Vaseline. They weaken latex condoms and may mask the signs of vaginal infections.

A longer-lasting lubricant alternative is a vaginal suppository (Lubrin) that melts in your vagina and lasts about three hours, so it simulates natural secretions. A better method is to restore the secretions themselves. In estrogen deficiency, your vagina produces fewer secretions, which alters the acid-base balance (pH) and reduces your normal acidity. You can restore normal acidity by using a vaginal moisturizer (Replens, Gyne-Moistrin), which stimulates production of natural secretions. These products are about the same consistency as hand lotion and have bio-adhesive qualities that make them last about three days (Notelovitz and Tonnessen 1993).

Hormones If You Need Them

You know that hormone production gradually declines during perimenopause. As we've discussed, perimenopausal women often wait to use HRT until late in the transition. Still, if you are plagued with perimenopausal symptoms that, in turn, are blunting your sexual desire, supplementing your flagging estrogen levels now may be helpful. Chapter 8 discussed the possibilities, which include low-dose birth control pills, patches, and hormonal creams. You may also need to take a testosterone supplement to enhance your sexual desire if you use the Pill.

Vaginal Conditioning

As a transitional women, you may be confronted with a sexual dilemma. On the one hand, your capacity for having sex may be robust, your ability for arousal undiminished, and emotional maturity may have given you confidence in initiating sex. On the other hand, in spite of this, your frequency of having sex may be diminishing. Studies show that the rates of having sex gradually decline for women and men from age twenty to forty. After forty, the decline accelerates. It is common for women in their late thirties to have sex about sixty times per year, but a decade later, the frequency is halved (Cone 1993).

The change from frequent to infrequent sex can sometimes create problems. The work of researchers like Masters and Johnson and others has demonstrated that the amount of vaginal moisture and sexual lubrication you produce are related to sexual frequency. As estrogen levels decrease, vaginal secretions diminish, but regular sexual stimulation prevents this, even without estrogen supplements. Women in their sixties who have had regular sexual stimulation about twice per week can often lubricate their vaginas naturally.

The keyword here is stimulation. It doesn't have to be intercourse; other techniques, such as masturbation and nonvaginal sex with your partner, can work just as well. (See the next section.) Using a dildo or vibrator can also stimulate secretions. Sexual excitement, regardless of its origin, stimulates blood flow to your pelvic organs, including your vagina. This keeps your ability to produce normal secretions intact. Because you utilize the same muscles whether sex consists of intercourse or an alternative technique, they benefit as well. Using a dildo can also prevent your vagina from losing its surface toughness. This helps prevent the kind of soreness you may notice when you resume having sex with a partner after a period of abstinence. The bottom line is that like other parts of your body, your vagina needs regular workouts to stay in shape; but you don't have to go to the health club to do it.

Kegel exercises are a good addition to your vaginal workout. These exercises were introduced in the early 1950s by Dr. Arnold Kegel, a urologist (Kegel 1951). The original purpose was to help control a type of involuntary urine loss called stress incontinence. Sex therapists soon discovered that it is also beneficial in improving sexual sensitivity and vaginal muscular control. Kegel exercises improve the strength of the pubococcygeus (PC) muscle that forms the floor of your pelvis and surrounds your urethra, vagina, and anus. You can teach yourself how to contract your PC muscle by stopping the flow during urination, or by placing two fingers in your vagina and contracting around them. The exercise consists of squeezing your PC for 5-10 seconds, then slowly relax it, wait 10 seconds and repeat. Do a set of about 10 15 repetitions and work up to 3-5 sets per day. Sexual improvement derives from doing "flutter" Kegels. Here you just squeeze, squeeze, squeeze as fast as your can during each set. You don't need to be passing urine or have your fingers in your vagina to do these exercises, of course, so you can work them into some of your daily routines: standing in line, on an elevator, at traffic lights, phone call on ignore, someone attractive happens by...you get the picture. Kegel exercises also help men to achieve firmer erections and maintain better control during sex; let your partner know.

Partner Availability

We all have lifelong needs for caring, sharing, and intimacy. These factors contribute to our normal desire for sex with a partner. Life circumstances, such as divorce, separation, disabilities associated with aging or illness, relationship problems, death, may result in your being without a suitable partner or with sharply reduced opportunities to have sex. These situations may not diminish your interest in sexual gratification. There are a number of methods to deal with this problem:

- **Masturbation:** Masturbation is a way to experience pleasure and discharge sexual tension if you do not have a partner or are not sexually active with your partner. You may have been brought up to feel guilty about self-arousal, but there are significant benefits to this healthy and harmless sexual practice. In addition to stimulating vaginal secretions, sexual release is well-known to dissipate the harmful effects of stress. Self-stimulation can also increase your understanding of your sensuality and promote better sex with a partner.

- **A change in partners:** In the transitional stage of life, many women experience a loss of partners, often as a result of death or divorce. Some women choose a new partner after events like these. A new partner can be a potent source of renewed sexual energy. If you decide to seek out another partner, your priorities in terms of choosing a partner may have changed. Social acceptability, financial stability, and suitability of the candidate as the father of your children may no longer be your primary concerns. You may simply be looking for someone whose company you enjoy and with whom you have pleasurable sex.

- **Nonvaginal sex:** If you and your partner are looking for alternatives to vaginal sex because of pain or discomfort, oral sex is a pleasurable method to both give and receive satisfaction. Mutual masturbation is another option that satisfies the need for closeness and relief of sexual tension.

Touching

We all need to hug and be hugged, to caress and be caressed, from infancy to advanced old age. Touching is thought to have a critical influence on mental health and our sense of well-being. Some researchers believe that this is mediated through the endorphins (Kaverne et al. 1989). So warm hugs (lots of them) are important to your health; and they say volumes about how you feel toward your partner. Tactile stimulation can certainly lead to great sex, but this does not need to be the goal or inevitable end point of the activity. Touching is satisfying on its own.

Timing Is Everything

Make time for sex. You may have children at home, a household to manage, a job to look after, a busy social schedule, community and political obligations, soccer players to transport . . . . Not only may you lack the energy for sex, you may not have the time for it. Just remember that when the frequency of sex declines, so does your desire for it. Try making an appointment—well, call it a date—with your partner. You may find yourselves "dating" a lot more after the first one or two. It also might be worth reexamining the responsibilities that keep you too busy for sex; you might want to rearrange your priorities.

Another useful technique is to try sex in the morning or midday. A good night's sleep will do a world of good for your fatigue, so you may have a lot more energy for sex in the early part of the day.

Sex Therapy

The common human trait of difficulty in discussing sexual matters has contributed to making sex therapy a growth industry in the U.S. If you have tried communicating, lubricating, masturbating, dating, hormones, and more, but nothing is working, now is the time to bring in some third-party help. A sex therapist can give you a whole new perspective. Most sex therapists are licensed psychologists, social workers, or psychiatrists (Landau et al. 1994). Being a sex therapist requires specialized education and licensure, so be sure to see someone who is properly credentialed. Many are not.

Before you decide on a sex therapist, take an honest look at the root of your problems as a couple. If bad sex seems to be resulting from poor

communication and disagreements about nonsexual issues, a marriage counselor may be a better choice for resolving your differences. If you still can't
agree, or are unable to decide the major source of your difficulties, a psychologist might be a better choice to help you sort it out. (Your psychologist
may even also be a sex therapist!)

Summary

Sexual activity and sexual pleasure are experiences for which you have
a lifelong capability. It is an inescapable fact that living your life will bring
change to your anatomy and to your physiology, which can also bring change
to your sexuality. It is also a true that the major controlling factor in sexual
enjoyment is your brain. (Your body may be the orchestra, but your brain
is the conductor.) With the cooperation of your brain, you can take advantage
of a number of well-proven techniques that favorably influence the anatomic
and physiologic changes that time imposes on your body and lead to enjoyable sex. With a healthy attitude, you can express this vital core of your
emotions and your humanity for as long as you live. You may experience
your sexuality as an expression of love, as a fountain of erotic pleasure, as
a means of communicating your desire for caring and intimacy, as a private
island where problems cease and pleasure is maximal, and/or as a time of
total acceptance., Regardless of how you experience it, there is no reason
your sexuality cannot flourish as the years pass. Good sex will not disappear
unless you allow it to.

○ ○ ○

14

Looking Good While Changing: Skin Care, Hair Care, and Cosmetic Surgery

Cultural demands often hold women to an unrealistic standard of youth and beauty. But don't worry—this is not one of those "how-to-stay-young-for-ever-no-matter-what" chapters. It simply offers suggestions for helping you present your best image—the one that makes you feel good—so you can move on to other matters in your life. If you're happy to let the natural signs of aging progress without interference (and many women are), feel free to skip this chapter.

Change has been the topic of this book, and that theme continues here, as we address changes in your appearance during perimenopause. The passage of time is unstoppable, of course, but there are ways of coping with it. Let's look at the causes and prevention of appearance changes that occur over time, as well as some treatment suggestions.

Skin

Alphabet Soup	
AHA	alpha hydroxy acids
MED	Minimal Erythema Dose
SPF	Sun Protective Factor
UV	Ultraviolet

The earliest visible signs of aging come in your body's largest and most public organ: your skin. You may not have known your skin is an organ, but it is, and it serves many important functions. Among other things, it contains one fourth of your entire blood supply, about two million sweat glands, and many more nerve endings.

First and foremost, though, it covers you up. Your intact skin is a barrier to invasion of microorganisms; it transmits sensations, both pleasurable and painful; and it is vital to regulating your body temperature. It also functions as part of your immune system and is replete with blood vessels, glands, nerve endings, connective tissue, and fat cells. Like other bodily organs, your skin changes with the years, but some of the adverse effects are avoidable and treatable. Let's start by considering its components.

A Bit of Biology

Figure 14-1 is a schematic of your skin's normal architecture. On the right side you will notice there are three layers bracketed: epidermis, dermis, and subcutaneous tissue. Skin consists of those first two layers. The third layer is made up mostly of fat. The epidermis is the layer you can see, and the dermis is the infrastructure, the dermis is the life support system for the visible part of your skin. Distributed through the dermis are blood vessels, nerves, oil (sebaceous) glands, sweat glands, and hair follicles, which are all supported by connective tissue fibers called collagen and elastin. The dermis transports nutrients to the epidermis; whatever happens there has an effect on your skin's surface appearance.

Your epidermis is made up of the five sublayers (each called a stratum or layer) noted on the upper-left side of Figure 14-1. These are the layers from which you get a continuous resupply of new skin cells. The new cells are generated by the germinal layer (also called basal layer), and gradually work their way to the surface where they die and are sloughed off. Transit time from the germinal layer to the stratum corneum takes on average about four weeks in adults. In children it only takes about two weeks. So you get a new skin about once per month. This means that whatever your skin looks like today reflects what you did for it, or to it, last month.

The appearance of your skin is influenced by both internal and external factors. The influence from within revolves around how well it's microcirculation of blood is working to bring necessary nutrients. Also by whether or not those nutrients are adequately supplied by your diet. Externally your skin is subject to various environmental influences such as ultraviolet damage from sunlight, weather conditions (hot, cold, humid, dry, windy), and pollutants. Fortunately, normal, healthy skin has many defenses for the hazards to which it may be exposed. It is constantly guarded by specialized cells that alert the general immune system to an invasion by bacteria, viruses, and other intruders. Your skin can also produce antioxidant molecules, which neutralize free radicals and prevent them from damaging skin cells and the collagen support matrix. In addition, your skin is a semipermeable structure that regulates the flow of water out of your body and helps prevent dehydration. In spite of these defenses, your skin is still a fragile organ and susceptible to major changes from the inevitable processes of aging.

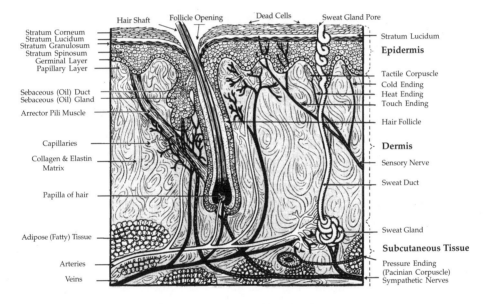

Source: Gerson, Joel, "Milady's Standard Textbook for Professional Estheticians." Rev. Ed. 1992; Milady Publishing Co.

Figure 14.1. Normal Skin Architecture

The Aging Process

Aging in cells throughout your body appears to be genetically programmed at birth. Each of your trillions of cells has DNA strands in its nucleus on which genes are located. The genes control a variety of cellular metabolic activities, including how frequently the cell will reproduce itself and how long it will live. For skin cells, as we mentioned, that's about one month. As aging occurs, genes are altered and the genetic messages are gradually changed. Cells throughout your body slow down the process of division into new cells. Cells throughout the body also diminish hormone production and production of the nearly three dozen growth factors necessary for new cell formation. (We discuss growth factors in a moment.)

What Causes These Changes?

There are several theories about what causes our bodies, including our skin, to age, including:

- **Genetic programming:** We just discussed this factor. Planned obsolescence seems to be part of the grand plan of nature. Plants and animals start from seeds, grow to maturity, reproduce, and then decline. Your skin is a reflection of this process.

- **Hormone and growth factor depletion:** Diminished production over time of hormones and other growth stimulators, called *growth factors*, slows cellular metabolism. (Aging cells have fewer receptor sites to which growth factors can attach, so the cells slow their metabolic activities.) The slower metabolism changes the appearance and function of tissues, including the skin. Hormones, as you know, are biologically active chemical messengers. Growth factors are also biologically active protein peptides; they act as intercellular messengers. At present, there are five known skin growth factors. They are produced by cells and accumulated on cells, where they direct the cell to perform certain functions, such as reproducing itself or increasing its metabolism. Like hormones, growth factors attach themselves to receptor sites on the cell surface and direct the action from there. The greatest drop in growth factor production is after age forty, and the most visible sign is in your skin (Notelovitz and Tonnessen 1993). As a result of diminished cellular activity, as well as the accumulation of photo damage, both of which diminish collagen and elastin, lines and wrinkles appear.

- **Free radical damage:** Free radicals are unstable molecules, and Chapter 10 discussed the mischief they cause. Exposure to free radicals over time causes damage not only to the cell membrane, but also to the DNA and genes in the cell nucleus. The DNA-damaged cells reproduce DNA-damaged daughter cells, and this leads to aging and malfunction, whether it is in your skin, brain, cardiovascular system, or any other part of your body. This can cause skin to visibly, and sometimes dramatically, age.

Actual Skin Changes

Visible skin changes actually begin slowly in your twenties, but the process speeds up and tends to be more noticeable in your mid-thirties (the start of your transitional years). It is finally out in the open that ultraviolet (UV) rays from the sun cause 75 to 90 percent of wrinkling, unnecessary aging, and dry skin with mottled pigmentation (Roenigk 1995). It is also a direct cause of skin cancer. The sun's UV rays penetrate through your epidermis into the dermis, much like an X-ray. The damage actually starts in childhood, but it is cumulative, and the damaging effect doesn't begin to be visible until you are in your late twenties to early thirties. The effect on your epidermis is overall thinning and creation of fine, dry lines, although the stratum corneum layer may vary in thickness with the development of solar keratoses. These are individual patches of skin thickening resulting from sun damage. In the dermis, UV radiation reduces your skin's collagen network, which makes your skin thinner. With less collagen, there is less space for your skin to hold water, and it loses its plumpness. UV light also damages elastin, resulting in skin that doesn't bounce back as well when stretched. As the damage continues, fine lines eventually become deep wrinkles.

It is now known that UV rays cause immunosuppression (a suppressed immune system) in your skin. In such an unprotected state, the free radicals released by the inflammation of sun exposure are unchecked in their attack on collagen, elastin, cell membranes, and the vital DNA elements of the cell nucleus. As a result of cellular damage in the basal layer, skin growth becomes irregular, which causes an uneven skin surface. Wrinkling, age spots, darker pigmentation, and enlarged and visible capillaries all become apparent in sun-damaged skin. As we mentioned in Chapter 2, this process is called photoaging. A suppressed immune system in the skin is also associated with melanoma (the most dangerous form of skin cancer) in 90 percent of people who develop it.

Chronic sun exposure causes a breakdown of the collagen fibers in your skin, which results in thinning of the epidermis. (Look at the difference in the skin thickness on your face and on a part of your body that doesn't get exposed to the sun.). Here's what happens:

- **Skin cells:** The number of cells in the basal layer of your epidermis decreases, and those still left are slower to divide; regeneration slows. It takes more time for cells to migrate from the basal layer of your epidermis to the surface. Sun damage reduces the overall thickness of your epidermis, but the number of dead cells in the outermost sublayer (stratum corneum) increases. These dead cells are therefore present for a longer period of time, which can dull your skin's appearance. More pigmentation accumulates, giving the skin a discolored look.

- **Oil and sweat glands:** These glands become less effective, so your skin becomes drier. It may get scaly or develop cracks.

- **Collagen and elastin:** The amount of collagen and elastin in your skin decreases. These connective tissues in the dermis comprise more than 90 percent of your skin's bulk between the ages of twenty to forty.

(Reichman 1996). Collagen gives your skin plumpness, and elastin gives it, you guessed it, elasticity. You can get a good idea of how these elements are working in your skin with a simple test: On the back of your hand, pinch some skin and raise it up. If your skin is young, when you release it, it springs back into position almost more quickly than you can see it. Older skin, with diminished collagen and elastin, takes much longer. (Another example is that as your skin loses some of its elasticity, your face doesn't bounce back as readily as it used to in the morning. If you slept all night on your face, those pillow lines won't disappear as quickly.) In addition, the loss of collagen and elastin contributes to thinner skin and one of the hallmarks of older skin: wrinkles!

- **Fatty tissue:** Fatty tissue under the dermis breaks down. This further reduces the thickness of your skin and may change the angles and contours of your face. Loss of fatty tissue combined with thinner skin can make your bony structures more prominent, in contrast to the rounder face of your youth, and make skin veins more prominent as well.

- **Microcirculation:** As microcirculation decreases, the blood supply to your skin is reduced. Skin can become less glowing and look less healthy. Your skin gets cold more easily because of the diminished circulation—unless you're having a hot flash, of course.

As these deteriorating conditions progress, the initial change is usually some fine smile lines about the eyes. Eventually, radial wrinkles, which some dermatologists and estheticians call lip stitches, form around the mouth. You've got about twenty-five years between smile lines and radial wrinkles, so there is plenty of time to take preventive measures.

Skin Abuse

In addition to the normal results of aging, there are many ways you can unintentionally abuse your skin. Pinching pimples may be a longtime habit, but it can leave scars. Scrubbing your face roughly or removing your makeup with wild abandon can also damage your skin; the same is true of tugging the skin around your eyes when you use eye pencils. Most facial tissues are made from wood pulp, which is abrasive. A better plan is to use a dry washcloth or cotton balls to remove your makeup. It treats your skin gently and still removes surface skin debris.

Neglecting your skin falls in the category of abuse. Failure to use a sunblock is a good example. Moisturizers are a must if you are to avoid drying and premature aging. (You'll find out more on these products later in the chapter.) Neglecting to remove makeup at night will cause clogged pores, skin eruptions, and unhealthy looking skin.

Habitual squinting and frowning can also cause wrinkles—the ones that make you look like you're squinting and frowning! You're going to get some wrinkles no matter what, so why not make them smile lines?

Skin Care from the Inside

The condition of your skin is a fair barometer of how well you are treating your body. If you have been neglecting your overall health, your skin may tell the tale.

Diet

You probably already know what we're going to say. Your diet should be balanced, which means rich in fruits, vegetables, whole grains, and complex carbohydrates, as we described in Chapter 10. On the other hand, a high animal fat intake is bad for your cardiovascular system; but contrary to popular belief, dermatologic research has shown that it has no negative effect on your skin. Neither a high-fat nor a low-fat diet in acne patients makes a difference in their acne (Fulton 1996). The same is true of a diet rich in sweets. On the other hand, chronic dieters who are not getting adequate fat or protein commonly experience dry skin and dull hair; your skin likes your diet balanced.

Fluids

Good hydration is essential for smooth, healthy skin. Fluids are stored in the spaces between collagen fibers in the dermis. This aids in maintaining the plumpness of your skin. It takes about two quarts of water consumption daily to meet your skin's needs (Eskin and Dumas 1995). You can buy commercial skin moisturizers, but you you'll achieve the same effect just by drinking water.

Alcohol

Alcohol dehydrates your body, which you now know is bad for your skin. Chronic alcohol abuse causes dilation of skin capillaries, particularly on the face and nose. Alcohol also interferes with your ability to absorb B vitamins, which are important to your skin's ability to heal itself.

Smoking and Drug Abuse

Smokers typically get radial wrinkles around the mouth and wrinkles on the outer part of the eyes. Nicotine causes blood vessel constriction, resulting in diminished oxygen and transportation of nutrients to your skin. That encourages wrinkles; cigarette smokers often have wrinkles equivalent to those of women more than a decade older. Smokers also have an earlier decline of estrogen production, which has a deleterious effect on collagen formation in the skin, leading to more wrinkles. Smokers also have poor healing of injured skin, which also contributes to the appearance of aging.

Drug abuse is one of the worst skin abusers because of the dietary and personal grooming neglect that may accompany such a lifestyle. It not only ages you faster, but you will look drawn and haggard while you age.

Skin Vitamins

Several vitamins are important to your skin:

- **Vitamin A:** This vitamin keeps your skin soft and prevents scaling and drying. It also is an antioxidant, so it protects your skin cells and collagen from free radical damage. In addition, vitamin A appears to be one of the co-factors necessary to collagen production (Ojeda 1995).

- **Vitamin C:** Because vitamin C is an antioxidant and is essential for healing, it has an important role in prevention of photoaging. Duke University researchers report that vitamin C plays a major role in prevention of sun damage by controlling the resulting inflammation (Darr et al. 1996). The inflammatory response to sun exposure causes release of free radicals, which damage skin constituents, including collagen and elastin. This effect has not been confirmed by other studies.

- **Vitamin E:** This is the main antioxidant vitamin for collagen protection.

- **B-complex vitamins:** The B-complex vitamins assist in tissue repair and prevent skin scaling and cracking.

Regular Exercise

Regular exercise is a major stimulant to blood flow, which contributes to vibrant-looking skin. Some experts believe that a vigorous workout does more to enhance blood flow and transport nutrients to your skin than the various creams, masks, and facials now available for these same purposes (Notelovitz and Tonnessen 1993). It is less expensive, too.

Skin Care from the Outside

There are some effective external techniques for improving your skin's health and for treating damage you may have already sustained. Some techniques involve making simple behavioral changes. There are also some new products on the market that do more than just cover up your skin problems cosmetically. These products stem from newer research in the late 1980s and early 1990s into the fundamental reasons that skin deteriorates and from a more pharmaceutical approach to dealing with the underlying causes (Leverette 1991). The goal of some of the new skin-care products is to prevent damage and to heal it. External skin care doesn't have to be time consuming, expensive, or complicated, but it should be consistent.

Protecting Against Sun Damage

Skin reactivity to sunlight exposure varies from person to person. Knowing which type of skin you have allows you to take appropriate protective measures when you are exposed to the sun:

- **Type 1:** Always burns easily, never tans; very fair skin, red hair

- **Type 2:** Always burns easily, sometimes tans; light skin, blond hair

- **Type 3:** Burns moderately, tans gradually; light brown skin, darker hair, like brunette

- **Type 4:** Burns minimally, always tans; olive skin, usually Asian or Mediterranean

- **Type 5:** Rarely burns, always tans; moderately pigmented brown skin, black hair

- **Type 6:** Never burns, heavily pigmented; black skin, black hair

Since skin damage from sun exposure occurs over the long term and is generally irreversible, sun protection is vital to prevention of photoaging. There are several steps you can take.

One of the simplest techniques is simply to avoid the midday sun. The most intense rays are from 10:00 A.M. to 3:00 P.M., from March to October. You can even get indirect exposure sitting in the shade, riding in a car, and on a cloudy day. Reflections of the sun on snow and water can also send UV rays your way. Another common-sense technique is to wear protective clothing. A broad-brimmed hat, long sleeves, and wide sunglasses offer good protection.

Using a sunscreen or sunblock is another important preventive measure. According to dermatologists, the words sunscreen and sunblock are interchangeable, no matter what the label claims. These products are rated by a system called Minimal Erythema Dose (MED). This refers to the length of time it takes for your skin to turn pink when exposed to the sun. Sun Protective Factor (SPF) is an indicator of how much increase in MEDs you get when using a particular product, the higher the SPF, the fewer MEDs reaching your skin. All sunscreen products absorb UV light, but some of it still gets through to your skin. Apply a sunscreen or sunblock about half an hour before you go out, or you will not be as protected as the product specifies. For everyday protection, an SPF of 15 is adequate, as long as you reapply it every two hours during sun exposure, no matter what it says on the label. The SPF you select should, of course, depend on which of the above skin types you have. Even heavily pigmented skin burns if exposed to sun for long periods of time. If you are near the water, at a high altitude, or close to the equator, double the strength of your sunscreen. A new field in sun protection is under investigation that involves the use of vitamin C. This will be discussed later.

Skin-Care Products

You skin is rather resistant to chemical penetration, but it is not impervious. Applying certain products to the skin can achieve internal effects. The estrogen skin patch, which we described in Chapter 8, is a good example. This bit of information has spawned a huge industry in skin-care products. When you select a product, read the label carefully. The first ingredients listed are the ones that will do you the most good. The farther down the list an ingredient appears, the less likely that the product supplies a significant amount of it. In general, the fewer ingredients the better. Try to avoid products that contain fragrances, artificial colorings, and especially, alcohol. Some of the claims made by manufacturers of skin products are simply hype, but many can be effective. Let's examine some of the choices.

Cleansers

Mild soap and water may be the only cleanser your skin needs. Some manufacturers of skin products would like you to believe that you need a cleanser, but you probably don't. If you have sensitive skin (such as eczema), that results in dry, flaky skin, a cleanser can help remove the excess skin debris. Manufactured cleansers in liquid, cream, bar, and gel form commonly contain varying combinations of water, allantoin, propylene glycol, urea, aloe vera, and other products to remove dirt, grease, and makeup. Some cleansers contain alpha hydroxy acids in varying strengths to assist in removal of dead skin debris. (You can find inexpensive nonsoap cleansers in pharmacies and department stores.)

Toners

A number of different toners are on the market, but you probably don't need to use a toner at all. Most of them are mildly astringent and recommended for use on oily skin, especially around the "T" zone of the nose. Toners can actually irritate your skin, and they cause a rash in some women with sensitive skin. Soap and water works just as well as a toner to degrease your skin and is a lot cheaper.

Moisturizers

Moisturizers can be very helpful for perimenopausal skin that has become somewhat thinned from collagen loss and therefore holds less moisture. Moisturizers are made up of two components: humectants, which are substances that attract and hold water (glycerin, glycol, sorbitol, gelatin), and occlusives (also known as emollients), which seal water in your skin (mineral oil, lanolin, petrolatum). Moisturizers have their effect on the epidermis, but their molecules are too large to penetrate the dermis, so no benefit is derived at that level except for helping to prevent water loss (Idson 1992). The available products vary in texture from light (slightly watery feel), to medium (lotion feel), to heavy (butter-like). The grade that works for your use depends, among other things, on the oiliness of your skin, the climate, and the season of the year. Cleanse your skin before applying a moisturizer. An ideal time for a moisturizer is after your bath or shower when your skin is still damp (McCallion and Li Wan Po 1993). Moisturizers can also be the base for your makeup since they last most of the day, and all you need is an occasional touchup (Hayman 1996).

Some moisturizers contain urea, a protein breakdown product that is a component of urine. Egyptians in ancient times used this substance as a moisturizer. (Just think, you and Cleopatra can have something in common—the same moisturizer!)

The existence of alpha hydroxy acids (AHA) has been known for many years, but in the late 1980s, skin researchers demonstrated their benefits to skin (Leverette 1991). AHAs are derived from fruits—for example, tartaric acid from grapes, malic acid from apples, citric acid from citrus fruit, and lactic acid from sour milk. A widely used AHA called glycolic acid comes from sugar cane. Most AHA products contain between 5 and 15 percent glycolic acid. If you use much higher concentrations, do so only under the direction of a dermatologist.

AHA products work by resurfacing your skin (Stiller 1996). Glycolic acid and other AHAs penetrate the stratum corneum of your skin and break up the buildup of dead skin cells that make your skin look dull and unhealthy. As your skin sheds these cells, areas of irregular pigmentation are also often reduced or eliminated, as well as irregularities in your skin contour, such as reduction in the depth of fine lines. This leaves a fresher-looking skin.

Glycolic acid also allows for more rapid regeneration of new cells, and it helps empty your pores of skin debris, which is an aid in acne control. When combined with sun protection, skin resurfacing with glycolic acid can aid in reversing some of the damage aging skin has suffered and in preventing further deterioration. Your interests are best served if you start a glycolic acid regimen under the supervision of a dermatologist or an experienced esthetician. Maintaining the improvements may require long-term use; you can implement a home treatment plan of glycolic acid in the strength your skin specialist recommends.

It may take three to six months to achieve maximum benefits with home use. At a 1995 meeting on cosmetic dermatology sponsored by Northwestern University, dermatologist Dr. Lawrence S. Moy confirmed his positive experience with glycolic acid at the UCLA Medical Center. When used in lower concentrations (5 to 20 percent), as in products for salon or home use, a longer period of use is necessary for improvement. The effect appears to be cumulative, though, so slow progress is okay. Dermatologists use higher glycolic acid strengths, of 50 to 70 percent to deal with deeper wrinkles and to allow the acid to penetrate into the dermis, where collagen formation is stimulated. Deep chemical peels, which we talk about a little later in the chapter, are one way to administer higher-strength glycolic acid. The results are more rapidly accomplished than with home use, but skin irritation is more severe.

Tretinoin

Tretinoin (Retin-A, Renova) is a vitamin A derivative applied in a lotion, cream, or gel directly to the skin to exfoliate (remove) dead cells from the stratum corneum. Its primary use has been for treatment of acne, but it also speeds up the turnover of dead surface cells, so it can also be helpful for perimenopausal skin (Eskin and Dumas 1995). Progress is slow, but it does provide cosmetic improvement after a few months. One drawback is that your skin may become irritated or extremely sun sensitive, which means you have to strictly avoid direct sunlight.

CAUTION! Do not take tretinoin during pregnancy. It has caused delayed fetal bone mineralization in laboratory animals. Studies on humans have not been conducted.

Topical Vitamin A

Vitamin A has well-known beneficial effects on the skin. Dietary vitamin A may be adequate; but if your skin's microcirculation is decreased, adequate amounts of the vitamin won't get there. Like hormones and other nutrients, vitamin A can be delivered through your skin in sufficient amounts to improve the skin's condition. Applied topically as a cream, it improves the microvascular (capillary) system and delivery of nutrients to your skin (Idson 1993). But vitamin A benefits do not stop there; vitamin A is an antioxidant, so it also prevents free radical damage to the collagen-elastin network, which prevents thinning of the skin. There is evidence that it stimulates the growth factor receptor sites on skin cell walls. This generates more rapid cell growth and thus a healthier skin, with less buildup of dead surface cells (Sies et al. 1992). Results are visible in three months, and you reach the maximum effect in about six to nine months.

CAUTION! High doses of vitamin A can be dangerous, as we discussed in Chapter 10. A toxic dose would be 12,000 IU of vitamin A per 25 pounds of body weight taken in a single dose, or 60,000 IU in a 130-pound woman. Toxic symptoms include dry, peeling skin, headache, blurred vision, altered mental status, jaundice, and possible hair loss (Olson 1994). Few investigators believe that enough vitamin A can be absorbed through your skin to do damage, but if you combine it with a daily vitamin supplement, you may exceed the safe levels of this vitamin (Notelovitz and Tonnessen 1993).

Topical Vitamin C

A number of researchers are studying skin application of vitamin C to understand its antiwrinkle benefits (Radd 1997). Oral vitamin C is known to promote collagen production by tissue cells, a major deterrent to wrinkling (McCallion 1993, Tajima 1996). Topically, vitamin C is absorbed and acts as a potent antioxidant to prevent oxygen free radicals from damaging skin cells and collagen (Idson 1993). According to one study, it also reduces photo-damage caused by both UVA (alpha) and UVB (beta) radiation in sunlight (Nakamura et al. 1995). When vitamin C is combined with vitamin E in a sunscreen, the photoprotective benefit may be even more enhanced (Darr 1996). More research is needed to determine how best to take advantage of this photoprotective effect if it truly does exist (Lewis 1996). Some companies are already using vitamin C in makeup and sunscreen lotions. If you use a vitamin C preparation on your skin, be sure it is L-ascorbic acid, the only form of vitamin C your body recognizes. Once it has penetrated into the skin, it lasts about three days and cannot be washed away.

Topical Vitamin E

Vitamin E's main value to your skin is its potent antioxidant effect, which protects collagen from free radical damage. It is available in some commercial skin creams, and you can buy it in capsules. Just penetrate the capsule with a pin and pat a few drops on fine wrinkles on a daily basis.

Topical Growth Factors

Growth factors are specialized protein polypeptide molecules, which are key elements of all living cells (Sporn and Roberts 1991). Growth factors attach to receptors on the cell membrane, and from that site they direct the cell to adopt new metabolic activities and to proliferate. The result is epidermal cell renewal and/or wound healing if the skin has been injured. In either situation, active cell division and formation of new collagen and elastin fibers are essential. There are thirty-five known skin cell growth factors. Five are known to be involved in skin growth and healing, including the epidermal growth factor (EGF). Researchers have been able to create EGF with bioengineering techniques, and it is now contained in a number of skin-care products. But a controversy exists as to whether just one or a complex of all five skin growth factors must be present for skin to benefit. Skin studies suggest that all the growth factors must be present in their natural homeostatic balance (MacKenzie and Sauder 1990). At this point, the necessary balance has eluded bioengineering capabilities; so most of the available products manufactured contain only EGF. At this point considerable doubt exists as to the usefulness of these products (Glick et al. 1994).

A Routine for Daily Care

You can incorporate a few simple practices into your daily schedule to ensure that your skin stays healthy over time.

Daily Facial Care

You can achieve good facial skin care in only a few minutes each day. In the morning there may be no necessity for cleansing your face, if you have done it before retiring. Just stimulate your skin with a cold washcloth and pat dry. Then apply a moisturizer if you have dry skin and put on any makeup you wear. During the rest of the day, you don't need to do anything but, perhaps, touch up your makeup. Remember to use a sunblock before putting on your makeup if you will be out of doors. In the evening, use a cleanser (a makeup-removing one if necessary), and apply a moisturizer before going to bed. Some skin experts recommend using a moisturizer with AHA for your bedtime application (Brumberg 1977).

Daily Hand Care

Even if you have a young-looking face, your hands can tell a lot of tales. If you wash them frequently or they are often wet during the day, the consequence can be dry skin. For washing, use a mild cleanser, such as Dove or Neutrogena transparent soap. Apply a hand cream every time after you wash your hands. (Lotions and oils are not as effective as hand creams.) Just keep some cream handy at all your sinks. Using a cream only takes a few seconds, and you should notice improvement in just a few days. At night, apply a moisturizer before you climb into bed. You can use the same one you use for your face, but cheaper ones, such as Lubriderm, Alpha Keri, and Neutrogena skin oil will also work quite well. If you have liver spots, those irregular brown pigmented areas, glycolic acid–laced moisturizers will help them fade, as long as you also use a sunscreen when you are outside (Leverette 1991). As discussed above, UV exposure is the primary cause of these discolored skin areas.

Daily Body Care

Taking a bath, especially a long hot soak, can dry your skin. Try to keep those luxurious soaks to a minimum; save them for when you especially need to relax or as a treat. Particularly if you have dry skin, try adding a half cup of sesame or almond oil or a capful of Sardo or Neutrogena bath oil. Caution is justified in using bath oils because they cause skin allergies in some women. Use a mild cleanser that is nonalkaline (meaning no mineral salts such as sodium bicarbonate): Dove, Neutrogena, Cetaphil, and Aquanil are examples. During your shower, try rubbing a loofah sponge (a coarse sponge made of horse hair) vigorously over your skin from the neck down to help remove dry and dead cells from the surface of your skin; using a loofah also increases circulation of blood and tones your skin. After your bath, pat your body dry and use a moisturizer all over your body, including your feet, while you are still slightly damp. This helps retain the moisture in your skin.

We tend to overwash in the U.S. (Hayman 1996). In the winter, when the weather is cold and blustery and you've turned up your heating system, your skin can become much drier than during the other seasons. Showering or bathing only adds to the problem. Try taking a shower every other day, with a sponge bath in between to minimize the drying effects of washing away your skin oils.

Hair

In your perimenopausal years, you can expect your hair to become thinner, drier, more brittle, and less shiny. To top it off, white and gray hair becomes coarse and doesn't reflect light the same as pigmented hair, so it can look dull. Why do these things happen?

Each of your hairs is made up of a number of plates, which are composed of hard keratin (called scleroprotein) that is also the primary constituent of nails. (Soft keratin is the main component of the dead surface cells of your skin.) The keratin plates are situated close to each other and give a hair shaft its strength. As you get older, the number of plates deposited in each growing hair declines, as cells in the hair follicle become less active. The plates don't adhere as well to each other, which makes your hair more brittle and inclined toward split ends.

Hormone changes also influence the condition of your hair. Normal estrogen levels make your hair lustrous by promoting oil production from skin glands, and androgen promotes hair growth. As estrogen declines, you secrete less oil in your scalp, resulting in drier hair that appears dull. During estrogen decline late in the perimenopausal years or after menopause, androgen production does not decrease at the same rate, so there is relatively more male hormone influence. This is the cause of increased facial hair. Hair loss at this time of your life is the result of loss of hair follicles due to aging, not to male hormones.

Another adverse influence is the cumulative effect of many years of perms, straightening, blow-drying, and coloring if peroxide is used as part of the coloring process. This contributes to a dry, brittle appearance. Fortunately, since you will grow six inches of hair every year, any damage done to your hair can be reversed with time.

To reverse or control these changes, estrogen replacement can be helpful if you are deficient in that hormone. Experts also recommend the following principles of routine hair care:

- Avoid washing daily if you blow-dry. Blow-drying your hair every day can be very drying. Every three to five days is usually sufficient, although daily washing of bangs is OK. If you have very oily hair, you may have to wash your hair each day to look presentable. Try to use lower heat, and hold the dryer farther from your head.

- Use a mild shampoo (no alcohol, and with emollients such as panthenol) that won't dry out your hair. Concentrate on using the shampoo on your scalp and the roots. If you avoid washing the ends, there is less drying. They will be adequately cleansed when you rinse.

- Use a conditioner or a cream rinse every time you shampoo. Conditioners penetrate the hair shaft, which softens your hair while adding nutrients and shine. Cream rinses are not as penetrating, but they provide a light conditioning, detangle your hair, and still give it shine.

- Dry your hair carefully. Use a wide-toothed, hard rubber comb (metal breaks the hair) to gently detangle your hair. Tangling is lessened if you brush out your hair before getting it wet. Ideally, you should allow your hair to at least partially dry on its own. If you towel dry, avoid vigorous rubbing, which can damage your hair. Hold your hair dryer at least six inches away from your head to avoid heat damage and dried-out hair shafts.

- Avoid harsh chemicals. Peroxide, ammonia, and alcohol are drying. Panthenol, a vitamin E extract, is a welcome addition to any hair product because it acts as a moisturizer. Many plant extracts, such as pectin, are good for your hair for the same reasons (Hayman 1996).

Gray Hair

As time passes, the pigment-producing cells in your hair follicles begin to falter, and graying gradually results. This is one of those immutable facts of living. If you decide to go gray, be aware that your hair is more coarse and brittle in this state, so be sure to use moisturizing conditioners. To prevent yellowing, a violet-toned shampoo is ideal. On the other hand, if you decide to defer having gray hair, a couple of options exist. A process called low-lighting (the opposite of highlighting) can accentuate the natural coloring of your hair. Low-lighting involves selective coloring of your natural hair in a deeper shade. Ask about it at your salon. With salt-and-pepper hair, low-lighting enhances the pepper aspect while improving texture (Hayman 1996).

The other option is total coloring. There are two types of coloring available: permanent and semi-permanent—the so-called rinse that washes out after a few shampoos. Before you decide to color your hair, it's a good idea to use a rinse to see whether you like the color. Coloring your gray hair changes its texture by changing the surface characteristics, making it more manageable.

If you choose to color your hair, try not to perm it as well. For coloring to work, the cuticle (outer coating) of the hair shaft is broken down to allow the coloring agent to penetrate into the center of the hair. This weakens hair. A perm works much the same way, and combining these two procedures can result in significantly weakened hair, which can break off at the scalp and leave you temporarily very short of hair, as in mainly bald. Some people develop allergies to the coal tar pigment in the dye, especially black dye, which seems to be much more allergenic than other colors (Fisher 1995). Color rinses, which are not as penetrating as total coloring, do not jeopardize your hair strength.

Unwanted Hair

As estrogen decline progresses and your androgen influence increases, you may notice more hair on your upper lip, chin, nipples, and abdomen below your navel. This occurs very gradually and is not harmful, but you may find it objectionable from a cosmetic standpoint. Estrogen replacement will help prevent this if you are deficient in that hormone, but there are other methods for dealing with it too:

- **Shaving:** The most basic way to remove hair. The problem is that you may need to shave every three or four days.
- **Bleaching:** Using over-the-counter preparations to bleach the hair can camouflage it.
- **Plucking:** Plucking out the unwanted hairs out by their roots lasts longer than shaving.
- **Waxing:** Waxing also pulls hairs out by the roots. Like plucking, it is somewhat painful, but it gets the job done faster than plucking one hair at a time.
- **Depilatories:** These are chemical creams for removing hair. They do a good job, but occasional skin allergies occur. It's best to test the cream on a small patch of skin before widespread use.
- **Electrolysis:** This process uses electrical current to destroy hair follicles. It is a tedious and painful process, but it lasts longer than other methods. If the unwanted hair is being caused by hormonal shifts, electrolysis is not a permanent solution, and you may need to repeat the procedure every few weeks or months.

Veins

Spider veins and varicose veins are common cosmetic complaints in transitional women. Spider veins are those bluish-reddish veins that appear just below the skin surface. They are flat to the surface, and harmless. If you want to remove them, though, you can take advantage of a technique called sclerotherapy, in which a concentrated solution of salt water or other irritant is injected into the vein to produce internal vein wall scarring and cessation

of blood flow. Sclerotherapy is usually done by dermatologists, general surgeons, and plastic surgeons. It leaves a whitish blemish less noticeable than
the original veins. New spider veins can still form, so you may need more
than one treatment.

Varicose veins result from the failure of small one-way valves in the
vein. These valves prevent backflow of blood between heartbeats and ensure
that blood flow continues back to the heart. When the vein loses its elasticity
and dilates, these valves become incapable of preventing backflow, and blood
tends to pool by gravity in dependent parts of your body, like your legs and
sometimes the vaginal labia. Varicose veins are raised, bulging, and serpen-
tine-shaped, with a bluish hue. In addition to a dull ache, they may cause
the rate of blood flow to decrease, which encourages clotting. When a clot
(thrombus) forms, it can become inflamed, resulting in a painful condition
called thrombophlebitis. The risk in this situation is that a portion of the clot
can dislodge and be carried to your lungs, resulting in a life-threatening problem called a pulmonary embolism (blood clot in the lung). Treatment for
thrombophlebitis involves heat, rest, elevation of the leg, and use of antico-
agulant (anticlotting) medications.

The tendency to develop varicose veins may run in some families. They
also tend to occur during pregnancy and with prolonged standing, as a result
of tight-fitting garments (like some knee-highs), in overweight people and
those with sedentary lifestyles, and from the habit of crossing your legs. Once
varicose veins have formed, there is no simple treatment. Surgical removal
is effective, but it leaves multiple small scars. Surgery does not prevent new
varicose veins from forming. Prevention is the best game in town, and you
can achieve it by following these guidelines:

- **Wear support stockings as often as you can:** If you are at risk for
developing varicose veins (family tendency, overweight, prolonged sitting and standing, multiple pregnancies), support garments can be
helpful. These days, support panty hose look sheer, so you can wear
them and still look fashionable. There are even summer-weight support
stockings for really hot days. Good-quality support knee-highs also
help and do not cut off your circulation.
- **Exercise:** Be sure to exercise your legs regularly (walking, cycling,
swimming, aerobic workouts).
- **Elevate your legs:** Raise your legs higher than your hips periodically
during the day.
- **Avoid prolonged sitting, standing, and crossing your legs:** Crossing
your legs obstructs circulation, as does prolonged sitting, and standing
allows blood to pool in your legs.
- **Avoid becoming overweight:** Extra weight puts extra pressure on
your veins.

Keep Smiling

By the time you become transitional, your teeth may show stains from years of coffee or tea drinking or from smoking. You may want to do something about getting rid of these stains. Tooth-brightening toothpastes may help a little, but some of them are very abrasive and can damage your tooth enamel. Cosmetic bonding by your dentist of new material over your teeth works well to hide the stains, but it is expensive. A less expensive technique involves the use of a whitening gel. Your dentist can make a plastic tray from impressions of your upper and lower teeth. The gel is placed in the trays, and you wear them in your mouth overnight for about a week.

Periodontal disease is the most common cause of tooth loss during perimenopause (Eskin and Dumas 1995). The problem is created by the build-up of plaque—a colorless film—on your teeth. If you don't remove plaque by flossing, using tiny brushes between your teeth (called proximate brushes), and/or visiting the dentist, the plaque hardens into tartar (calculus). Bacteria in your mouth become incorporated in the hardened plaque and irritate your gums. This results in loss of gum tissue and the supporting structures of your teeth. Pockets of infected tartar eventually develop below the gum lines and start destroying the bone tissue. With less and less support, your teeth start loosening and can eventually fall out. Don't forget to visit your dentist twice a year; having your teeth cleaned professionally reduces your risk of tooth loss and gum disease.

An additional important dental precaution during perimenopause is to make certain your calcium intake is sufficient. Your jaw bones can become osteoporotic, just like bones elsewhere in your body. (Chapter 5 describes your calcium requirements.)

Cosmetic Surgery

More and more American women are opting for the "last resort" procedure of plastic surgery. Women with smile lines, frown lines, wrinkled necks, protruding tummies, and broad hips are hearing the siren call of the quick fix. Record numbers of Americans are undergoing facelifts, eyelid revisions, facial resurfacing, tummy tucks, breast implants, and body contouring with liposuction. The American Academy of Cosmetic Surgery (Podolsky and Streisand 1996) estimates the number at more than 1.5 million annually. A wide array of procedures is available. These procedures often work; but they are expensive and not without risk. The cost can be very dear both financially and in terms of the effects of potential complications. The overall complication rate is low, in the range of 2 percent, but this is just an average. As with any other surgery, when you have cosmetic surgery you are at risk for complications from anesthesia, infection, bleeding, allergic reactions, and scarring; these operations are not a simple quick fix. In addition, most cosmetic surgery is not covered by health insurance; check with your insurance carrier or HMO before you decide to have any procedure.

If you are considering having a doctor perform plastic surgery on you, be sure to get answers to these questions:

- **Are you board certified in plastic surgery?** You can get this information by examining the doctor's diploma on the wall or by asking. You can also call the American Board of Medical Specialties at (800) 776-2378. Certification requires special training and completion of a rigorous examination by peers who are qualified in the specialty.

- **What are the possible complications?** This information should be laid out to you explicitly and in terms you understand.

- **How many operations such as mine have you done?** Experience with the proposed procedure is some assurance that you will obtain the desired result.

- **Is it likely I will need more surgery?** Touch-ups and redoing an undesirable outcome are common. Find out if there is a charge for it.

- **Do you have before-and-after pictures?** The results on other patients may be important to you in making your decision. Just remember that good results on someone else are no guarantee for your own outcome.

- **Will you be doing my surgery?** Don't settle for a conference with an associate or an office nurse. In teaching hospitals, resident doctors in training may be scheduled to do your surgery under the supervision of your doctor. If this is objectionable to you, say so.

- **Where do you have hospital privileges?** The answer to this question not only tells you what type of hospital, it tells you that this doctor has been reviewed by peers on the hospital staff. Such reviews look at a doctor's record of competence and proper indications for the surgery performed.

- **Will this be an office operation?** If so, find out whether the office operating suite has been accredited for ambulatory surgery. Ask your doctor, or call the American Association for Accreditation of Ambulatory Surgery Facilities at (847) 949-6058.

According the to American Academy of Cosmetic Surgery, women who ask for plastic surgery mostly want to be rid of varicose and spider veins and have smoother faces and trimmer bodies (Podolsky and Streisand 1996). The remainder of this section gives you a brief look at the menu of cosmetic options. As you read it over, keep in mind that many of the procedures we describe are not permanent. The initial benefit may last for only a few years or, in some cases, only months. If general anesthesia is involved, you run the same risks as for any other operation. Further, if your surgery turns out to be disappointing, you may be stuck with it. The only answer is more surgery, again with no guarantees. The benefits can be astonishing, but do not take lightly the decision to try it.

Chemical Peels

The purpose of a chemical peel is to remove the outer layers of skin from the face, neck, chest, hands, arms, and legs with acids (Chemical Peeling 1994). In the process, fine wrinkles are also removed. Estheticians do peels with mild concentrations of glycolic acid, which we talked about earlier in this chapter. A series of treatments is usually required. For severe acne or sun-damaged skin, stronger concentrations of glycolic acid are necessary. Deep wrinkles require stronger acids, such as phenol, salicylic acid, or trichloracetic acid. Dermatologists and plastic surgeons can perform these peels. It takes three to five days to recover from the skin redness of a superficial peel with low concentration acids, and up to a month from a deeper peel because of swelling, blistering and crusting that occur with stronger concentrations of acid. Your face will be reddened after deeper peels, and this may take three months or more to fade. A chemical peel makes your skin very sensitive to the sun, so be very careful about sun exposure until your skin returns to normal. Stronger peels occasionally result in permanent lightening of the skin and can lead to irregular pigmentation.

Chemical peels do not remove loose or sagging skin. (That's what a face lift does.) They also do not remove deep scars and may not change pore size in skin. The cost varies from $1,000 to $6,000.

Dermabrasion

Dermabrasion, or removal of the top skin layers using high-speed rotary wheels, can also remove fine wrinkles and soften acne scars wherever they appear on your body (Epps and Stuart 1995). Recovery takes about two weeks, and redness fades in three months. You must observe strict sun avoidance for several months, until the pigment has returned to your skin. The effect is permanent—until new wrinkles form. Plastic surgeons and dermatologists perform dermabrasion. Costs run from $900 to $5,000.

Plumping

Plumping involves injections of commercially prepared collagen from pig skin or from fat (removed from your hips or thighs) beneath the skin to fill out wrinkles and depressions. The procedure is also used on lips to make them fuller (Epps and Stuart 1995). These injections do a good job cosmetically, but they only last a few months to a year, so they don't take the place of good skin care. Risks include allergic reactions, lumpiness, and infection. Costs for collagen range from $300 to $1,500, and for fat from $200 to $2,000.

A plumping method introduced in 1991 involves mixing collagen with your own plasma to create a substance called plasmagel or Fibrel. Some are reluctant to try this method because of fears associated with the need to have their blood processed and reinjected into their body. The effect is said to last 1 to 2 years (Brumberg 1977).

Botulinum Toxin Injection

Botulinum toxin is the same toxin seen in the type of food poisoning known as botulism. It has been used since 1991 to treat frown lines and furrows in people who habitually scowl (Brumberg 1997). If you scowl habitually, your facial skin eventually adopts permanent furrows. The botulinum toxin paralyzes your frown muscles for about three to six months. During this time you are unable to frown or raise your eyebrows. Extremely tiny doses of the toxin are used, so there is no systemic effect elsewhere in your body. During the paralysis, some women have their frown creases treated with laser resurfacing (discussed below). Costs range from $250 to $500. It's probably better just to concentrate on keeping your face more relaxed.

Laser Resurfacing

Laser resurfacing is a newer alternative to the chemical peel or dermabrasion. It uses a carbon dioxide laser beam (Brumberg 1997). The beam vaporizes the first few layers of skin, and they are replaced with new skin. This procedure also causes some collagen shrinking, which produces a tightening effect. Laser vaporization is effective in removing fine lines and smoothing out deeper wrinkles (Alster and Garg 1996). It is also used to treat stretch marks, birth marks, acne scars, sun-damaged skin such as in the cleavage area, and to remove tattoos. Like peels and dermabrasion, laser resurfacing does not take the place of a face lift; it cannot deal with sagging muscles. Following treatment, your skin will be swollen and reddened for up to a month, and three months may be necessary for a complete return to normal.

If the vaporization is too aggressive, scarring can result (a 1 to 4 percent risk). Weekly cortisone injections soften the scarring if started immediately upon its appearance. Pigment changes may leave you with a raccoon appearance if the treatment is confined to your eyes. According to Dr. Thomas L. Roberts III, a plastic surgeon at the University of South Carolina who introduced this technique in 1995, around 10 to 20 percent of patients develop dark skin patches about a month after treatment. If started early, Retin-A treatment can clear up these patches in about six weeks (Podolsky and Streisand 1996).

Since laser resurfacing is a relatively new modality for cosmetic skin improvement, qualified plastic laser surgeons may be hard to find. For a referral to a board-certified laser surgeon, call the American Society for Dermatologic Surgery at (800) 441-2737. You can also write to the American Society for Laser Medicine and Surgery at 2404 Stewart Square, Wausau, Wisconsin 54401.

Eyelid Lift (Blepharoplasty)

A blepharoplasty is a surgical procedure to correct droopy lids and remove puffy bags. It removes excess skin and fat and repairs sagging muscles (Eyelid Surgery: Blepharoplasty 1993). The procedure generally takes between one and three hours.

An eyelid lift will not remove your smile lines, eliminate dark circles under your eyes, or lift sagging eyebrows. Incisions are made along the natural creases of your upper lids and just below the lashes in the lower lids. Bruising and swelling afterward make you look like you've been in a brawl. Most people can use makeup to disguise residual bruising and be back in public in one to two weeks. Avoid strenuous activity for three weeks after surgery to reduce the risk of bleeding and disruption of the operation. If the drooping is not severe, consider using laser vaporization instead, to treat fine wrinkles.

Certain medical conditions can make blepharoplasty riskier. These include hypothyroidism, hyperthyroidism (Grave's disease), insufficient tearing, high blood pressure, cardiovascular disease, and diabetes. Complications can include temporarily blurred or double vision, asymmetry, difficulty closing your eyes, and rarely, damage to the eye with blindness. If the repair is too aggressive on lower lids, you may have more exposure of your sclera (whites of the eye), creating an unnatural, staring look.

Upper lid surgery can only be done once because of the limited amount of skin available for removal, but occasionally a repeat operation can be done on the lower lid. Results last several years, and for many people the results are permanent. Costs range from $2,500 to $5,000.

Forehead Lift

A forehead lift is a one- to two-hour operation designed to raise drooping brows, minimize forehead lines, soften frown lines above the nose, and improve drooping skin at the outer part of your eyes (Podolsky and Streisand 1996, Face Lift 1994). The classic method uses an incision across the top of the head, a few inches inside your hairline, but another technique, endoscopic surgery, is also available. Gynecologists have used the endoscopic technique (called laparoscopy) for years to do pelvic operations, and general surgeons use it when removing a gallbladder or an appendix. This technology has recently been expanded to apply to cosmetic surgery. The endoscope is a hollow tube with fiber-optic lighting that is inserted beneath the skin of your forehead through a tiny incision inside your hairline. Surgical instruments are introduced through other small incisions. The surgeon can either look through the endoscope to do the operation or attach a small video camera and view it on a monitor. When the skin is freed up from beneath, it is pulled up, excess skin is removed, and the remainder is attached by sutures or to nonmetallic screws embedded above the incision which are removed in the office after a week or so. A forehead lift lasts about five to ten years.

Post-operative bruising can persist for two to three weeks, but you can get back to everyday activities, such as going to work, in seven to ten days. (Avoiding strenuous activity prevents postoperative bleeding or breakdown of the operation.) You may also have temporary numbness and swelling of your forehead. Risks include injury to the facial nerve, which can cause muscular weakness or an asymmetrical appearance. If you have had previous eyelid surgery, a forehead lift may not be a good procedure for you; it can result in stretching your upper lids, preventing you from being able to completely close your eyes. The cost can range from $3,000 to $6,000.

Face Lift

A face lift is a two- to four-hour operation that eliminates sagging skin and jowls by removing excess fat, tightening muscles, and rearranging the skin (Face Lift 1994). It is commonly said that a facelift takes five to ten years off your facial appearance, but it is probably more realistic to say that it will make you look good for your age. The usual incision starts just inside the hairline in the temple area, passes in front of the ear, and extends backward to the nape of the neck. The facial skin is pulled upward and backward, and the excess is removed. Endoscopic techniques eliminate the large incisions that used to be necessary. A face lift does not eliminate lip lines or smile lines around your eyes. Additional methods like laser resurfacing must be employed for those improvements, but they can possibly be done at the same time as a face lift. Postoperative bruising and swelling fade in two to three weeks, which is about the time you will need to be off work. You must avoid strenuous activity during the recovery period to prevent disruption of the operation. The results last about five to ten years.

Facial nerve injury is a risk, with resultant muscle weakness. This is usually temporary, although it can be permanent. A face lift may also change your hairline. Costs range from $5,000 to $12,000.

Liposuction

Liposuction is a method of contouring the body by removing fat deposits from various areas (Podolsky and Streisand 1996). The procedure involves inserting a tube through small incisions and vacuuming the fat away. It can be used on the face, abdomen, thighs, buttocks, and many other places where you have stored fat. Swelling and bruising may take one to six months to fade, but return to normal nonstrenous activities can be in one to two weeks. (Vigorous activity too soon after liposuction may cause bleeding under the skin.) Blood loss can be quite heavy with liposuction, so some women donate their own blood prior to surgery in case replacement is needed.

Results can be excellent; the fat is gone for good—unless you replace it with a high-fat diet. (You manufacture new fat cells if your diet overloads your existing cells with fat.) However, liposuction is fraught with such problems as skin numbness, rippling skin surfaces, baggy skin, lumpiness, uneven pigmentation, scarring, and asymmetry. Depending on the operation, it can cost from $2,500 to $9,000.

Tummy Tuck

Pregnancies and significant weight loss can create a droopy belly. A tummy tuck removes fat, tightens up your abdominal muscles, and removes excess skin (Surgery of the Abdomen 1993). The conventional incision is a large one running from hip to hip below the bikini line, but once again, the new endoscopic techniques avoid large incisions. Fat is removed by liposuction, and muscles are tightened through the endoscope. If you are planning to lose weight, it is a good idea to do so before your surgery because there will be less need for liposuction and because your good recovery requires good nutrition. You will also tolerate your surgery better and recover more quickly if you are in good physical condition.

This operation takes about two to five hours and requires about a month of recovery. Major complications, such as accumulation of blood clots and thrombophlebitis, occur in 1 percent. About half are plagued with minor problems, such as prolonged fluid accumulation under the skin, lumpiness where not enough fat was removed, temporary numbness, or a navel that is slightly out of position (Wilson 1992). Touch-up procedures to get it all right are common. The results of a tummy tuck are permanent. It will cost about $5,000 to $8,000.

Breast Implants

The issue of breast implants is extremely controversial, from both medical and legal standpoints. You are probably aware of class action lawsuits involving a wide array of claims of bodily harm resulting from implants, but not everyone agrees that they are to blame. With so many contradictory claims, deciding on whether to have breast implants is not an easy decision.

The operation involves placing saline-filled silicon sacs under your breasts, or under your chest muscles, to augment the size of your breasts (Breast Augmentation 1993). Other fillers, such as safflower oil, are also being used on an investigational basis. Newer methods utilize small incisions in the armpits or navel to insert deflated sacs, which are then filled when in position. Breast implantation is an outpatient operation that requires two or three days of recuperation.

A common complaint is hardening around the implant from scar tissue, called a capsular contracture. Also, implants sometimes rupture from trauma or leak and deflate. After a few years, most implants must be removed or replaced. If your breasts are also sagging, a breast lift may be recommended in addition to the implants. Cost of the breast implants varies from $4,500 to $8,500.

Breast Lift

Sagging of your breasts is an inevitable consequence of time and gravity. Altitude can be restored by a breast lift (Breast Lift 1993). The best candidates for a breast lift are women who have small breasts. Heavier breasts can also be lifted, but the result is not as long lasting. In this 1½- to 3½-hour operation, an anchor-shaped incision is made that follows the natural contour of your breast. The nipple is isolated, excess skin is removed, and the nipple is replaced at a higher position. Suturing the incision edges together raises your breasts and makes them firmer. There will be stitches around your nipples, as well in a vertical line below them and along the crease beneath your breasts. You can resume normal activities in about one week, except for strenuous activity, which you should avoid for a month. Breast lifts are not recommended for women who intend to breast-feed in the future because milk ducts may be damaged by the surgery.

The scars are initially quite visible but fade in about a year. Potential complications include loss of nipple sensitivity, asymmetrical breasts or nipples, and skin loss if healing is not normal. Permanence of the result varies with such subsequent events as pregnancy, weight gain, and effects of the aging-gravity duo. Cost is $3,000 to $9,000.

Breast Reconstruction after Mastectomy

Women who have suffered the loss of a breast to cancer sometimes choose breast reconstruction for cosmetic reasons (Love 1995). The operation relocates muscle tissue to the mastectomy site to create a breast mound. The muscle used is a broad back muscle called the *latissimus dorsi* or an abdominal muscle called the *rectus abdominis.* The operation detaches the end of the muscle farthest from the mastectomy site and draws it under the skin to the proper location on the chest wall, where it is formed to resemble a breast. A nipple is then made from skin of the leg or labia and attached. When the abdominal muscle is used, a tummy tuck is sometimes done at the same time to strengthen the abdominal wall. In spite of the strengthening, some women have postoperative problems with abdominal wall hernias. Breast reconstruction is a bigger operation than implant surgery, but it avoids the issue of silicon implants, and the resulting breast mound of living tissue has a more normal feel and appearance. Breast reconstruction for replacement following cancer is not considered cosmetic and is therefore covered by insurance.

Summary of Cosmetic Surgery

Before you invest your money and subject your body to cosmetic operations, think it over carefully. Surgery won't cure your depression or solve problems with self-esteem. On the other hand, if there is something you really hate about the way you look, like droopy eyelids or your breast size, consider the options we've described, but be a smart consumer. Do some reading about the various ways your problem can be fixed. Have a consultation with someone qualified to do your surgery, and don't forget to ask the questions we suggested earlier. You may be offered a "blue plate special," that includes not only a basic face lift operation, but also adjustments to smile lines, a lid lift, and reshaping your cheek bones with implants. If so, turn it down and find a plastic surgeon who is more attuned to incremental progress. You may be happy with the result of just a single procedure and save yourself the prolonged recovery and expense of a big reconstructive overhaul. Think of yourself as a person who is going to have a serious surgical operation; you are not a lump of clay that just needs to be nudged into better shape.

Summary

This chapter has dealt extensively with the cosmetic effects that aging and lifestyle may have on your body. It has given you suggestions and tools to modify or modulate the changes to which you may be subjected. You can pick and choose among them or ignore them entirely; just make sure your choice makes you feel good about yourself.

○ ○ ○

15

Gynecologic Surgery and Medical Treatment: When the Unexpected Happens

You're finally ready. You've had every lesson you could take. You can finally ski down the fall line (that's "straight down the hill," for you nonskiers) with your skis parallel. You can shift your weight to the downhill ski without thinking about it. You face downhill all the time. You can take the bumps with your legs, without moving your body. You move your body in a C shape, ever focusing on the hill below. You've made it! But suddenly, out of nowhere, a snow snake appears, grabs your skis, and down you go.

For those of you who don't ski, a snow snake is what causes you to fall just when everything is going well. It could be a branch that suddenly works its way to the surface of the snow pack, or simply be an uneven patch that catches you unaware. Sometimes it's just because the snow gods are angry with you. Whatever it is, it's similar to what happens to you when things start to go wrong in perimenopause. It might be bleeding through your clothes without warning. It might be wetting your pants when you cough or sneeze or even *think* about having to go to the bathroom. Whatever it is, it trips you up and you unexpectedly fall flat on your face—a snow snake got you.

Unexpected changes like these often require surgery or a major lifestyle change—just when everything else in your busy life is going well. When symptoms occur, you may be reluctant to take time out for such bodily "inconveniences." This chapter is about the unplanned changes that can occur during perimenopause, and describes a variety of surgical and nonsurgical strategies that are available to manage these problems.

Abnormal Uterine Bleeding

During perimenopause, irregular menstrual bleeding is a common accompaniment to the decline of ovarian hormone production. For the most part, these changes are not serious. They can usually be managed with hormone supplements or even weathered without any treatment at all. Sometimes uterine bleeding gets out of control, however, and becomes truly abnormal. The medical term for this condition is *dysfunctional uterine bleeding.*

What Causes Dysfunctional Uterine Bleeding?

The first half of your normal menstrual cycle is dominated by the production of estrogen. Estrogen causes your endometrium to regenerate after you have shed it in a menstrual period. During this regeneration, your growing endometrium is supported by blood vessels arranged in fairly straight lines. At midcycle, ovulation takes place and you begin to produce progesterone in large quantities. Progesterone thickens your endometrium, preparing it to receive a fertilized egg. (Your body wants to get pregnant, even if you don't!) Progesterone changes those straight blood vessels to corkscrew shapes. When you shed this lining at your next menstrual period, uterine contractions (cramps) squeeze these corkscrew vessels closed to limit the amount of blood loss.

If you don't ovulate, you don't produce progesterone. If progesterone is not available to convert your straight vessels to the corkscrew type, your vessels don't close completely, so your bleeding is heavier when you menstruate. This is called dysfunctional uterine bleeding,

Most of the time dysfunctional uterine bleeding begins when your period is due; but it can also occur earlier or later in your cycle. It often begins without warning. You may be at a meeting, walking through the mall, teaching a class, or running a Brownie meeting when you feel warmth between your legs. You know you haven't wet your pants. You look down and, to your great embarrassment, see a patch of bright red blood.

During perimenopause you may begin to ovulate less frequently. As you get closer to menopause, you usually stop ovulating, so dysfunctional bleeding may occur monthly. The embarrassment is bad enough, but you may also become anemic from blood loss. Menstrual bleeding is the main source of iron loss in women, and the most common cause of iron deficiency anemia in the developed nations (Fairbanks and Bentler 1995). Chronic anemia can impair your body's immunity, increase the frequency of serious infection, and even cause you to bleed even more heavily. It's time to see your doctor.

Tell Me What's Wrong!—Diagnosis

You and your doctor need to know exactly what's causing your abnormal bleeding so it can be treated effectively. The reason for dysfunctional uterine bleeding is purely hormonal, but abnormal bleeding may be caused by other factors. To determine the cause of your bleeding, your doctor will perform an office procedure called an *endometrial biopsy*. A small amount of tissue is removed from the uterine cavity and evaluated microscopically. Almost all biopsies will confirm the diagnosis of dysfunctional uterine bleeding. Occasionally, the biopsy reveals polyps or fibroids (these are described later in this chapter). The biopsy is also used to screen for uterine cancer, which is rare in perimenopause (Brill 1995).

In the past, physicians obtained endometrial tissue by doing a *dilation and curettage* (D & C). A D & C is performed in an operating room, under anesthesia. In recent years, gynecologic surgeons have largely supplanted the D & C with an endometrial biopsy. In a 1982 study, Grimes established the advantages of an endometrial biopsy over a D & C based on several factors: convenience, adequacy of tissue sample, complications, diagnostic accuracy, and cost. The D & C remains a useful surgical procedure, but it has been relegated to certain therapeutic treatments rather than diagnosis.

CAUTION! Make sure your health provider has a microscopic diagnosis before treating your abnormal bleeding. Although uterine cancer is rare in your age group, it is cured 93 percent of the time when a timely biopsy is done at the onset of abnormal uterine bleeding (Cramer 1994).

Medical Treatment of Dysfunctional Uterine Bleeding

When your doctor has diagnosed abnormal uterine bleeding and surgery is not required, you need medical treatment. A variety of medications are helpful in controlling this bleeding. These medications make up for the progesterone you lost when you didn't ovulate; they include both male and female hormones, as well as nonhormonal treatments. Herbal medicine and creams can be used to replace progesterone (discussed in Chapters 8 and 9), but they don't work consistently to control this bleeding problem.

Female Hormones

Progesterone therapy is targeted at women who are not ovulating and bleeding heavily. Both natural progesterone and synthetic progestins can be used (see Chapter 8 for more about these two drugs). Oral progestins such as medroxy-progesterone (Provera, Cycrin) and norethindrone (Micronor, Nor-QD), given in large enough doses, simulate ovulation. The progestins cause the blood vessels in the lining of your uterus to corkscrew. When you stop the progestin, the vessels constrict, returning your menstrual bleeding to normal.

After several months of progestin therapy, your blood loss can be reduced by as much as 20 percent (Cameron et al. 1990). Women who have progestin intolerance can use micronized progesterone or the new progesterone vaginal cream approved by the FDA in 1997. This cream prevents the development of an abnormal uterine lining without increasing your blood levels of progesterone.

Birth control pill therapy is targeted at women who are still ovulating but experiencing heavy bleeding. Your endometrial biopsy may be normal but you are bleeding heavily anyway. The Pill contains both estrogen and progesterone. This combination of hormones prevents the uterine lining from thickening, which decreases menstrual bleeding by as much as 50 percent (Brill 1995). Birth control pills are contraindicated in certain perimenopausal women. If you smoke or have migraine headaches, high blood pressure, a history of blood clots in your legs, or fibroid tumors, you can't take the Pill. It is also contraindicated for women who don't tolerate progestins (Leventhal 1996).

The progesterone-impregnated IUD is targeted at all women who bleed heavily—those who ovulate and those who don't. After your doctor places this IUD within your uterus, your bleeding will be reduced by 65 percent over the 12-month period it is in place (Brill 1995). Your uterine lining is affected by direct contact with the progesterone in the IUD, and progesterone levels within your uterus are much higher than can be achieved by taking a progestin by mouth. The endometrial lining becomes very thin, so you bleed very little during your menstrual period. The greatest reduction in bleeding from any nonsurgical method is seen with the use of the progesterone-impregnated IUD (Brill 1995).

The blood level of progesterone isn't increased with this IUD, so you can use it even if you have a progestin intolerance. It must be replaced every year.

A new IUD containing levonorgestrel, a very powerful synthetic progestin, is in use in Finland. It has shown an even greater benefit, reducing bleeding by 86 percent after three months of use and by 97 percent after

twelve months. This IUD is still in Food and Drug Administr
is not yet available in the United States (Brill 1995, Grimes

Nonhormonal Treatment

Nonsteroidal anti-inflammatory drugs (NSAIDs) also work to control dysfunctional uterine bleeding. Mefenamic acid (Meclomen, Ponstel) has been shown to reduce abnormal bleeding by 50 percent (Brill 1995, Cameron et al. 1990). It also decreases menstrual cramps, which is a bonus. Mefenamic acid even reduces bleeding in some women with known fibroids (Brill 1995).

Ibuprofen (Motrin, Advil) and naproxen (Anaprox, Naprasyn, Alleve) are also NSAIDs; they reduce bleeding but are not as effective as mefenamic acid. In addition, there's a downside to taking these medications. If you have a history of ulcer disease, are allergic to aspirin, or bruise easily, you won't like what the NSAIDs do to you. You may have an upset stomach, reactivate your ulcers, and increase your bruising. If you have diabetes, asthma, kidney, or liver disease, NSAIDs should not be used because they may increase the complications associated with these diseases.

Male Hormone

Danazol, a derivative of the male hormone testosterone, dramatically reduces your menstrual blood loss when taken daily in doses of 200 to 800 mg (Brill 1995). Taking danazol also reduces menstrual cramps. Lower dosages are associated with irregular bleeding, and higher dosages have bothersome side effects. Since the drug is a derivative of testosterone, it may lower your voice, so don't use danazol if you use your voice professionally. The medication may also decrease your breast size, increase your weight, and cause acne.

Surgical Treatment of Dysfunctional Uterine Bleeding: Endometrial Ablation

In addition to the medical treatments we've discussed so far, surgery is sometimes used to stop abnormal uterine bleeding. Until 1981, a hysterectomy was often performed when medical management was unsuccessful in controlling such bleeding.

When your abnormal bleeding is associated with progesterone intolerance, severe cramps, migraine headaches, premenstrual syndrome, prolapsed (fallen) uterus, or involuntary urine loss, a hysterectomy is still your first choice to stop heavy menstrual bleeding. However, if you don't have any other problems associated with your abnormal bleeding, an alternative treatment has emerged: *endometrial ablation* (Goldrath et al. 1981). This surgical procedure destroys your uterine lining (endometrium) and stops the bleeding. Your doctor may pretreat you with danazol, depo-medroxy progesterone, or a GnRH agonist to thin your endometrium so its deepest layers can be destroyed (Goldrath 1990). Once they are destroyed, they can't regenerate, and voilá! Your problems are solved.

Your doctor will perform the endometrial ablation in an operating room under general or spinal anesthesia. Because it is an outpatient procedure, most women can return to normal activities within a week. There may be some slight bleeding for about six weeks; but from then on bleeding is either minimal or stops altogether for 50 to 80 percent of women (Brill 1995). Ten to 40 percent of women continue to have normal to light periods. About 10 percent of women have no change in their bleeding patterns whatsoever. These women will still need a hysterectomy to control their bleeding.

As with any surgical procedure, there are certain risks associated with an endometrial ablation. The procedure destroys most of the endometrial lining, forming a scar. The scarring prevents remaining cells from bleeding but not from developing into cancer cells after menopause. Women who have had an endometrial ablation must take progesterone along with estrogen for hormone replacement once they reach menopause, to prevent those remaining cells from becoming endometrial cancer. If you cannot tolerate progesterone, you shouldn't have an endometrial ablation.

Your menstrual period may reappear two to three years following an ablation because your endometrial lining has grown back. Occasionally, scar tissue may block the *cervical canal* (the channel between the endometrium and vagina). Your menstrual blood remains trapped within your uterus causing severe pain and requiring a hysterectomy to cure the pain (Margos et al. 1991).

Fewer than 3 percent of women who have had endometrial ablation have serious complications (Lefler et al. 1991). Fraser reported in 1993 that of the three ablation techniques currently in use, the rollerball method has the fewest complications.

Researchers are developing newer methods to destroy the endometrium. One uses radio waves (microwave); another places hot saline solution in the uterus to destroy the endometrium with heat. To date, neither of these has been shown to be as safe as an ablation (Brill 1995, Baggish 1995).

Let's turn now to some physical causes of abnormal bleeding: polyps and fibroids.

Polyps and Fibroids

Polyps and fibroids are the two most common nonhormonal causes of dysfunctional uterine bleeding. Often the doctor detects fibroids during an initial pelvic examination. Polyps are more difficult to diagnose. Let's start by looking at the diagnosis and treatment of polyps and then at the somewhat more complicated issues involved in the treatment of fibroids.

Polyps: Diagnosis and Treatment

Endometrial polyps are teardrop-shaped glandular growths of the endometrium. They hang into the uterine cavity and are not sloughed off during menstruation. Instead, they remain attached to the uterus, which causes prolonged and sometimes heavy bleeding. Polyps are not abnormal cells and are not considered to be tumors.

If you have abnormal bleeding caused by endometrial polyps, a biopsy of your uterine lining usually appears normal. The diagnosis can be made if your doctor gets a piece of the polyp. More often, however, the biopsy fails to detect polyps.

Polyps do not respond to the various hormonal drug therapies. Physicians diagnose and treat polyps with surgical procedures. Surgeons often remove polyps with a D & C, and a fiber-optic instrument called an *operative hysteroscope* may help find polyps and remove them.

What Are Fibroids?

Except for the thin glandular endometrium, your uterus is composed exclusively of muscle. (Most women are aware of this because of the two "Big Cs"—cramps that come with your periods, and contractions when you deliver your babies. A *fibroid* (the medical term is leiomyoma) is a benign muscle tumor of the uterine wall. Fibroids are hereditary. They usually begin to grow when a woman is in her early forties, and estrogen is the catalyst that makes them grow. W. H. Parker estimated that 30 percent of all women have fibroids sometime during their lifetime, but only one-fifth of these women have symptoms and need to be treated (Parker 1995 Myomectomy).

Fibroids can occur at various places in your uterus. The only ones which will cause you trouble are those that grow on the inside wall of the uterus and push their way into the uterine cavity (endometrial cavity). They cause abnormal bleeding in two ways. First, they interfere with the corkscrewing of the blood vessels in the endometrium during the second half of the menstrual cycle, simulating dysfunctional uterine bleeding. Second, they push into the cavity, causing pressure on the opposite wall, making the endometrium abnormal there also. Fibroids that grow into the uterine cavity are called *submucous* fibroids. Some submucous fibroids grow on a pedicle (like serosal fibroids) and hang down into the cavity itself. These *pedunculated* fibroids cause abnormal bleeding, and lots of it. Unfortunately, progestins do not stop the bleeding caused by submucous fibroids. In some women, mefenamic acid or ibuprofen can decrease the bleeding by constricting the blood vessels, but most women will eventually need surgery to stop the abnormal bleeding caused by their fibroids.

In a 1995 study, Brill noted that fibroids were rarely the source of infertility unless they were located inside the uterine cavity. Pregnancy is unaffected by the presence of fibroids, except for a slightly higher rate of cesarean section births (Parker 1995 Myomectomy).

Fortunately, fibroids are never cancerous. (There is a rare cancer that resembles a fibroid in the early stages, but it's extremely uncommon in perimenopausal women.)

Treating Symptomatic Fibroids with Medication

Alphabet Soup	
FSH	Follicle stimulating hormone
GnRH-a	Gonadotropin-releasing hormone agonist
LH	Leuteinizing hormone

Your doctor can't *cure* fibroids with medications; but you *can* take a medication that works nicely to shrink them and stop them from bleeding: gonadotropin-releasing hormone agonists (GnRH-a).

GnRH is the hormone your hypothalamus sends to the pituitary gland. It tells your pituitary to release FSH (follicle stimulating hormone) and LH (leuteinizing hormone), and they in turn stimulate your ovaries to make estrogen and progesterone. A GnRH agonist is a drug that blocks your GnRH, interrupting your ovarian hormonal cycle. You stop producing estrogen and progesterone. Sounds like menopause, doesn't it? That's right; a GnRH agonist causes a temporary menopause and stops uterine bleeding. Not surprisingly, then, side effects of GnRH agonists include hot flashes, vaginal dryness, skin aging, and possibly osteoporosis if the medication is used for too long.

Treating fibroids with GnRH agonists (by injection or with a nasal spray) is only a short-term measure to control bleeding, clear up anemia, and shrink fibroids. The next step in treatment is either a hysterectomy or the surgical removal of the fibroids, because once you stop the medication, the fibroids grow back to their previous size and your bleeding problems return.

You can reduce the side effects of a GnRH agonist by taking low-dose estrogen and progesterone—called *add-back therapy*. Add-back therapy does not negate the benefits of the GnRH agonist, but it controls hot flashes, usually stops your menstrual period, menstrual cramps, and PMS. Doctors do not prescribe GnRH agonists for longer than six months because of risks of osteoporosis.

Physicians are also using RU-486 (mifepristone) to shrinks fibroids Grimes (1997). reported that RU-486 reduced fibroid size by 50 percent and without the side effects of GnRH agonists, so add-back therapy was not needed. Like treatment with GnRH agonists, however, once the RU-486 is stopped, the fibroids return to their former size. And you should have corrective surgery before discontinuing the medication, just as is necessary with GnRH agonists.

The Food and Drug Administration has not yet approved RU-486 for use in the United States.

Surgical Treatment of Symptomatic Fibroids

There are two surgical approaches to dealing with symptomatic fibroids: hysterectomy and *myomectomy*. In a hysterectomy, your uterus is removed, as well as all your fibroids. (Hysterectomies are performed for other reasons besides fibroid removal, as you'll find out later in this chapter.) In a myomectomy, your individual fibroids are removed but not the uterus. A myomectomy can be performed in several ways.

The appropriate operation for removing fibroids is based on your fertility status, your desire for future pregnancies, your age, and surgical feasibility. You and your doctor will make these choices together.

Let's start with a look at the types of myomectomy.

Intrauterine Myomectomy

An *intrauterine myomectomy* is the removal of fibroids located inside the uterus. The operation is nearly identical to an endometrial ablation.

Surgical risks for this procedure increase when the uterus is enlarged because of the fibroids. These risks include fluid overload, the chance of incomplete removal of the fibroids (which could require additional surgery), and uterine perforation. For women with a large numbers of fibroids, the safest surgery is a hysterectomy or, as described next, a myomectomy through an abdominal incision.

Extrauterine Myomectomy

An *extrauterine myomectomy* is the removal of the cauliflower-shaped fibroids on the outside of the uterus through an abdominal incision. The doctor uses a large incision (abdominal myomectomy) to remove very large fibroids or when future childbearing is desired. Each fibroid is cut out individually, and then the space left in the uterus is sutured and closed. When childbearing is no longer an issue and the fibroids are small (less than 2 inches in diameter) and the uterus smaller than a three month pregnancy, a smaller incision and a laparoscope (laparoscopic myomectomy) are used to remove or destroy small fibroids.

The following complications are associated with an abdominal myomectomy (less frequently with a laparoscopic myomectomy):

- **Adhesions:** Tulandi found that 92 percent of women developed adhesions between the uterus and bowel following an abdominal myomectomy (Tulandi et al. 1993), but only 46 percent of the time following a laparoscopic myomectomy (Parker 1995 Myomectomy). Adhesions are scar tissue that bridges the gap between the uterus and the bowel, tubes, and ovaries. Adhesions can prevent an egg from reaching the tube, causing infertility; block the intestines, causing bowel obstructions; and be a cause of chronic pelvic pain. Adhesions are caused by the heavy blood loss during this operation.

- **Blood loss:** Fibroids have an abundant blood supply. When they are removed, the typically heavy blood loss can be reduced by injecting a drug called vasopressin directly into the fibroid (before removal) or by placing a tourniquet or clamps around the uterine vessels. In spite of these efforts, however, postoperative bleeding can be a complication. Blood transfusions or reopening the abdomen to stop the bleeding may be necessary. Sometimes a hysterectomy is the only option at this point. There is less blood loss with a laparoscopic myomectomy because the fibroids are smaller. Parker summarized three studies of laparoscopic myomectomy—all done on women with small fibroids—and reported that there was only one case requiring blood transfusion, and that none needed a hysterectomy (Parker 1995 "Myomectomy. . ." p398).

- **Infertility:** You may become infertile because of adhesions following an abdominal myomectomy. Adhesions form between your ovaries and fallopian tubes 56 to 93 percent of the time following an abdominal myomectomy (Tulandi et al. 1993). These adhesions may prevent the egg from reaching the fallopian tube or the sperm from reaching the egg. The myomectomy may also cause scar tissue within the uterus, making the endometrial lining inhospitable to the fetus, compromising your ability to successfully complete a pregnancy.

Even if you have surgery to remove fibroids, you have a one in four chance of growing more and needing a repeat operation at a later date (Malone,1969). Due to the risks involved, physicians typically recommend a hysterectomy instead of a multiple myomectomy if you have completed your child-bearing. The laparoscopic myomectomy used for smaller fibroids is a less invasive operation because fiberoptic technology is used instead of an open incision. You have less pain and usually go home the same day.

When pregnancy is still part of your plans, another aspect of the laparoscopic procedure must be considered. Surgery weakens the uterine wall. When a women does get pregnant following a myomectomy, she has a small risk that her uterus will rupture (Harris 1992, Garnet 1964). The risk of uterine rupture is greater when a woman has had a laparoscopic myomectomy than when she has had the traditional abdominal procedure (Harris 1992). As a result, doctors are reluctant to remove fibroids with a laparoscope in women desiring pregnancy. However, if you don't want more children and have only one or two small fibroids, a laparoscopic myomectomy may be your best choice.

Myolysis

Another procedure performed through the laparoscope is called *myolysis*. In this operation, the doctor heats (or cauterizes) the base of the fibroid until the blood supply is destroyed. You benefit from the same short recovery time as with the laparoscopic myomectomy. The procedure causes the fibroid to shrink. Since no cutting is involved, adhesion formation is less than for a myomectomy. This relatively recent procedure was first described in 1990 (Gallinat 1990), and there are no statistics on pregnancy outcome following this procedure. Because myolysis is a lengthy operation, surgeons will usually recommend an abdominal myomectomy if there are four or more fibroids larger than three inches, if the fibroids are in deep in the uterine wall, or if the location of the fibroid makes it difficult to reach. Four to six months are usually required to totally recover from the operation.

On the Horizon—Fibroid Embolization

In 1995, J.H. Ravina, M.D. and other French radiologists, using an X-ray technique called *embolization*, reported that they had successfully stopped massive bleeding from fibroids in sixteen French women who were too weak to withstand a hysterectomy. Radiologists frequently use an embolization technique to stop bleeding, but this was the first time embolization was used for women with bleeding fibroids. Using artery catheters, and X-ray dye as a visual aid, small (500 micron) poly-vinyl-alcohol particles were injected into the uterine arteries. These particles traveled to the bleeding vessels, clotted them, and stopped the bleeding. The fibroids supplied by these small vessels then died. However, the particles were too big to block the vessels in the endometrium. And because two other arteries supply blood to the uterus, the uterus didn't die.

Following the embolization, 80 percent of these patients didn't need a hysterectomy; their fibroids shrank in size and their heavy bleeding stopped. Since the 1995 report, these doctors have embolized over 400 French women, with similar results. The same procedure is now being used by radiologists in radiology centers around the United States (McLucas and Goodwin 1996).

We see the advantages of this new technique as follows:

- No general anesthetic; the procedure is done under sedation.
- No surgery; this is an X-ray procedure done with the aid of an X-ray machine.
- No adhesions or other postsurgical risks.
- At least a 50-percent decrease in fibroid size; the bigger they are, the smaller they get.
- All fibroids die, not just the ones the doctor can see or feel.

- Lower chance than with a myomectomy or myolysis of fibroid re-growth. Ravina reported only 20 percent of his patients needed a hysterectomy because bleeding recurred.

Unfortunately, fibroid embolization does creates some problems.

- The sudden decrease in the fibroid's blood supply causes pain equivalent to the pain of a mild heart attack. The pain continues until the whole fibroid dies off.
- The bigger the fibroid, the more it hurts.
- Flulike symptoms result from the inflammatory reaction to the dying fibroid.
- A smelly and profuse discharge develops as the fibroids inside the uterus die and are discharged through the vagina. You just have to wait it out.
- You may need hospitalization because of the pain and fever.
- There are no statistics on pregnancy complications, but doctors worry that there will be a decrease in the blood supply to a fetus because of the embolization. This procedure is not recommended for women who wish future pregnancies.
- A small risk of pulmonary embolis or stroke is associated with any arterial catheterization procedure.

As with any procedure, embolization doesn't work every time. One patient out of five failed to respond and needed a hysterectomy or myomectomy anyway.

Hysterectomy

Alphabet Soup	
TAH & BSO	Total abdominal hysterectomy and bilateral salpingo-oophorectomy
LAVH	Laparoscopically assisted vaginal hysterectomy

We've already mentioned two valid indications for doing a hysterectomy: uncontrollable bleeding and symptomatic fibroids. Other indications for a hysterectomy that will be discussed in this chapter include cancer and precancerous conditions, infection, severe endometriosis, pelvic pain, and uterine prolapse. First, though, it will be helpful to know more about the operation itself, the various ways it can be carried out, and the reasoning behind choosing one technique over another.

According to the National Center for Health Statistics over 600,000 hysterectomies are performed each year in the United States. Drs. Carlson,

Nichols, and Shiff reported in a 1993 article that by age sixty, one-third of American women will have had a hysterectomy. Hysterectomies are the second most common major female operation after cesarean sections. The five-billion-dollar annual cost to our health care system for hysterectomies has stimulated efforts to find alternatives. The newer medical and surgical technologies discussed earlier in this chapter have reduced the number of hysterectomies by 20 percent.

If your doctor recommends a hysterectomy, making your decision will be easier if you understand some of the terminology surrounding this procedure. In other words, as the saying goes, if you want to walk the walk you got to talk the talk. The following list of definitions will help. In addition, Figure 15-1 illustrates normal pelvic anatomy; and Figure 15-2 illustrates the structures removed in the various operations.

- **Total hysterectomy:** Removal of the entire uterus, including the cervix (the opening into the vagina), but not the ovaries or the fallopian tubes.

- **Total abdominal hysterectomy and bilateral salpingo-oophorectomy (TAH & BSO):** An abdominal operation that removes the entire uterus, fallopian tubes, and both ovaries.

- **Subtotal abdominal hysterectomy:** Removal of the main body of the uterus but not the cervix.

- **Vaginal hysterectomy:** Removal of the entire uterus through the vagina, with no abdominal incision.

- **Laparoscopically assisted vaginal hysterectomy (LAVH):** The laparoscope and other necessary instruments are inserted through several

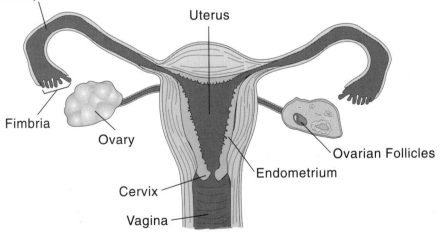

Figure 15.1.   Normal Pelvic Anatomy

small abdominal incisions to help the surgeon remove the uterus vaginally.

- **Oophorectomy:** An abdominal or laparoscopic operation to remove one or both ovaries. Immediate menopause occurs only if both ovaries are removed.
- **Salpingectomy:** An abdominal or laparoscopic operation to remove one or both fallopian tubes.

Dark outline = structures removed

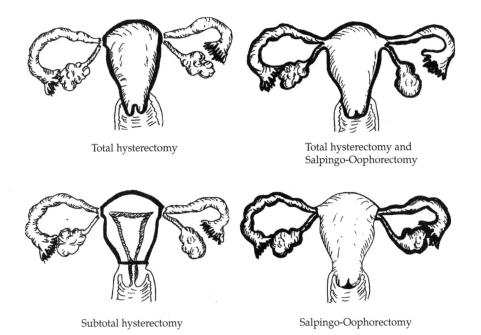

Total hysterectomy

Total hysterectomy and
Salpingo-Oophorectomy

Subtotal hysterectomy

Salpingo-Oophorectomy

Figure 15.2.   Pelvic Operations

Why Should You Have a Hysterectomy?

Hysterectomies generally fall into two categories: nonelective and elective. A nonelective hysterectomy is required when you have invasive cancer of the endometrium, ovary, or cervix; life-threatening uterine hemorrhage; or uncontrollable life-threatening infection. There are alternatives to hysterectomy in only two conditions: Invasive cervical cancer is sometimes treated with radiation instead of surgery, and uterine hemorrhage due to fibroids can be treated with embolization. But don't delay your operation if you have any of these problems. Time has run out to try alternative therapies.

Elective hysterectomies are performed when the indications are less urgent. You have more time to plan for your surgery or to try alternative therapies. Indications for an elective hysterectomy include persistent abnormal uterine bleeding and symptomatic fibroids, both of which we've already discussed. Other indications are

- **Endometriosis:** A portion of your menstrual blood flows backward through the fallopian tubes into your abdomen. Most women's bodies destroy this blood and tissue, but some do not. In these women, the endometrial tissue becomes implanted in sites outside the uterus, commonly on the ovaries, fallopian tubes, peritoneum (abdominal lining), and intestines. This condition is called *endometriosis*. Every time you have a menstrual period, the endometriosis implants bleed also. This results in painful adhesions, menstrual cramps, and painful intercourse. Your doctor may treat your endometriosis with a GnRH agonist, danazol, or birth control pills, but the treatment is effective only as long as the medication is taken. Hysterectomy with removal of the ovaries cures this disease; but it is a last-ditch therapy after medical treatment fails.

- **Precancerous conditions of the uterus:** Cryosurgery, LEEP, and a cervical conization (described in Chapter 7) can be used to treat precancerous lesions of the cervix. Progestin therapy can often treat precancerous lesions of the endometrium. A hysterectomy always cures both precancerous conditions.

- **Chronic pelvic pain:** The source of pelvic pain is often difficult to diagnose, and treatment of the pain itself is difficult. Causes range from nerve damage, endometriosis, and adhesions from sexually transmitted diseases or previous surgery, to psychological sexual trauma. Hysterectomy is an absolute last-ditch treatment for chronic pelvic pain.

- **Prolapse of the uterus:** As a perimenopausal woman, you are not likely to have a prolapse (sagging) of the uterus, but the condition does occur. It is more commonly found in postmenopausal women, and the uterus sometimes protrudes outside of the vagina. As an alternative to hysterectomy, methods such as pessaries (a plastic or soft rubber device placed in your vagina to keep the uterus in place) can help. Prolapse is a nuisance, so many women opt for a hysterectomy.

Half of all hysterectomies are done for abnormal uterine bleeding, and one-half of these uterine specimens are determined in pathology to be free of disease (Brill 1995), There has been so much negative press about unnecessary hysterectomies that many women feel they have somehow "failed" if they agree to have this operation (West et al. 1994). But that the tissue was pronounced "free of disease" does not mean these hysterectomies were performed needlessly. Many women opt for a hysterectomy because the alternative therapies are not well tolerated or are simply not working.

Study after study has shown that women who opted for hysterectomy were more satisfied with the outcome than women choosing other forms of alternative therapy (Alexander et al. 1996; Dwyer et all 1993). This is true even though the other treatments are less invasive, have fewer complications, and involve quicker recovery.

Now let's take a closer look at the various types of hysterectomies.

Types of Hysterectomy

All hysterectomies involve detachment of the five ligaments that support the uterus, tying off the blood vessels, and pulling the ligaments together to prevent a later vaginal prolapse. This can be done with an abdominal, vaginal, or laparoscopically assisted vaginal (LAVH) procedure.

Abdominal Hysterectomy

Currently, 70 percent of all 600,000 hysterectomies done in North America each year are done through an abdominal incision (Munro and Deprest 1995). Prior to 1950, the majority of hysterectomies done in North America were subtotal abdominal hysterectomies, leaving the cervix in place. Antibiotics of that era were not as effective as they are now. Removal of the cervix required opening the vagina. The vagina has bacteria in it; the abdominal cavity does not. Opening the vagina caused a higher incidence of postoperative infection. Since 1950, physicians have favored removal of the cervix along with the uterus—a total hysterectomy. The cervix was removed to prevent cervical cancer, which we discussed in Chapter 7.

Today, the thinking on this subject is changing again. An intact cervix can preserve bladder function, maintain sexual pleasure, and prevent vaginal prolapse after a hysterectomy (Lyons and Parker 1996). Cervical cancer is caused by HPV (genital warts), and if you don't have HPV you may be able to keep your cervix. Most subtotal hysterectomies (removal of the body of the uterus but leaving the cervix behind) are performed abdominally rather than vaginally.

What are the disadvantages of abdominal hysterectomy? For one thing, a large abdominal incision is necessary. The recovery period is longer and more painful than for either a vaginal hysterectomy or LAVH. The incision may become infected, and blood may collect under the skin. For these reasons, only the most difficult hysterectomies are done abdominally. Women with invasive cancer of the female organs (with the exception of some very early cervical or endometrial cancers) have abdominal hysterectomies because the surgeon needs to remove diseased tissue other than the uterus (Montz and Schlaerth 1995). Other reasons for an abdominal hysterectomy include large fibroids, severe endometriosis, severe adhesions from multiple prior operations, and multiple cesarean births.

Abdominal hysterectomies usually require a three- to four-day hospitalization and then six weeks of recuperation. This compares with a one- to two-day hospitalization and a two-week recuperation for a vaginal hysterectomy or LAVH.

Vaginal Hysterectomy

A vaginal hysterectomy is an option for women who have a relatively small uterus, some relaxation of uterine supporting structures, and a large-enough vagina to allow the instruments in and the uterus out. Typically, women who have had at least one vaginal birth, have a uterus smaller than a three-month pregnancy, and have none of the problems requiring an abdominal hysterectomy can have a vaginal hysterectomy. There are no external incisions, so postoperative pain is strikingly less than with an abdominal hysterectomy. This translates to a shorter hospital stay and full recovery in two to three weeks (VanDenEeden et al. 1997).

One common complication with vaginal hysterectomies (and LAVHs) is an inadvertent incision in the bladder during the surgical removal of the uterus. This incision is easily recognized and easily repaired; but if it happens to you, you'll need to wear a catheter for seven to ten days while your bladder heals. The chance of this complication is much lower with abdominal surgery.

Laparoscopically Assisted Vaginal Hysterectomy (LAVH)

The laparoscopically assisted vaginal hysterectomy (LAVH) was first described in 1989 by Dr. Harry Reich and others. This operation combines abdominal surgery through a laparoscope with vaginal surgery. By operating through a laparoscope, the surgeon can cut scar tissue that would otherwise prevent the uterus from being removed vaginally. The uterus is freed from its attachments with instruments inserted through three or four small incisions in the abdomen. Once it is detached, the uterus is removed through the vagina.

The advantage of an LAVH is the conversion of an abdominal hysterectomy to a vaginal one. Length of hospital stay and recovery time for an LAVH are about the same as for vaginal hysterectomies. An LAVH takes a little longer to perform than either a vaginal or abdominal hysterectomy, but it is worth the effort.

Many critics, who are not concerned with pain and the timely return to normal activities, say that the greater operating room expenses associated with an LAVH more than offset the savings of an extra two or three days in the hospital. These expenses include a longer operation and costly disposable instruments. VanDenEeden et al. in 1997 disagree. They found the LAVH to be less costly than an abdominal hysterectomy. There is no denying, however, even by the critics, that you feel better and return to your normal lifestyle much more quickly—in about three weeks—if you have an LAVH instead of an abdominal hysterectomy.

Hysterectomy Complications

Minor complications of hysterectomies include bladder and incision infections, skin edge separations, anemia, and in rare cases, a drug reaction (usually a rash and itching).

Most studies show *major* complication rates to be low. In 1995, Munro and Deprest summarized nine studies by different surgeons and including over 600 patients. They reported major complications from abdominal hysterectomies occurred less than 1 percent of the time. Major complications occurred in 4.5 percent of vaginal hysterectomies and 2.5 percent of LAVHs.

The more serious complications from abdominal hysterectomy include injury to the bladder, intestine, and ureter (the tube from the kidney to the bladder). Major postoperative complications include significant bleeding, infection with abscess formation, total wound separation, and adhesions. For vaginal hysterectomies and LAVH, major complications were injury to the bladder (as mentioned for the abdominal procedure), but also included significant bleeding and abscess formation. Dicker et al. (1982) showed vaginal hysterectomies to have a lower overall complication rate than abdominal hysterectomies. Liu's series of seventy-two LAVHs compare to the Munro and Deprest summary, which included eighty-eight LAVHs. Out of seventy-two patients having an LAVH, Lui had no major and only two minor complications. In other words, most complications of hysterectomy are minor ones. The major complications deserve a closer look.

Heavy Bleeding

All patients lose blood during any surgery. You can take iron pills for three or four weeks to correct the minor blood loss from a hysterectomy. Heavy bleeding during surgery is rare, but when it does occur doctors often can return your own blood with the help of a *cell saver*. A cell saver is a machine that collects and filters the blood you lose during surgery. Your doctor returns your own blood to you, often avoiding the need for a blood-bank transfusion. When there is a possibility of a blood-bank transfusion, you can give one or more units of your own blood prior to surgery, which can then be given back to you during or after the operation.

Adhesions

As explained earlier in the chapter, adhesions are scar tissue that develops during the normal healing process after most hysterectomies. They are your body's way of protecting itself from major insults. Adhesions rarely cause problems. Infrequently, however, they can be dense and cause tissues and organs to stick together. When organs are immobilized by adhesions, normal body movement may cause pain. Future surgery may be complicated by the presence of adhesions, and the organs themselves (most commonly, the bladder and intestines) may be damaged in the process of separation.

If you have had several cesarean sections, you may have dense adhesions between your bladder and uterus. Your surgeon may have difficulty separating the two during a hysterectomy, and it's possible the bladder may be injured. Your doctor can easily repair this injury, but you will have to wear a catheter for the seven- to ten-day healing period.

Ureteral Injury

The ureters—the two tubes that carry urine from your kidneys to your bladder—pass within a quarter-inch of your uterus. This close proximity puts the ureters in harm's way during all kinds of hysterectomies. In rare cases, a ureter may be damaged, requiring corrective surgery to restore normal function.

Serious Infection

You have a significant risk of serious infection after a hysterectomy because your surgeon enters the vagina, which is teeming with bacteria. Your vagina exists in perfect harmony with its normal bacterial flora, but when these same organisms are transported into the abdominal cavity during a hysterectomy, serious infections may result. When your doctor gives you preoperative prophylactic antibiotics, your risk of serious infection is reduced by 50 percent for all types of hysterectomies (Reggiori et al. 1996; Tanos and Rojansky 1994). Although there is some debate over the use of antibiotics to prevent disease, especially with the emergence of "superbugs," there is no disagreement at all about the use of these drugs in hysterectomies. Without antibiotics, there is a high risk of infection (The Medical Letter 1995).

Damage to a Major Blood Vessel

In an LAVH, instruments are inserted through the abdomen, in an area close to major blood vessels. The vessels may be inadvertently torn during the operation, causing heavy bleeding that can be stopped by pressure and several stitches. Occasionally, a larger incision is needed to visualize the vessels and stop the bleeding.

Long-Term Complications

Some problems resulting from a hysterectomy occur months to years after the surgery. You may develop bladder dysfunction, a hernia of the intestines into the vagina, vaginal prolapse, bowel obstruction, and sexual dysfunction (Lyons and Parker 1996). When they are feasible alternatives, an endometrial ablation, fibroid embolization, or subtotal hysterectomy are all procedures that decrease the risk of long-term complications.

Elective Removal of Ovaries as Part of the Hysterectomy

Should you have your ovaries removed when you have your hysterectomy? There is no easy answer to this question. Your ovaries produce the hormones that keep things running smoothly, and if they're removed you experience instant menopause. Why not leave them alone to do their job? On the other hand, removal of your ovaries at the time of your hysterectomy, prevents ovarian cancer. That's a compelling reason to have them removed. Let's take a closer look at this debate.

What About Cancer?

Ovarian cancer (discussed in Chapter 7), while rare in perimenopause, remains the leading cause of death from gynecologic malignancy, and the fourth most frequent cause of death from cancer for women in the United States (Maiman 1995; Cramer 1994).

Approximately three-quarters of malignant ovarian tumors are detected only after the disease has spread throughout the abdominal cavity (Maiman 1995). The continued high risk for ovarian cancer is the main reason ovarian removal is recommended when a hysterectomy is being performed.

When Gilda Radner died in 1989 from ovarian cancer, following extensive infertility treatment, the foundation that bears her name publicized the existence of a blood test (CA-125) that could detect ovarian cancer. Unfortunately, CA-125 is not specific for ovarian cancer in perimenopausal women unless levels are extremely high—and by then it's too late. Women who have fibroids, endometriosis, certain ovarian cysts, cirrhosis of the liver, other cancers, are pregnant, and also having their menstrual periods produce high levels of CA-125 (Parker 1995 ". . . Adenexal mass" p364). Most elevated CA-125 levels will be false positives in perimenopausal women (Maiman 1995). And 25 percent of women with ovarian cancers will have a normal CA-125 value (Creasman 1997).

Berchuck has recently discovered a *tumor-suppresser gene* (named *gene p53*) that is responsible for two-thirds of all ovarian cancer. Uninterrupted ovulation of many years' duration causes mutations of this gene, which results in ovarian cancer. Women who have had fewer than three children or who have had a tubal ligation instead of using the Pill are known to be at higher risk for ovarian cancer. Women who have taken the Pill for ten years or longer cut their risk for ovarian cancer in half (Schildkraut 1997). This discovery opens up the exciting possibility for prediction of ovarian cancer in two-thirds of women at risk. To date, though, there is no reliable method to detect ovarian cancer early, which is the only time when it matters. Even when the genetic test for the altered p53 gene is available, it will only detect in two-thirds of women at risk.

Contributing Factors

Now let's look at some specific factors to consider in terms of whether you should have your ovaries removed (oophorectomy).

- **Hereditary ovarian cancer:** For certain familial cancers, doctors recommend an oophorectomy when a woman has finished her family. When you need a hysterectomy for other reasons, having your ovaries removed at the same time may prevent ovarian cancer.

- **Limited remaining ovarian function:** If you are close to menopause, your ovarian function will soon be dramatically reduced. Based on your individual risk factor, you may consider your risk of developing ovarian cancer too great to justify keeping your ovaries for the few years they will continue to function.

- **Shortened ovarian life:** If your uterus is removed, some of the blood supply to your ovaries is lost. Studies (Loft 1993) have shown that many perimenopausal women who retain their ovaries after a hysterectomy will be menopausal within a few years—a significant factor in making your decision.

- **Ovarian cysts:** Ten percent of women who have a hysterectomy will develop painful recurrent ovarian cysts during the remaining years before menopause (Mancuso et al. 1991). These cysts are not cancer, but they hurt and often need to be removed, which means a second operation. Ovaries can usually be removed using a laparoscope, but cysts may be hidden in scar tissue after a hysterectomy and impossible to remove without a large abdominal incision.

The removal of normal ovaries at the time of a hysterectomy is not foolproof; however, it does reduce your chance of developing ovarian cancer by 90 percent. Cancer of the ovary can develop in ovarian cells that exist outside the ovary. These cells are too few in number to be visible at the time of a hysterectomy, but they can later develop into ovarian cancer even if your ovaries have been removed.

The other primary reason to keep your ovaries is their continued production of hormones in just the right amount and at just the right time.

The Bottom Line

When you need a hysterectomy for any number of reasons, we find that most gynecologists recommend that you keep your ovaries if you are less than forty years old. Between age forty and forty-five, if you have severe PMS symptoms, menstrual migraines, or significant endometriosis and you are having a hysterectomy, your symptoms will decrease or disappear with the removal of your ovaries (Casper and Hearn 1990). If you are close to menopause or postmenopausal and you are having a hysterectomy, your doctor will usually recommend that you have your ovaries removed.

When you are pondering the question of ovarian conservation or removal, ask and get answers to these three questions:

- Are my ovaries still functioning? How long can I expect that to continue?

- If I choose to keep my ovaries, how likely is it that I will need future ovarian surgery?

- Do I have familial cancer risk factors that may shorten my life if I keep my ovaries?

Elective Hysterectomy Accompanying Removal of the Ovaries

Should you have a hysterectomy when you have your ovaries removed? If you choose to have your ovaries removed because of a strong family history of hereditary ovarian cancer, or if you have ovarian cysts or tumors, should you have your uterus out as well? The answer is maybe. Let's consider the factors involved.

Once your ovaries are removed, you will need hormone replacement (HRT). If your uterus is removed at the same time, you won't need to take progesterone to prevent endometrial cancer and so you won't ever have to have another menstrual period—which means no more PMS, menstrual migraines, or anything else associated with your periods.

There is a much higher complication rate from a hysterectomy than from an oophorectomy. In a study of 200 women who had their ovaries removed, 100 women kept their uterus and 100 did not. Twenty-three of the 100 women who had hysterectomies also had serious complications (Gambone 1992). The only complication in the 100 women who did not have hysterectomies was a wound infection. If you can take progesterone without adverse side effects, the removal of your ovaries without the removal of your uterus lowers your risk of complications.

You Needed That Hysterectomy and You Don't Miss Your Uterus—So Why Are You So Sad?

Post-hysterectomy sadness is a common effect; 25 percent experience it (Alexander et al. 1996). It is also a short-lived effect of the operation.

An element of that sadness may have to do with a woman's loss of childbearing capability or her relationship to her sexual partner. Women who regard menstrual periods as a monthly affirmation of their femininity, believe them to be a time of cleansing, or have other strongly held beliefs about them, may find their absence unsettling. In North America, the importance of childbearing is implanted early. Most young girls play with dolls and plan to have children. The loss of this ability can and does have a psychological impact on most women. It is not inevitable, however.

In 1996, Alexander and others studied 204 women who needed treatment for abnormal bleeding. Ninety-nine had had a hysterectomy, and the rest an endometrial ablation. The researchers found no lasting psychiatric illness in either group. In addition, both groups experienced the same degree of sexual interest and intensity of orgasm as they had prior to surgery. During the first six postoperative months, the women who had undergone the hysterectomy had significantly more anxiety and depression; but this was gone by twelve months.

The degree of sadness following a hysterectomy is negligible for women who have had a tubal sterilization. We believe this may be because they have already come to terms with the loss of their ability to have children. Women with a strong family history of depression and those who have a hysterectomy following unsuccessful treatment of infertility are more often depressed postoperatively (Hendricks-Matthew 1991). Typically, though, the sadness following a hysterectomy passes quickly. Your new sexual freedom and liberty from the pain and embarrassment of out-of-control periods more than make up for any sadness you feel.

Summary of the Treatment for Abnormal Uterine Bleeding

When you have abnormal uterine bleeding, your doctor must determine the cause. When a hormonal imbalance is the diagnosis, you can take various medications, or have an endometrial ablation which obliterates your endometrium—the source of your bleeding. When the bleeding is due to a structural change such as polyps or cancer, surgery is necessary to correct the abnormal bleeding. Fibroids can be treated by various operations, including the removal or destruction of the fibroids themselves or by a hysterectomy, depending on your desire for future childbearing. You may choose to have a radiologist embolize your fibroids instead of having surgery at all. Hysterectomies do save lives and remain the most common treatment for dysfunctional uterine bleeding as well as genital cancer. Hysterectomies are the second most common operation in the United States today. A higher percentage of women are satisfied with their hysterectomy than with any other procedure used to correct similar problems (Dwyer et al. 1993).

Your doctor can remove the uterus through the vagina when your uterus is small and your vagina is pliable enough to accommodate the delivery. A women who has cancer, whose uterus is markedly enlarged due to fibroids, or who has significant endometriosis or adhesions must have an abdominal incision to remove the uterus; this procedure comes with increased risk of complications and prolonged recovery time.

To have your ovaries removed while having a hysterectomy is a difficult decision and must be based on your assessment of the risk of ovarian cysts or cancer, as well as your desire for continued natural hormonal production.

Loss of your uterus is rightly regarded as a significant event and a major life change. You and your doctor must address many complex issues before deciding on this or any other operation. You are a valuable and necessary part of the decision-making process. Being informed is a good way to begin.

Ovarian Cysts

A *cyst* is any closed cavity lined with cells that contains liquid or semi-solid material. Cysts are painful in perimenopause, but rarely malignant (Maiman 1995). Often the pain occurs upon deep penetration during sex. A pelvic examination will usually detect an enlarged ovary, but not whether the enlargement is caused by a fluid-filled cyst or a solid tumor. An ultrasound examination gives your doctor more information; it differentiates between a cyst with clear fluid, a cyst with particles in the fluid, and a solid tumor. Your doctor will usually advise the immediate removal of a solid tumor of the ovary. When you have an ovarian cyst, the ultrasound can be used in the doctor's clinical evaluation to help you decide on the correct treatment.

Several types of ovarian cysts are common to perimenopausal women.

Functional Ovarian Cysts

Perimenopausal women's cysts are almost always *functional cysts:* smaller than a golf ball, filled with clear fluid, occurring in one ovary at a time, and almost never cancerous. These cysts are painful, but they usually disappear over two to three months without any therapy except watchful waiting.

There are various types of functional ovarian cysts. In general, only when a cyst is larger than a golf ball does it require drainage or surgical removal. In this case, it may not be a functional cyst and won't go away without treatment. Herrmann studied 185 women with ovarian masses and found that when they were purely cystic and smaller than four inches in diameter, they were all benign (Herrmann et al. 1987).

Age is on your side in this matter. Even when a cyst has particles within the fluid, is larger than a golf ball, or doesn't disappear on its own, it is rarely cancerous in perimenopause. Mecke and others operated on 773 women under forty-five years of age with enlarged cystic ovaries; only 11 (or 1.4 percent) of the masses were ovarian cancers (Mecke et al. 1992).

Nonfunctional Ovarian Cysts

Ovarian cysts larger than four inches are usually nonfunctional and won't be reduced with hormonal therapy or watchful waiting. They need to be removed by laparoscopic or abdominal surgery. Nonfunctional cysts are diagnosed by the pathologist after surgery.

These cysts are rarely malignant. If your ovary is larger than a tennis ball and a nonfunctional cyst is the cause of the enlargement, your doctor may remove the ovary and sometimes the fallopian tube. Again, age is on your side. In only 0.04 percent of 13,739 premenopausal women with apparently benign ovarian cysts did the result turn out to be ovarian cancer (Maiman et al. 1995).

Endometriomas

Endometriomas are endometriosis of the ovary; they are also called "chocolate cysts" and they may prevent conception.

As described earlier in the chapter, endometriosis tissue located in the pelvis bleeds during the menstrual period (endometriosis). When endometrial tissue is located in the ovary, this bleeding results in an ovarian cyst which is full of old blood. This blood becomes very thick and turns brown. These cysts are called *endometriomas* or "chocolate cysts" because the fluid in them looks just like chocolate syrup.

The blood cyst (endometrioma) elevates the CA-125 blood test so your doctor will advise removal. These cysts are now removed routinely by laparoscopic surgery with a subsequent pregnancy rate approaching 40 percent (Marrs 1991). The advantage of laparoscopic removal over an open operation is a lower chance of adhesion formation and a much quicker recovery. If the accompanying pelvic endometrosis is already extreme, with dense adhesion formation, removal of endometriomas may require a larger abdominal incision.

Summary of Ovarian Cysts

When smaller than a golf ball, ovarian cysts, including endometriomas, can be managed with a laparoscopic operation. When they are the size of a tennis ball or don't meet the clinical or ultrasound criteria for laparoscopic removal, they must be removed by a larger abdominal incision.

Ectopic (Tubal) Pregnancy

An ectopic pregnancy is a pregnancy that implants itself outside the uterus. The large majority of ectopic pregnancies occur in the fallopian tube, less frequently in the ovary, and very rarely in the abdomen.

When the fallopian tube has been damaged, the journey to the uterus can be interrupted; the fertilized egg nestles in the tube and results in a tubal, rather than a uterine pregnancy. The growing fetus strains the confines of the fallopian tube until it can stretch no further and ruptures, causing serious and potentially life-threatening internal hemorrhage. Without early diagnosis and medical treatment, tubal rupture and internal bleeding requiring emergency surgery occurs in approximately two-thirds of women who have ectopic pregnancies.

Lund's study published in 1955 reported statistics for 215 women who experienced ectopic pregnancies. In 96 of these women, tubes ruptured and required emergency surgery because of internal bleeding. The other 120 women were simply observed; they were put in bed, given pain medications, and had pregnancy tests and blood counts every week. Bed rest was continued until their pregnancy tests became negative and their pain subsided. Forty-five percent of the 120 women being observed eventually needed surgery to treat their ectopic pregnancies; but 68 out of the original 215, about one-third, resolved the ectopic pregnancies without an operation. Most doctors aren't willing to wait for an ectopic pregnancy to disappear on its own, however, and will treat you as soon as the diagnosis is made, hoping to prevent tubal rupture. Treatment includes medication to terminate the pregnancy before the tube ruptures, or early laparoscopic surgery which also saves the tube.

There has been a fourfold increase in the incidence of ectopic pregnancies over the last twenty-five years, unfortunately; a high percentage of these occurred in perimenopause (Jaffe and Jewelewicz 1991). Following are contributing factors to this condition:

- **Endometriosis.** Women with endometriosis have gradually increasing damage to their tubes and ovaries. If they choose not to have children or to postpone pregnancy, they are more likely to have endometriosis in the fallopian tubes, resulting in an increased risk of ectopic pregnancy.

- **Early treatment of sexually transmitted diseases early in life.** When STDs are diagnosed and treated early, the result is damaged but not blocked fallopian tubes, causing a higher incidence of ectopic pregnancy. Perimenopausal women have had more years to contract an STD than have younger women, so the incidence of a previous STD is greater in perimenopause.

- **Corrective tubal surgery.** Today's infertility specialists are opening previously blocked tubes, resulting in an increased incidence of tubal pregnancies

Diagnosis of Ectopic Pregnancy

If you are at high risk for developing an ectopic pregnancy, you are encouraged to call your physician as soon as you miss your first period. Risk factors include a prior ectopic pregnancy, prior pelvic inflammatory disease (PID), a history of endometriosis, and previous tubal surgery. Your doctor will order a series of blood tests to measure the exact amount of hCG (*human Chorionic Gonadotropin*, the hormone of pregnancy) in your blood. Your hCG rises 60 percent every two days and doubles every three days when you have a normal uterine pregnancy. If your hCG level hasn't risen by 100 percent in three days, a tubal pregnancy will be suspected. Your doctor will then order repeated testing of hCG levels and an ultrasound scan of your uterus when the hCG levels continue to lag. If the radiologist doesn't see the pregnancy in your uterus, ectopic pregnancy is diagnosed. Treatment is then either medical or surgical.

When your physician diagnoses your ectopic pregnancy before six weeks' gestation, he or she may be able to treat you with medication instead of surgery and prevent tubal rupture.

Medical Treatment of Ectopic Pregnancy

Methotrexate, an anticancer drug, effectively destroys ectopic pregnancy in the fallopian tube. Your doctor will give this drug by injection. Then you will have hCG blood levels drawn weekly until this test indicates that your pregnancy is gone.

The success rate for medical treatment is quite high. Gomel reviewed ten studies that reported a 94 percent success rate using methotrexate (Gomel 1995). Ninety percent are cured with a single dose of methotrexate; 4 percent needed a second dose to dissolve the pregnancy (Stovall 1995); in 6 percent the fallopian tube ruptured anyway and required surgery (Gomel 1995;

Stovall 1995). Methotrexate doesn't work when the pregnancy is larger than 3.5 centimeters or the radiologist detects a heartbeat in the fallopian tube; surgery then becomes the only treatment.

Methotrexate is almost always given in a single low dose, so side effects are minimal. Stovall believes that nearly 100 percent of women who take methotrexate will have some pain, usually controlled with a nonsteroidal anti-inflammatory such as ibuprofen or naproxen. Only one woman out of 120 patients treated by Stovall had other side effects—nausea and vomiting (Stovall 1995). Subsequent successful pregnancy rates in women treated with methotrexate are as high as they are with surgical intervention: 89 percent had an 11-percent incidence of recurrent ectopic pregnancy, as compared with 60 percent of women who had surgery experiencing a 13-percent incidence of recurrent ectopic pregnancy (Stovall et al. 1991; Langer et al. 1990; Silva et al. 1993). Both doctors and patients prefer the medical treatment of ectopic pregnancy when the diagnosis is made early.

Surgical Treatment of Ectopic Pregnancy

Surgery remains the only method for treating women with ectopic pregnancies that are not candidates for medical therapy. Laparoscopic surgery has largely supplanted the larger abdominal incision in all instances except life threatening emergencies. The type of tubal surgery is dependent on the extent of damage to the tube. Minor tubal damage may be repaired while greater damage may require removal of a portion of the tube or the entire tube. All three can be accomplished with a laparoscope or an open abdominal incision. Let's take a look at those options:

- **Removing the ectopic pregnancy itself, leaving the tube behind**. When the pregnancy is removed by surgery and the tube is left intact, some of the ectopic tissue remains in the tube (15 percent after laparoscopy, 2 percent after an abdominal incision). These women need methotrexate therapy or a repeat operation to cure them (Seifer et al. 1993).

- **Removing the affected portion of the tube**, allowing future reattachment of the two severed ends.

- **Removing the entire tube** when it is seriously damaged.

Summary of Ectopic Pregnancies

An ectopic pregnancy is a life-threatening event that, when recognized early, can be treated either medically or with laparoscopic surgery. Either treatment can result in the retention of some of the pregnancy tissue, but this is infrequent. This small risk seems more than offset by the ease of treatment and the speed of recovery. In the past, traditional management of ectopic pregnancies has been open abdominal incision, but this surgery has been relegated to handling life-threatening internal hemorrhage due to tubal rupture.

Urinary Incontinence

Significant urinary incontinence occurs in 25 percent of all women in their reproductive years and in 50 percent of all postmenopausal women. Some degree of incontinence occurs in 85 percent of women over age eighteen (Lyons 1995). Over $16 billion is spent annually on treatment of incontinence, including the cost of protective garments (Brown 1996). To help you understand the causes and treatment of incontinence, let's take another brief look at your anatomy.

The Genito-Urinary System

The reproductive organs (genitals) and the urinary organs form your *genito-urinary system*. Problems with both the genital and the urinary systems often coexist, so they are usually diagnosed and treated together. When urinary incontinence occurs, the following parts of your body are involved:

- **Kidneys:** Your kidneys filter wastes out of your blood and make urine, which is passed to the bladder by the ureters.
- **Bladder:** The bladder is simply a reservoir to store urine until it is convenient to empty it. When your bladder fills to a certain amount, the *detrusor* (bladder muscle) contracts to expel the urine.
- **Urethra:** This is the tube connecting your bladder to the outside world. Your urethra is only about three inches long. It is surrounded by muscles that maintain their strength with the help of your estrogens. The urethra and the muscles around it lose tone with age and with estrogen depletion. In addition, the urethral muscles may have been damaged during childbirth (Brown 1996). During perimenopause, when your tissues begin to lose their tensile strength, your damaged urethra may lose strength as well. The urethra may not be strong enough to keep urine from running out of your bladder when you cough or sneeze. During and after menopause, prolonged estrogen depletion further damages the urethra and it may remain open, acting as a siphon from the bladder to the outside.
- **Bladder neck:** This is the area where your bladder joins the urethra. It is surrounded by muscles that automatically keep the bladder neck closed so urine stays in your bladder. When you urinate, the bladder neck opens, and urine enters the urethra. Age, estrogen depletion, and childbirth trauma cause these muscles to lose strength, resulting in urine loss.

- **External urethral sphincter:** Vaginal muscles support your bladder, bladder neck, and urethra. The external urethral sphincter is a portion of the vaginal muscles near the opening of your vagina. The sphincter prevents urine from escaping. It is under voluntary control. Unable to do the job alone, this sphincter needs help from its neighbors, the urethra and bladder neck. When your bladder neck and urethra can not control urine loss, neither can your sphincter, no matter how tightly you squeeze it.

- **Pelvic floor muscles:** One of the pelvic floor muscles, the *pubococcygeus*, circles your vagina and acts as a sling to suspend your uterus, bladder, bladder neck, and urethra. It is a voluntary muscle that helps the structures it supports to function correctly. Pregnancy, childbirth, and decreased estrogen states all cause the pelvic floor muscles to lose some of their strength. The organs it supports start sagging downward. If your bladder is one of these organs, incontinence results.

Continence—The Way It Ought to Be

When your bladder is full, it sends messages to your brain: "I have to go now!" Your brain sends a message back to your bladder giving it permission to empty. Sometimes, it isn't convenient to empty your bladder.

You may at the time be the referee in the middle of a soccer game, for instance, and are pretty sure emptying your bladder in center field doesn't fit the referee image. Instead of giving your bladder the "all ahead, full throttle" directive, you send the message to "hold it." Your external sphincter tightens for all it's worth, the bladder muscles relax and the bladder neck remains closed, and your urge to urinate subsides. Once you get to the bathroom at halftime, though, your bladder sends a more urgent message to your brain: "Are you folks up there aware that we have a problem down here?" Your brain answers, "Affirmative, detrusors. We have you punched up on our monitor. Let it go." Your external sphincter relaxes, your detrusor muscles contract, your bladder neck opens, and . . . RELIEF!

Types of Incontinence

Our description of normal continence may sound funny to you—but it's no fun when something goes wrong, causing you to lose urine when you don't want to. Depending upon which part of the body has a problem, you develop one (or more) types of incontinence: stress incontinence, urge incontinence, or siphon incontinence. More than 65 percent of all urinary incontinence is a mixture of these types (McGuire and Cespedes 1996).

Type I, Stress Incontinence

Stress incontinence is also called Type I incontinence. You can lose urine with any activity that increases the pressure (stress) on your bladder, including sneezing, laughing, coughing, jogging, lifting, and even sex. The increased pressure on the bladder puts added pressure on your bladder neck to open. If your external sphincter is not strong enough to compensate, urine escapes.

Stress incontinence occurs mainly in women who have had babies. Only 4 percent of childless women have stress incontinence (Brown 1996). (Note: Although women athletes sometimes lose urine with exercise, usually this is due to a bladder infection rather than true stress incontinence.)

According to Brown, for 22 to 32 percent of women, the first experience with incontinence is during pregnancy when the baby's head is pressing on the bladder. Immediately after birth, 6 percent of these women are still incontinent, but by one year only 3 percent still lose urine. The time spent pushing a baby out in the second stage of labor is related to the development of incontinence: The longer a woman pushes during delivery, the greater her chance of developing incontinence when she reaches her mid- to late forties and beyond. The type of delivery also has an effect on how often stress incontinence occurs (Brown 1996). Forceps deliveries have a higher incidence of stress incontinence than do vacuum extraction deliveries. Women who have had a vacuum extraction have a higher incidence of incontinence than do women who had spontaneous vaginal deliveries. These results are deceiving, however, because women who have either forceps or vacuum deliveries have been pushing longer than women who have had spontaneous deliveries. Two large studies proved that the early intervention with forceps and episiotomy decreased the damage to the vaginal muscles and resultant incontinence (Gainey 1955; Ranney 1990). Of all methods of delivery, Cesarean births have the lowest incidence of incontinence.

You may find the cause of your incontinence interesting indeed, but chances are you're more interested in fixing it. You've already had your last baby and you are dealing with incontinence *now*. You can't go back and change the way your children were delivered. What can you do today to help stop this embarrassing problem? Here are the medical treatments that work:

- **Kegel exercises:** Fifty percent of women can eliminate or decrease their incontinence by doing pelvic floor exercises called *Kegel exercises.* Mouritsen and others studied 80 women with documented anatomical stress incontinence who had been referred for corrective surgery. They were all treated with Kegel exercises. By the end of one year, 50 percent didn't need the operation! (Mouritsen et al. 1991) showed that performing fifteen repetitions of Kegel exercises three or four times a day restores continence. The technique is to tighten the muscles that control urination (Elia and Bergmann 1993; Hahn et al. 1993; Mouritsen et al. 1991). Another way to identify these muscles is to place two fingers in your vagina and press on your rectum from inside the vagina. Try to tighten the muscles you can feel with your fingers. Kegel exercises also help Type II urge incontinence (see the next section).

- **Vaginal cones:** You can use gradually increasing weights to learn to contract your pelvic muscles. You place the 20 gram cone in your vagina and keep it in place by contracting your muscles. Once you are able to keep it there twice a day for fifteen minutes, you change to the next heavier cone. Seventy-five percent of women who use the cones improve their stress incontinence significantly (Ostergard 1997).

- **Electrical stimulation:** Low-voltage electrical current applied to the pelvic muscles treats both Type I and Type II incontinence. The stimulation is delivered either through the vagina or rectum and teaches you to recognize the contraction of your pelvic muscles and strengthen them. There is a 50-percent improvement in two-thirds of women who use this method, and 30 percent are cured of their incontinence (Ostergard 1997).

- **Biofeedback:** With the help of biofeedback, women with stress and urge incontinence can learn to distinguish the contraction of their pelvic muscles from their abdominal muscles. This method requires one-hour sessions for four to eight weeks, but it achieves an 81-percent success rate (Ostergard 1997).

- **Obstructing devices:** There are several devices that mechanically close off the urethra, stopping urine from leaking out (like a cork in a bottle). The most popular of these devices is a short catheter that fits through the urethra into the bladder and has a small inflatable balloon which blocks the urethra. The catheter/balloon device completely prevents stress incontinence and can be worn for six hours, but 30 percent of the time there is complication of repeated bladder infections (Ostergard 1997, Reliance package insert).

CAUTION! Some women are so afraid they will lose urine that they contract their vaginal muscles all the time. As a result, the muscles are in a state of constant fatigue. They can't tighten anymore because they are already tight. When the urge hits, these women lose urine anyway.

Type II, Urge Incontinence

Urge incontinence is also called Type II incontinence, tiny bladder syndrome, and detrusor instability. In Type II incontinence, your brain perceives the urge to urinate even though your bladder is only partially full, so your bladder contracts. Even when you can successfully keep your external sphincter closed and prevent passage of urine, your bladder continues to contract and the urge to void continues. You can lose urine when your bladder is full, or when you hear water running, or at any other time when you think you have to urinate—your bladder has taken control!

If you give in to urge incontinence, the bladder contracts even sooner the next time, and then sooner again, until you are spending your day running from bathroom to bathroom. You may be up several times every night passing dribs and drabs of urine, ending up exhausted and upset about the loss of control. The good news is, you can fix this problem. The first step is to identify the cause.

There are many possible causes of urge incontinence:

- **Urinary tract infections,** both acute and chronic, keep the bladder inflamed and irritated, leading to spasms of the detrusor muscle. You need a full urological evaluation if you have frequent urinary tract infections, not just repeated antibiotic therapy.

- **Estrogen deficiency** leads to thinning (atrophy) of the lining of your urethra and bladder. In this situation, your resistance to infection is lowered.

- **Uterine enlargement** puts pressure on the bladder and can cause urge incontinence. Fibroids are the most common source of uterine enlargement in perimenopausal women. A simple pelvic exam will reveal this.

- **Nerve damage** from a spinal cord injury, or spinal nerve-root pressure from a ruptured disc can result in poor muscle control of the bladder wall.

- **Chemotherapy** treatment may damage neurological control of the bladder or the muscles themselves.

- **Emotional stress** may increase your adrenaline (ephinephrine) levels causing your bladder to contract more frequently with smaller and smaller amounts of urine present each time. Counseling may help you deal with your stress, your epinephrine levels will lower and so will the frequency of bladder spasms.

- **Cigarette smoking, alcohol, and caffeine** (even the amount in decaffeinated coffee) all irritate the bladder and worsen the symptoms of urge incontinence.

- **Some antihypertensive medications** cause urge incontinence.

If you have urge incontinence, treatment also involves behavior modification techniques to retrain your out-of-control bladder. Retraining is a very successful remedy but requires a great deal of effort on your part.

If you have urge incontinence, your doctor will prescribe an antispasmodic medicine such as oxybutynin or propantheline to help you gain control of your bladder. When these drugs don't work, your doctor may prescribe a low dose of imipramine, a tricyclic antidepressant (Appell 1997). You will also need to use an estrogen cream or ring to increase your vaginal collagen strength (Fantl et al. 1994).

The treatment of urge incontinence also involves behavior modification techniques to retrain your out-of-control bladder. Retraining is a very successful remedy but requires a great deal of effort of your part. Your retraining program should start with a regular schedule of urination every two hours, even if you don't need to go. In addition, it is most important that you do not give in to the urge to empty your bladder before the scheduled time. (It's okay to lose a little urine.) Once you can hold it for two hours, increase the time to two hours and ten minutes. Over a period of weeks, slowly increase the time between voidings until you can hold your urine for four hours. At this time you can usually go off the medication and retain control of your bladder.

A hypnotist can cure urge incontinence 58 percent of the time and improve incontinence 30 percent of the time. An acupuncturist can improve incontinence by 85 percent (Ostergard 1997).

TIP! When you feel you have to go, stop what you are doing, sit down if you can, and do six quick Kegel exercises. The Kegel exercises relax your bladder's detrusor muscle so it stops contracting. You can then take a leisurely walk to the bathroom.

Gynecologists can cure stress incontinence 80 percent of the time with a variety of surgical procedures (Cosiski-Marana et al. 1996). If you have a combination of urge incontinence and stress incontinence, however, you must acquire control of your urge incontinence before having surgery for stress incontinence (McGuire and Cespedes 1996), because the stitches used to repair stress incontinence will make urge incontinence worse.

CAUTION! The stitches add an extra irritant to an already irritable bladder. It is therefore important that you be completely evaluated before undergoing any bladder surgery. Many doctors use a trial of oxybutynin or imipramine before agreeing to do any surgery. These bladder relaxants help determine what portion of your incontinence, if any, is due to an irritable bladder. If urge incontinence is the only type of incontinence you have, medical treatment is the only way to cure your problem.

Type III, Siphon Incontinence

Type III siphon incontinence is due to a weak urethra. This condition is also called "stove-pipe urethra" because the urethra has become a rigid straight tube instead of a pliable structure. Type III incontinence is not common in perimenopausal women; it occurs as the result of multiple surgical repairs or prolonged estrogen depletion.

Surgical Options for Incontinence

When you need surgery, several diagnostic tests are needed to help your doctor decide which operation to perform. First, a laboratory technician will culture your urine to make sure incontinence is not due to a bladder infection. Then a urologist or gynecologist will insert a fiber-optic equipped cystoscope inside the urethra and bladder to evaluate local causes of incontinence. During this procedure, the surgeon can add water or gas which distends your bladder and allows visualization of your entire bladder and urethra. The surgeon can measure the pressure your bladder can withstand before it begins to contract. This information helps your doctor determine which type of incontinence you have and what operation, if any, is best for you.

Your surgeon can repair Type I and Type III incontinence by either a vaginal or abdominal operation, but surgery will not correct Type II incontinence.

Vaginal Repair of Incontinence

The first vaginal repair for incontinence was described by Kelly in 1913 and it is still used today. The Kelly repair tightens the connective tissue beneath the urethra by suturing the tissue along the sides of the urethra, raising the bladder neck to its original position. The Kelly repair has an immediate success rate of 84 percent, but only 60 percent of the patients were continent five years after their surgery. A variety of vaginal suspension operations have since been designed but have proved no more successful over the long run than the original Kelly repair.

A Kelly repair or another urethral suspension operation remains the treatment of choice for incontinence in conjunction with extensive vaginal surgery to repair the bladder (cystocele) and rectum when they have ballooned into the vagina (the rectal hernia is called *rectocele*).

Abdominal Surgery for Incontinence Repair

The original abdominal repair to correct stress incontinence was described by Marshall, Marchetti, and Krantz in 1949. The MMK operation suspends the bladder neck by stitching it to the covering of the pubic bone. The success rate with this operation over five or more years is greater that 85 percent. However, sometimes the stitches cause an infection in the pubic bone, which is difficult to treat (Marshall, Marchetti and Kranz 1949).

For this reason, the MMK has been largely replaced by the Burch procedure. In the Burch procedure, two permanent stitches are placed along each side of the urethra and attached to an abdominal ligament, rather than anchored to the pubic bone as in the MMK procedure. The success rate with the Burch procedure over five or more years is between 88 and 90 percent when Type I incontinence is present (Burch 1961; Bergman and Elia 1995; Kjolhede and Ryden 1994).

Neither the Burch nor the MMK procedure restores the bladder to its original position. And when there is a large cystocele or rectocele present, the surgical success rate of these operations is reduced to 60 percent (Cosiske-Marana et al. 1996). Unfortunately, there is a 17 to 50 percent incidence of herniation of intestines into the vaginal space (*enterocele*) following a Burch procedure (Nichols 1991); this may require future corrective surgery.

Note that the Burch procedure is also being done through the laparoscope, with long-lasting results similar to those seen with an abdominal incision (Lyons 1995).

Even if incontinence persists after Kegel exercises and the removal of caffeine and alcohol from your diet, by employing these measures your tissues are in much better shape when you do have an operation (Brown 1996). Healing is improved, as are the chances of long-term success. And the retraining can do wonders for your continence and sex life even if your vaginal muscles have been seriously damaged in childbirth.

The Estrogen Connection

Estrogen deficiency contributes to urinary incontinence. Loss of estrogen translates to loss of collagen anywhere in your body where collagen exists: the breasts, face, neck, abdomen, vagina, and bladder. Supplementation of estrogen during these years, in the form of pills or vaginal cream or both, can help avert these difficulties.

A new method of delivering estrogen, the vaginal estrogen ring, came on the market in February 1997. The ring delivers a slow, steady dose of estrogen to the vagina and bladder, with only small amounts getting into general circulation. Unfortunately, the ring is contraindicated when you have a cystocele, rectocele, or uterine prolapse, because in this case the device will continually fall out or may cause a vaginal ulcer (Ayton et al. 1996; Henriksson et al. 1996). In women who can use this product, however, the ring will help prevent problems due to long-term estrogen deprivation.

Summary

Anatomic and functional changes in your gynecologic organs may never become a problem for you. If they do, though, these pages will serve as a guide to current thinking about surgical management and nonsurgical alternatives.

Pharmaceutical and technological advances continue to be made, offering welcome alternatives to traditional surgical intervention. Nevertheless, surgery is sometimes the only alternative. The primary goal is always to restore function and return you to a normal lifestyle.

○ ○ ○

Conclusion

As your post-WWII baby boomer generation has moved through its various stages of life, it has made fundamental changes in many aspects of American culture. Because of your sheer size, you changed the number of schools in existence and even how they were built. Mickey Mouse Clubbers, Howdy Doody devotees, and Captain Kangaroo watchers changed children's television. Bell-bottom pants, miniskirts, and long hair became the norm for many years. Sexual liberation from long held social standards of propriety was a mark of your generation, although this may not have been one of your best moves. You embraced Elvis and the Beatles to change contemporary music. As you began to marry, an enormous housing boom blossomed and so did suburbs with connecting freeways. You changed childbirthing with natural childbirth, and made it a family event with fathers in attendance. One of you was elected President in 1992 and reelected in 1996. Yours is an energized and energizing group. Unlike your predecessors, you have always taken control of challenges and events facing you, rather than being controlled by them. All generations have changed their times in varying degrees; but you boomers *changed* yours.

This book has been about another change facing you . . . perimenopause. It certainly isn't anything new in life's scheme; but it is new to you. It is the old age of your youth and the gateway to mid-life. The four or five decades of your life to this point have been blatantly oriented toward youthfulness. Look young, act young, stay young. Social bias and commercialism have favored your youth, and curried your favor every step of the way. You grew up thinking that youth is perpetual and that aging and death are only theoretical considerations. For that matter, so did we all. We aren't worried about you though. We have every faith in you and your peers that you will not fall into a "lost youth" funk. You have seized the moment in every other phase of your life, and perimenopause should be no exception.

We hope we have convinced you that perimenopause is a watershed time in your life. It is a transition from the wonderful years of your youth to the fantastic years of your second half of life. Our purpose has been to inform and educate you about certain changes you can expect, and to empower you to deal with them successfully. To do this, we have heaped a lot of good news-bad news concepts on you. Some of our advice may have been welcome; and we regretfully acknowledge that some of it was not. Still, we hope you are charitable enough to recognize that we have been in your corner when it came to things that can benefit you.

We do not want you to dwell on perimenopause and the changes it may impose on your body and in your life. Once you are aware of what is required to protect yourself from adverse changes, and once you have woven the protective techniques into the fabric of your life, move on. Life and living it are much too precious to be subverted by daily preoccupation with burdensome details of techniques, treatments, and menus. This isn't a dress rehearsal you are going though, it's an authentic life and we want you to live it that way. Our hope for you as our reader is for you to have increased your fund of knowledge about perimenopause; but our fondest and most fundamental wish for you as a woman is for you to stay focused on your journey.

Appendix A

Information Resources

Aging

National Council on Aging
409 Third Street, SW, 2nd Floor
Washington, DC 20024
(800) 424-9046

National Institutes of Health
National Institute of Aging
900 Rockville Pike
Bethesda, MD 20892
(800) 222-2225

Alternative Medicine

Chinese Medicine
AAAOM Referrals
4101 Lake Boone Trail, Suite 201
Raleigh, NC 27607
(919) 787-5181

National Center for Homeopathy
810 North Fairfax, Suite 306
Alexandria, VA 22314
(703) 548-7790

National Institutes of Health
Office of Alternative Medicine
6120 Executive Blvd.
Executive Plaza South, Suite 450
Rockville, MD 20892
(301) 402-2466

Cancer

American Cancer Society
1599 Clifton Road NE
Atlanta, GA 30329
(800) 227-2345

American Lung Association
1740 Broadway
New York, NY 10019
(212) 315-8700

American Gastroenterological
Association
7910 Woodmont Avenue
Bethesda, MD 20814
(301) 654-2055

National Cancer Institute
Bethesda, MD 20205
(800) 422-6237

Society of Gynecologic Oncologists
401 North Michigan Avenue
Chicago, IL 60611
(312) 644-6610

The Skin Cancer Foundation
245 Fifth Avenue, Suite 2402
New York, NY 10016
(212) 725-5176

Diet and Nutrition

American Dietetic Association
216 W. Jackson Blvd., Suite 800
Chicago, IL 60606
(312) 899-0040

Human Nutrition Information Service
U.S. Department of Agriculture
Hyattsville, MD 20782
(301) 436-7725

Exercise

American College of Sports Medicine
P.O. Box 1440
Indianapolis, IN 46202
(317) 637-9200

Fertility and Pregnancy

The Alan Guttmacher Institute
111 Fifth Avenue
New York, NY 10063
(212) 254-5656

American College of Obstetricians and
Gynecologists
Office of Public Information
409 12th Street SW
Washington, DC 20024-2188
(202) 484-3321

American Fertility Society
1209 Montgomery Highway
Birmingham, AL 35216
(205) 978-5000

American Society for Reproductive
Medicine
(617) 623-0744
Fax 617-623-0254

National Center for Education in
Maternal and Child Care
2000 15th Street, North, Suite 701
Arlington, VA 22201
(703) 524-7802

National Down Syndrome Society
666 Broadway
New York, NY 10012
(800) 222-4602

National Society of Genetic Counselors
233 Canterbury Dr.
Wallingford, PA 19086

RESOLVE (Info for Infertile Couples)
1310 Broadway
Somerville, MA 02144-1731
(617) 623-0744
FAX (617) 623-0254

Serono Laboratories
Patient Education Library on Infertility
100 Longwater Circle
Norwell, MA 02061
Hotline for infertility 1-800-860-4134

Heart Disease

American Heart Association
7320 Greenville Avenue
Dallas, TX 75231
(800) 242-8721

National Cholesterol Education
 Program
At National Heart, Lung and Blood
 Institute Information Center
4733 Bethesda Ave., Suite 500
Bethesda, MD 20814-4820
(301) 951-3260

Medicines

American Pharmaceutical Association
2215 Constitution Ave.
Washington, DC 20037
(800) 237-2742
Food and Drug Administration (FDA)
8800 Rockville Pike
Bethesda, MD 20852
Chicago, IL 60610
(301) 295-8228
(800) 262-3211

Menopause

North American Menopause Society
4074 Abingdon Road
Cleveland, OH 44106
(216) 844-3334

Mental Health

American Psychiatric Association
1400 K Street, NW
Washington, DC 20005
(202) 682-6000

American Psychological Association
750 First Street, NW
Washington, DC 20002
(202) 336-5500

Anxiety Disorders Association of
 America
600 Executive Blvd.
Rockville, MD 20852

Mind/Body Medicine

Deaconess Hospital
Division of Behavioral Medicine
1 Deaconess Road
Boston, MA 02215
(617) 632-9530
Tapes on relaxation available

Osteoporosis

National Osteoporosis Foundation
2100 M Street NW
Washington, DC 20037
(202) 223-3336

Physicians Organizations

American Board of Medical Specialities
1-800-776-2378

American College of Obstetricians and
 Gynecologists
Office of Public Information
409 12th Street SW
Washington, DC 20024-2188
(202) 484-3321

American Medical Association
515 North State Street
Chicago, IL 60610

American Society for Dermatologic
 Surgery
930 North Meacham Road
Schaumburg, IL 60137-6016
(847) 330-9830

American Society for Laser Medicine
 and Surgery
244 Stewart Square
Wausau, WI 54401

American Society of Plastic and
 Reconstructive Surgeons
444 East Algonquin Road
Arlington Heights, IL 60005-4664
(708) 228-9900

Sexuality

American Association of Sex
Educators, Counselors, and
Therapists
435 Michigan Avenue, Suite 1717
Chicago, IL 60611
(312) 644-0828

Council for Sex Information and
Education
2272 Colorado Blvd., #1228
Los Angeles, CA 90041

Sexually Transmitted Diseases

Centers for Disease Control and
Prevention
Division of STD Prevention
1600 Clifton Road, NE
Atlanta, GA 30333
(404) 639-3311

National AIDS Hotline
(800) 342-AIDS

National Sexually Transmitted Disease
Hotline
(800) 227-8922

Specialty Pharmacies
(For Natural Hormones)

Belmar Pharmacy
Lakewood, CO
(800) 525-9473

Madison Pharmacy
Madison, WI
(800) 558-7046

Women's International Pharmacy
5708 Monona Drive
Madison, WI 53716-3152
1-800-279-3708 Fax (608) 221-7819

Substance Abuse

Al-Anon Family Group Headquarters
P.O. Box 862, Midtown Station
New York, NY 10018
(800) 356-9996 for free pamphlets
(800) 344-2666 for USA meeting dates
(800) 443-4525 for Canada

Alcoholics Anonymous
General Service Office
Box 459, Grand Central Station
New York, NY 10016
(212) 686-1100

Cocaine Anonymous
3740 Overland Avenue, Suite G
Los Angeles, CA 90034
(800) 347-8998

Narcotics Anonymous
World Services Office
P.O. Box 9999
Van Nuys, CA 91409

National Clearinghouse for Alcohol
and Drug Information
P.O. Box 2345
Rockville, MD 20847-2345
(800) 729-6686 or (301) 468-2600

Women for Sobriety
P.O. Box 618
Quaker Town, PA 18951
(800) 333-1606

Urinary Incontinence

American Urological Association
1120 North Charles Street
Baltimore, MD 21201
(401) 727-1100

Help for Incontinent People (HIP)
P.O. Box 544
Union, SC 29379
(800) BLADDER

The Simon Foundation for Continence
P.O. Box 835
Wilmette, IL 60097
(800) 23-SIMON

Women's Health

The Endometriosis Association
8585 North 76th Place
Milwaukee, WI 53223
(800) 962-ENDO

National Institutes of Health Office of
    Research on Women's Health
Building 1, Room 201
9000 Rockville Pike
Bethesda, MD 20892
(301) 402-1770

National Self-Help Clearinghouse
25 W 43rd Street, Room 620
New York, NY 10036
(212) 642-2944
Databank for self-help groups

National Women's Health Network
1325 G Street, NW
Washington, DC 20005
(202) 347-1140

Women's Health Initiative
Federal Building, Room 6A09
9000 Rockville Pike
Bethesda, MD 20892
(800) 548-6636

Appendix B

Recommended Reading

Alternative Medicine

Bienfield, H., and E. Korngold. 1991. *Between Heaven and Earth: A Guide to Chinese Medicine.* New York: Ballantine Books.

Lockie, Andrew, 1989. *The Family Guide to Homeopathy.* New York: Fireside.

O'Brien, P. 1995. *Yoga for Women.* New York: Harper Collins.

Ullman, D., 1991. *Discovering Homeopathic Medicine For the 21st Century.* North Atlantic Books.

Wolfe, H. L., 1990. *Second Spring: A Guide to Healthy Menopause Through Traditional Chinese Medicine.* Boulder, CO: Blue Poppy Press.

Cancer

Karnicky, Lydia, M.D., Anne Rosenberg, M.D., Marian Betancourt, 1995; *What To Do If You Have Breast Cancer.* New York: Little, Brown & Company.

Love, Susan, M.D., 1995. *Dr. Susan Love's Breast Book.* Rev. ed. New York: Addison-Wesley.

Spiegel, David, M.D. 1997. *Living Beyond Limits.* New York: Times Books.

Contraception

Harlap, S, F. Frost, J. D. Forrest, 1991. *Preventing Pregnancy, Protecting Health*. New York: Alan Guttmacher Institute.

Exercise and Fitness

Alter, Michael J., 1990. *Sport Stretch*. Champaign, IL: Human Kinetics.

American College of Sports Medicine, 1992. *ACSM Fitness Book*. Champaign, IL: Human Kinetics.

Bailey, Covert, 1994. *Smart Exercise: Burning Fat, Getting Fit*. New York: Houghton Mifflin.

Fertility and Pregnancy

American College of Obstetricians and Gynecologists, 1992. *Planning For Pregnancy, Birth and Beyond*. New York: Dutton

Berger, Gary S., M.D., Mark Goldstein, M. D., Mark Fuerst, 1995. *The Couples Guide To Infertility*. New York: Doubleday.

Heart Disease

Legato, Marianne J., M.D. and Carol Colman, 1992. *The Female Heart: The Truth About Women and Coronary Artery Disease*. New York: Simon and Schuster.

Ornish, Dean, M.D., 1992. *Dr. Dean Ornish's Program For Reversing Heart Disease*. New York: Ballantine Books

Mental and Emotional Health

Benson, Herbert, M.D. and Eileen M. Stuart, R.N., M.S., 1993. *The Wellness Book: The Comprehensive Guide to Maintaining Health and Treating Stress-Related Illness*. New York: Fireside.

Domar, A. D. and H. Drayer, 1996. *Healing Mind, Healthy Woman*. New York: Henry Holt.

Drayer, H. 1995. *The Immune Power Personality: 7 Traits You Can Develop To Stay Healthy*. New York: Dutton.

Gold, M., 1990. *The Good News About Panic, Anxiety and Phobias*. New York: Bantam.

Kass, Frederick T., M.D., John M. Oldman, M.D., Herbert Pardes, M.D., and Lois B. Morris, ed., 1992. *The Columbia University College of Physicians and Surgeons Complete Home Guide to Mental Health*. New York: Henry Holt.

Khalsa D. H., 1997. *Brain Longevity*. New York: Warner.

Klein, A., 1989. *The Healing Power of Humor*. Los Angeles: Jeremy P. Tarcher.

Nuland, S. B., 1997. *Wisdom of the Body*.

Midlife Health

Doress-Worters, Paula B., and Diana L. Siegal, 1994. *The New Ourselves, Growing Older*. New York: Simon and Schuster.

Foley, D, E. Nechas, ed. 1993. *Women's Encyclopedia of Health and Emotional Healing.* Emmas, PA: Rodale Press.

Landau, Carol, PhD., Michele G. Cyre, M.D., Anne M. Moulton, M.D., 1994. *The Complete Book of Menopause: Every Woman's Guide to Good Health.* New York: G.P. Putnam's Sons.

Notelovitz, Morris, M.D. and Dianna Tonnessen, 1993. *Menopause and Midlife Health.* New York: St. Martin's Press.

Reichman, Judith, M.D., 1996. *I'm Too Young To Get Old: Health Care For Women After Forty.* New York: Times Books.

Mind/Body Medicine

Chopra, Deepak, M.D., 1990. *Quantum Healing: Exploring the Frontiers of Mind/Body Medicine.* New York: Bantam.

Goleman, D. and J. Gurin, ed. 1993. *Mind/Body Medicine.* Yonkers, NY: Consumer Reports Books

Kabat-Zinn, J., 1990. *Full Catastrophe Living: Using the Wisdom of Your Body and Mind To Face Stress and Illness.* New York: Delacorte Press.

Khalsa, D. H., M.D., 1997. *Brain Longevity.* New York: Warner.

Nuland, S.B., 1997. *Wisdom of the Body.* New York: Alfred A. Knopf.

Nutrition and Diet

American Heart Association, 1995. *American Heart Association Brand Name Fat and Cholesterol Counter*, 2nd ed. New York: Viking.

American Heart Association, 1995. *American Heart Association Low-Fat, Low Cholesterol Cookbook.* New York: Times Books.

American Heart Association, 1995. *American Heart Association Low-Salt, Low-Cholesterol Cookbook,* New York: Times Books

Brody, Jane, 1990. *Jane Brody's Good Food Gourmet.* New York: W.W. Norton.

Connor, Sonja L., M.S., R.D., and William E. Connor, M.D., 1991. *The New American Diet System.* New York: Simon & Schuster.

Griffiths K., and H. Aldercretz, 1996. *Nutrition and Cancer.* New York: Mosby.

Messina, Mark, PhD., Virginia Messina, Ken Setchell, Ph.D., 1994. *The Simple Soybean and Your Health.* Garden City Park, NY: Avery Publishing Group.

Ojeda, Linda, PhD., 1995. *Menopause Without Medicine.* Alameda, CA: Hunter House.

Somer, E., 1993. *Nutrition For Women,* New York: Henry Holt.

Waterhouse, Debra, 1993. *Outsmarting the Female Fat Cell.* New York: Hyperion.

Wotecki, Catherine E. and P.T. Thomas, ed., 1993. *Eat For Life: The Food and Nutrition Board's Guide to Reducing Your Risk of Chronic Disease.* New York: Harper Perennial.

Osteoporosis

ACOG Technical Bulletin No. 167, 1992. *Osteoporosis.* Washington, DC: American College of Obstetricians and Gynecologists.

American Medical Association, 1995. *American Medical Association Pocket Guide to Calcium.* New York: Random House.

Peck, William A., M.D., 1988. *Osteoporosis: The Silent Thief.* Glenview, IL: AARP Books.

Sexuality

Masters, William H. and Virginia Johnson, 1986. *Master and Johnson on Sex and Human Loving.* New York: Little Brown.

Michael, Robert T., John H. Gagnon, Edward O. Laumann, Gina Kolata, 1994. *Sex in America: A Definitive Survey.* Boston: Little, Brown.

Rosenthal Saul H., M.D., 1987. *Sex Over 40.* New York: Tarcher, Putnam.

Stoppard, Miriam, M.D., 1991. *The Magic of Sex: The Book That Really Tells Men About Women and Women About Men.* New York: Dorling Kindersly, Inc.

Surgery

Harris, Dena E., M.D. and Helene MacLean, 1992. *Recovering From a Hysterectomy.* New York: Harper Collins.

Wilson, Josleen, 1992. *The American Society for Plastic and Reconstructive Surgery's Guide to Cosmetic Surgery.* New York: Simon and Schuster.

References

Chapter 1: What Changes? An Overview

Eskin, B., and L. Dumas. 1995. *Midlife Can Wait: How to Stay Young and Healthy After 35*. New York: Ballantine Books.

Friegenbaum, Seth. Head of Reproductive Endocrinology, Kaiser Permanente of Northern California. Personal communication, March 14, 1997.

Henderson, B. E., R. K. Ross, A. Pagannini, and T.M. Mack. 1986. "Estrogen Use and Cardiovascular Disease." *American Journal of Obstetrics and Gynecology* 154:1181.

Speroff, Leon, R. H. Glass, and N. G. Kase. 1989. *Clinical Gynecologic Endocrinology and Infertility*. Baltimore: Williams and Wilkins.

Graham, Ellen. 1995. "The Baby Boom Hits 50." *Wall St. Journal*, October 31.

Chapter 2: Changes You Can See and Feel: Symptoms and Signs of Perimenopause

Avis, N. E. 1997. "Hormones and Mood Among Menopausal Women." *Menopausal Medicine* 5 (1):1–5.

Brown, J. 1996. "Episiotomy and Pelvic Floor Exercise For Incontinence." *Audio Digest, Obstetrics and Gynecology*. Volume 43.

Campbell, S., and M. Whitehead. 1977. "Estrogen Therapy and the Menopausal Syndrome." *Clinical Obstetrics and Gynecolology* 4 (3):94–99.

Kronenberg, Fredi. 1990. "Hot flashes: Epidemiology and Physiology. *American Journal for the Academy of Science* 6:56–58.

Kronenberg, Fredi. 1993. "Menopausal Hot Flashes." Paper presented at *Annual Meeting of the North American Menopause Society* May 21, 1993

Nachtigall, Lila E., and Joan Rattner Heilman. 1995. *Estrogen: The Facts Can Change Your Life.* New York; Harper Collins.

Sheehy, Gail. 1991. *The Silent Passage.* New York: Random House.

Chapter 3: Fertility Changes: Pregnancy, Infertility, and Contraception

"Folic Acid and Neural Tube Defects" (editorial). 1991. *Lancet* 338:153–54

"Folic Acid to Prevent Neural Tube Defects" (letters to the editor). 1991. *Lancet* 338:505–506.

ACOG Committee Opinion. March 1993. "Folic Acid for the Prevention of Recurrent Neural Tube Defects." No. 102:1–3.

Alexander, D. A., A. A. Naji, S. B. Pinion, J. Mollison, H. C. Kitchner, E. E. Parkin, D. R. Abramovich, and I. T. Russell. 1996. Randomized Trial Comparing Hysterectomy with Endometrial Ablation for Dysfunctional Uterine Bleeding: Psychiatric and Psychosocial Aspects. *British Medical Journal* 312 (7026):280–284.

American College of Obstetricians and Gynecologists. April 1991. "Alpha-Fetoprotein." *ACOG Guide to Preconception Care, Technical Bulletin no. 154.* Washington, D.C.: ACOG.

Amino, N., M. Hidemitsu, Y. Iwatane, O. Tanizawa, M. Kawashima, T. Tsuge, K. Ibaragi, Y. Kumahara, and K. Miyal. 1982. "High prevalence of transient post-partum thyrotoxicosis and hypothyroidism." *New England Journal of Medicine* 306:849–852.

Asch, R. H, and R. P. Marrs. 1993. *Assisted Reproductive Technologies :Serono Patient Education Library.* Norwell, Mass.: Serono Laboratories, Inc.

Bogart, M. H., O. W. Jones, R. A. Felder, R. G. Best, L. Bradley W. Butts, B. Crandall, W. MacMahon, F. H. Wians, Jr., and P. V. Loeh. 1991. "Prospective Evaluation of Maternal Serum Human Chorionic Gonadotropin Levels in 3428 Pregnancies." *American Journal of Obstetrics and Gynecology* 165:663–667.

Brill, A. I. 1995. "What Is the Role of Hysteroscope in the Management of Abnormal Uterine Bleeding?" *Clinical Obstetrics and Gynecology* 38:319–345.

Brown, J. R., H. Ye, R. T. Bronson, P. Dikkes, and M. E. Greenberg. 1996. "A Defect in Nurturing in Mice Lacking the Immediate Early Gene fosB." *Cell* 86:297–309.

California Department of Health Services, Genetic Disease Branch. 1995. "Prenatal Testing Choices for Women 35 Years and Older" (monograph). Berkeley: California Department of Health Services.

Center for Disease Control. 1977. "MMWR Morbidity and Mortality Weekly Report: Immune Globulines for the Protection against Viral Hepatitis." U.S. Department of Health, Education and Welfare/Public Health Service.

Centers for Disease Control and Prevention. 1993. "Recommendations for Use of Folic Acid to Reduce Number of Spina Bifida Cases and Other Neural Tube Defects." *Journal of the American Medical Association* 269:1233.

Chard, T., L. Lowings, and M. J. Kitau. 1984. "Alphafetoprotein and Chorionic Gonadotropin Levels in Relation to Down's Syndrome. *Lancet* 2 (8405):750.

Collaborative Group for the Study of Stroke in Young Women. 1975. "Oral Contraceptives and Stroke in Young Women." *The Journal of the American Medical Association* 231:718-722.

Cuckle, H. A., N. J. Wald, and S. C. Thompson. 1987. "Estimating a Woman's Risk of Having a Pregnancy Associated with Down's Syndrome Using Her Age and Serum Alpha-Fetoprotein Level." *British Journal of Obstetrics and Gynaecology* 94:387.

Dale, P. O., T. Tanbo, O. Lunde, and T. Abyholm. 1993. "Ovulation Induction with Low Dose Follicle-Stimulating Hormone in Women with Polycystic Ovarian Syndrome." *Acta Obstetrica and Gynecologica Scandinavica* 72:43–46.

Darney, P. D. 1996. "Oral Contraceptives and Upcoming Slow-Release Hormones. *Audio Digest Obstetrics and Gynecology* 43:(16)

Dodson W. C., D. K. Walmer, C. L. Hughes, and S. E. Yancy, B.S.N., A. F. Haney. 1991. "Leuprolide Therapy Does Not Improve Cycle Fecundity in Controlled Ovarian Hyperstimulation and Intrauterine Insemination of Subfertile Women." *Obstetrics and Gynecology* 78(92) 187–190.

Dodson, W. C., and A. F. Haney. 1991. "Controlled Ovarian Hyperstimulation and Intrauterine Insemination for Treatment of Infertility." *Fertility and Sterility* 55:457–467.

Dorris M. 1990. *The Broken Cord.* New York: Harper Collins.

Dwyer, N., J. Hutton, and G. M. Stirrat. 1993. "Randomized Controlled Trial Comparing Endometrial Resection with Abdominal Hysterectomy for the Surgical Treatment of Menorrhagia." *British Journal of Obstetrics and Gynaecology* 100:237–43.

Edge, V. L., and R. K. Laros. 1993. "Pregnancy Outcomes in Nulliparous Women Aged 35 or Older." *American Journal of Obstetrics and Gynecology* 168 (6), Part 1:1881–1885.

Emerson, C. H. 1991. "Thyroid Disease During and After Pregnancy." Chapter 93 in Braverman, L. E. and R. D. Utiger. *Werner and Ingbar's The Thyroid,* 6th ed. Philadelphia: J. Lippincott.

Fraser, I. S., and G. J.Dennerstein. 1994. "Depo-Provera Use in an Australian Metropolitan Practice." *The Medical Journal of Australia* 160:553–556.

Garner, C., and G. W. Patton. 1995. *Pathways to Parenthood: Serono Patient Education Library.* Norwell, Mass: Serono Laboratories Inc.

Gindoff, P. R., and R. Jewelewicz. 1986. "Reproductive Potential in the Older Woman." *Fertility and Sterility* 46:989–1001.

Grimes, D. 1997. "Sense and Sensuality: Contraceptives." *Audio-Digest Obstetrics and Gynecology* 44 (2).

Harris, B. S., S. Othman, J. A. Davies, G. J. Weppner, C. J. Richards, R. G. Newcombe, J. H. Lazarus, A. Hayslip, C. C., H. G. Fein, V. M. O'Donnell, D. S. Friedman, T. A. Klein, and R. C. Smallridge. 1988. "The Value of Serum Antimicrosomal Antibody Testing in Screening for Symptomatic Post Partum Thyroid Dysfunction." *American Journal of Obstetrics and Gynecology* 159:203–209.

Helstrom, L., P. O. Lundberg, D. Sorbom, and T. Bäckström. 1993. "Sexuality After Hysterectomy: A Factor Analysis of Women's Sexual Lives Before and After Subtotal Hysterectomy." *Obstetrics and Gynecology* 81:357–62.

Henzel, M. R., S. L. Corson, K. Morghissi, V. C. Buttram, C. Berqvist, and J. Jacobson. 1991. "Administration of Nasal Nafarelin As Compared with Oral Danazol for Endometriosis: A Multicenter Double-Blind Comparative Clinical Trial." *New England Journal of Medicine* 318:485–514.

Hook, E. G. 1983. "Chromosome Abnormalities and Spontaneous Fetal Deaths Following Amniocentesis: Further Data and Associations With Maternal Age." *American Journal of Human Genetetics* 35:110–116.

Hook, E. G., P. K. Cross, and D. M. Schreinemachers. 1983. "Chromosomal Abnormality Rates at Amniocentesis and In Live-Born Infants." *Journal of the American Medical Journal* 249:2034-2038.

Jaffe, S. B., and R. Jewelewicz. 1991. "The Basic Infertility Investigation." *Fertility and Sterility* 56:599–613.

John, E. M., D. A. Savitz, and D. P. Sandler. 1991. "Prenatal Exposure to Parents' Smoking and Childhood Cancer." *American Journal of Epidemiology* 133:123-132.

Kaunitz, A. M. 1996. "Long-Acting Contraceptive Options." *International Journal of Fertility and Menopausal Studies* 41:69–76.

Keye, W. R., R. J. Chang, R. W. Rebar, and M. R. Soules. 1995. *Infertility Evaluation and Treatment.* Philadelphia: W. B. Saunders.

Leventhal, J. April 1, 1997. "Libido and Menopause." Lecture given to the Women's Health Department, Kaiser, Walnut Creek, CA.

Marrs, R. P, and A. Domar. 1995. *Assisted Reproductive Technologies: Serono Patient Education Library.* Norwell, Mass.: Serono Laboratories, Inc.

Masters, W. H., and V. E. Johnson. 1966. *Human Sexual Response.* Boston: Little, Brown and Co.

Menken, J., J. Trussel, and U. Larson. 1986. "Age and Infertility." *Science* 233:1389.

MRC Vitamin Study Research Group. 1991. "Prevention of Neural Tube Defects: Results of the Medical Research Council Vitamin Study.: *Lancet* 338:131–37.

Nathorst-Boos, J., B. von Schoultz, and K. Carlstrom. 1993. "Elective Ovarian Removal and Estrogen Replacement Therapy—Effects on Sexual Life, Psychological Well-Being, and Androgen Status." *Journal of Psychosomatic Obstetrics and Gynaecology* 14:28393.

Nelson, A. L. 1996. "Norplant and Depo-Provera." *Audio Digest Obstetrics and Gynecology* 43:(16).

Norton, D. L. 1997. "Rezulin (Troglitazone)." Drug information handout. Morris Plains, N.J.: Parke-Davis.

Palomali, G. E., J. E. Haddow, G. J. Knight, N. J. Wald, A. Kennard, J. A. Canick, D. N. Saller, Jr., M. G. Blitzer, L. H. Dickerman, and R. Fisher. 1995. "Risk-Based Prenatal Screening for Trisomy 18 Using Alpha-Fetoprotein, Unconjugated Oestriol, and Human Chorionic Gonadotropin." *Prenatal Diagnosis.* 15:713–723.

Parkes, R. Hall, and D. I. W. Phillios. 1992. "Association Between Postpartum Thyroid Dysfunction and Thyroid Antibodies and Depression. *British Medical Journal* 305:152–156.

Ransom, M. X., N. C. Doughman, and A. J. Garcia. 1966. "Menotropins Alone Are Superior to a Clomiphene Citrate and Menotropin Combination for Superovulation Induction Among Clomiphene Citrate Failures." *Fertility and Sterility* 65:1169–1174.

Reichman, J. 1996. *I'm Too Young to Get Old: Health Care For Women After Forty.* New York: Times Books.

Rose, N. C., G. E. Palomaki, D. B. P. Goodman, and M. T. Mennuti. 1994. "Maternal Serum Alpha-Fetoprotein Screening for Chromosomal Abnormalities: A Prospective Study in Women Aged 35 and Older." *American Journal of Obstetrics and Gynecology* 170:1073–80.

Scott, R. T., M. S. Opsahl, M. R. Leonardi, G. S. Neall, E. H. Illions, and D. Navot. 1995. "Life Table Analysis of Pregnancy Rates in A General Infertility Population Relative to Ovarian Reserve and Patient Age." *Human Reproduction* 10:1706–10.

Serhal, P. F., M. Katz; V. Little, and H. Woronowski. 1988. "Unexplained Infertility—The Value of Pergonal* Superovulation Combined with Intrauterine Insemination. *Fertility and Sterility* 49:602–606.

Silberstein, S. D. 1992. "The Role Of Sex Hormones In Headache." *Neurology* 42 (2):37–42.

Soares, C. J. 1996. "Learning in the Fast Lane: Making the Most of Your Evolving Brain." *Perspectives* May/June 1996:33–41.

Society for Assisted Reproductive Technology and the American Society for Reproductive Medicine. 1996. "Assisted Reproductive Technology in the United States and Canada: 1994 Results Generated from the American Society for Reproductive Medicine/Society for Assisted Reproductive Technology Registry." *Fertility and Sterility* 68:697–704.

Stewart, D. E., A. M. Addison, G. E. Robinson, R. Joffe, G. N. Burrow, and M. P. Olmsted. 1988. "Thyroid Function in Psychosis Following Childbirth." *American Journal of Psychiatry* 145:1579–1581.

Stjernfeldt, M., K. Berglund, J. Lindsten, and J. Ludvigsson. 1986. "Maternal Smoking During Pregnancy and Risk of Childhood Cancer." *Lancet* 1 (8494): 1350–1351.

Teufel, A. E., and K. J. Trimmer. 1992. "HBV Screening and Routine Vaccination in Pregnancy. *Clinical Advances in the Treatment of Infections. A KSF Group Publication* 6 (5):1–3.

U.S. Department of Health, Education and Welfare/Public Health Service. 1977. "Immune Globulins for the Protection Against Viral Hepatitis." *Morbidity and Mortality Weekly Report* 26:425–442.

University of Minnesota Office of Continuing Medical Education. April 19,1997. "New Developments and Practice Guidelines: OCs and IUDs" (video satellite conference, San Francisco).

Virtanen, H., J. Makinen, T. Tenho, P. Kiilholma, Y. Pitkanen, and T. Hirvonen. 1993. "Effects of Abdominal Hysterectomy on Urinary and Sexual Symptoms." *British Journal of Urology* 72:868–72.

Werler, M., M. S. Shapiro, and A. Mitchell. 1993. "Periconceptional Folic Acid Exposure and Risk of Occurrent Neural Tube Defects." *Journal of the American Medical Association* 269:1257–93.

Chapter 4: PMS Can Change You: Premenstrual Syndrome in Your Transitional Years

Alvir, J., S. Thys-Jacobs. 1991. "Premenstrual and Menstural Symptom Clusters and Response to Calcium Treatment." *Psychopharmacology Bulletin* 27:145.

American Psychiatric Association. 1994. *Diagnostic and Statistical Manual of Mental Disorders,* 4th ed. Washington, D,C,: American Psychiatric Association.

Andersch, B. 1986. "Premenstrual Complaints: I. Prevalence of Pre-Menstrual Symptoms in a Swedish Urban Population. *Journal of Psychosomatic Obstetrics and Gynecology* 5:39–49.

Ayers, J. W., and G. P. Gidwani. 1983. "The 'Luteal Breast': Hormonal and Sonographic Investigation of Benign Breast Disease in Patients with Cyclic Mastalgia." *Fertility and Sterility* 40 (6):779-784.

Backstrom, T., Y. Hansson-Malmstrom, B. A. Lindhe, B. Cavalli-Bjorkman, and S. Nordenstrom. 1992. "Oral Contraceptives in Premenstrual Syndrome: A Randomized Comparison of Triphasic and Monophasic Preparations." *Contraception* 46 :253–68.

Bancroft, J., and D. Rennie. 1993. "The Impact of Oral Contraceptives on the Experience of Premenstrual Mood, Clumsiness, Food Craving and Other Symptoms." *Journal of Psychosomatic Research* 37:195–202.

Barnhart, K. T., E. W. Freeman, and S. J. Sondheimer. 1995. "A Clinician's Guide to the Premenstrual Syndrome." *Medical Clinics of North America* 79:1457–1473.

Becker, H. 1990. "Supportive European Data on a New Oral ContraceptiveContaining Norgestimate." *Acta Obstetrica and Gynecologica Scandinavica Supplementum* 152:33–39.

Burkman, Jr., R. T., M. E. Kafrissen, W. Olsen, and J. Oaterman. 1992. "Lipid and Carbohydrate Effects of a New Triphasic Oral Contraceptive Containing Norgestimate." *Acta Obstetrica and Gynecologica Scandinavica Supplementum* 156:5–8.

Brown, C. S., F. W. Ling, R. N. Andersen, R. G. Farmer, and K. L. Arheart. 1994. "Efficiency of Depot Leuprolide in Premenstrual Syndrome: Effect of Symptom Severity and Type in Controlled Trial." *Obstetrics and Gynecology* 84:779–786.

Casper, R. F., and M. T. Hearn. 1990. "The Effect of Hysterectomy and Bilateral Oophorectomy in Women with Severe Premenstrual Syndrome." *American Journal of Obstetrics and Gynecology.*162 (1):105-109.

Condon, J. T. 1993. "The Premenstrual Syndrome: A Twin Study." *British Journal of Psychiatry* 162:481-486.

Cullberg J. 1972. "Mood Changes and Menstrual Symptoms with Different Gestagen/Estrogen Combinations. A Double Blind Comparison with a Placebo." *Acta Psychiatrica Scandinavica* 236 (Supplement):1–86.

Dalton, K. 1959. "Menstruation and Acute Psychiatric Illness." *British Medical Journal* 1:148–149.

Dalton, K., and M. J. Dalton. 1987. "Characteristics of Pyridoxine Overdose Neuropathy Syndrome." *Acta Neurologica Scandinavica* 76:811.

Dennerstein, L., C. Spencer-Gardner, G. Gotts, J. B. Brown, M. A. Smith, and G. D. Burrows. 1985. "Progesterone and the Premenstrual Syndrome: A Double-Blind Crossover Trial. *British Medical Journal* 290:617–1620.

Derzko, C. M. 1990. "Role of Danazol in Relieving the Premenstrual Syndrome." *Journal of Reproductive Medicine* 35 (Supplement):99–102.

Ekholm, U. B., and T. Backstrom. 1994. "Influence of Premenstrual Syndrome on Family, Social Life, and Work Performance." *International Journal of Health Services* 24:629–647.

Elks, M. L. 1993. "Open Trial of Flouxetine Therapy for Premenstrual Syndrome." *Southern Medical Journal* 86:503–7.

Facchinetti, F., P. Borela, G. Sances, L. Fioroni, R. Nappi, and A. R. Ganassane. 1991. "Oral Magnesium Successfully Relieves Premenstrual Mood Changes." *Obstetrics and Gynecology* 78:177.

Forrest, A. R. W. 1979. "Cyclical Variations in Mood in Normal Women Taking Oral Contraceptives." *British Medical Journal* 1:1410–1410.

Frank, R. T. 1931. "The Hormonal Causes of Premenstrual Tension." *Archives of Neurology and Psychiatry* 26:1053.

Freeman, E., K. Rickels, and S. Sondheimer. 1990. "Ineffectiveness of Progesterone Suppository Treatment for Premenstrual Syndrome." *Journal of the American Medical Association* 264:349.

Freeman, E. W., E. Schweizer, and K. Rickels. 1995. "Personality Factors in Women with Premenstrual Syndrome." *Psychosomatic Medicine* 57:453–459

Freeman, E. W., and S. Sondheimer. 1993. "Menstrual Cycle, Diet, and Premenstrual Syndrome." In: *Encyclopedias of Food Service, Food Technology, and Nutrition.* London: Academic Press.

Freeman, E. W., K. Rickels, S. J. Sodheimer, and M. Polansky. 1995. "A Double Blind Trial of Oral Progesterone, Alprazolam, and Placebo in Treatment of Severe Premenstrual Syndrome." *Journal of the American Medical Association* 274 :51–57.

Halbreich, U., N. Rojansky, and S. Palter. 1991. "Elimination of Ovulation and Menstrual Cyclicity (with Danazol) Improves Dysphoric Premenstrual Syndromes." *Fertility and Sterility* 56:1066–69.

Halbreich, U., and H. Tworek. 1993. "Altered Serotonergic Activity in Women with Dysphoric Premenstrual Syndrome." *International Journal of Psychiatry in Medicine* 23 (1):1–27.

Harvard Medical School. June 1995. "Natural Progesterone." *Women's Health Watch. Information for Enlightened Choices from Harvard Medical School* II (10):1.

Hsia, L. S.; and M.H. Long, 1990. "Premenstrual Syndrome: Current Concepts in Diagnosis and Management." *Journal of Nurse Midwifery* 35:351–357.

Huber, J. 1991. "Clinical Experience with a New Norgestimate-Containing Oral-Contraceptive." *International Journal of Fertility* 36 (supplement):25–31

Kamen, B. 1996. *Hormone Replacement Therapy Yes or No: How to Make an Informed Decision About Estrogen, Progesterone and Other Strategies for Dealing with PMS, Menopause and Osteoporosis.* Novato, Calif: Nutrition Encounter.

Kendler, K. S., J. L. Silberg, M. C. Neale, R. C. Kessler, A. C. Heath, and L. J. Eaves. 1992. "Genetic and Environmental Factors in the Aetiology of Menstrual, Premenstrual and Neurotic Symptoms: A Population-Based Twin Study. *Psychological Medicine* 22:85–100.

Khoo, S. K., C. Munro, and D. Battistutta. 1990. "Evening Primrose Oil and Treatment of Premenstrual Syndrome." *The Medical Journal of Australia* 153: 189–192.

Kleijnen, J. 1994. "Evening Primrose Oil: Currently Used in Many Conditions with Little Justification." *British Medical Journal* 309:824–825.

Kleijnen, J. 1994. "Comments to the Editor." *British Medical Journal* 309:1437.

Lanka, L. D., and J. Klingman. Research in Progress on Ongoing Evaluation of the Use of Testosterone Pellets in the Treatment of Recalcitrant Menstrual Migraines. Kaiser Foundation Hospital, Walnut Creek, CA.

Lee, J. R., and V. Hopkins. 1996. *What Your Doctor May Not Tell You About Menopause.* New York: Warner Books.

Leventhal, J. October 15, 1996. "Premenstrual Dysphoric Disorder." Lecture given to the Women's Health Department, Kaiser, Walnut Creek, CA.

Leventhal, J. April 1, 1997. "Libido and Menopause" Lecture given to the Women's Health Department, Kaiser, Walnut Creek, CA.

London, R. S., L. Bradley, and N. Chiamor. 1991. "Effect of Nutritional Supplement on Premenstrual Symptomatology in Women with Premenstrual Syndrome: A Longitudinal Study." *Journal of the American College of Nutrition* 10:494–499.

Magos, A., and J. Studd. 1985. "Progesterone and the Premenstrual Syndrome: A Double-Blind Crossover Trial," correspondence. *British Medical Journal* 291:213.

Mauvais-Jarvis, P., N. Sterkers, F. Kuttenn, and J. Beauvais. 1978. ["The Treatment of Benign Pathological Conditions of the Breasts with Progesterone and Progestogens."] *Journal de Gynecologie, Obstetrique et Biologie de la Reproduction* 7:477–484.

Moline, L. 1993. "Pharmacological Strategies for Managing Premenstrual Syndrome." *Clinical Pharmacology* 12:181–196.

Mortola, J. F. 1994. "A Risk-Benefit Appraisal of Drugs Used in the Management of Premenstrual Syndrome." *Drug Safety* 10:160–169.

Mortola, J. F. 1992. "Issues in the Diagnosis and Research of Premenstrual Syndrome." *Clinics of Obstetrics and Gynecology* 35:587–598.

Parker, P. D. 1994. "Premenstrual Syndrome." *American Family Physician* 50:1309–1317.

Parry, G., and D. Bredesen. 1985. Sensory Neuropathy with Low Dose Pyridoxine. *Neurology* 35:1466–1468.

Pearlstein, T. B. 1995. "Hormones and Depression: What Are the Facts About Premenstrual Syndrome, Menopause, and Hormone Replacement Therapy?" *American Journal of Obstetrics and Gynecology* 173 (2):646–653.

Pearlstein, T. B., A. Rivera-Tovar, and E. Frank. 1992. "Nonmedical Management of LLPDD: A Preliminary Report." *Journal of Psychotherapeutic Practice and Research* 1:49–55.

Physician's Desk Reference, 51st ed. 1997. Montvale, NJ: Medical Economics.

Reid, R. L., and S. S. C. Yen. 1981. "Premenstural Syndrome." *American Journal of Obstetrics and Gynecology* 139:85–104.

Revlin, M. E., J. C. Morrison, and G. W. Bates 1990. *Manual of Clinical Problems in Obstetrics and Gynecology*, 3rd ed. Boston: Little Brown.

Riggs, L., and L. J. Melton. 1986. "Involutional Osteoporosis." *New England Journal of Medicine* 314:1676–1686.

Rosenstein, D. R. Elin, J. Hosseini, G. Grover, and D. Rubinow. 1994. "Magnesium Measures Across the Menstrual Cycle in Premenstrual Syndrome." *Society of Biological Psychiatry* 35:557–561.

Rubinow, D. 1992. "The Premenstrual Syndrome: New Views." *Journal of the American Medical Association* 268:1908.

Sarno, Jr., A. P., E. J. Miller, Jr., and E. G. Lundblad. 1987. "Premenstrual Syndrome: Beneficial Effects of Periodic, Low-Dose Danazol for the Treatment of Premenstrual Tension." *Obstetrics and Gynecology* 70:30–36.

Schagen van Leeuwen, J. H., E. R. te Velde, H. P. F. Koppeschaar, W. J. Kop, J. H. H. Thijssen, J. M. van Ree, and A. A. Haspel. 1993. "Is Premenstrual Syndrome an Endocrine Disorder?" *Journal of Psychosomatic Obstetrics and Gynaecology* 14:91–109.

Schaumburg, H., J. Kaplan, A. Windebank, N. Vick, and M. J. Brown. 1983. "Neuropathy from Pyridoxine Abuse: A New Megavitamin Syndrome." *New England Journal of Medicine* 309:445–490.

Schmidt, P. J., G. N. Grover, and D. R. Rubinow. 1993. "Alprazolam in the Treatment of Premenstrual Syndrome. A Double-Blind, Placebo-Controlled Trial." *Archives of General Psychiatry* 50:467–73.

Schmidt, P. J., L. Nieman, G. N. Grover, K. N. Nuller, G. R. Merriam, and D. R. Rubinow. 1991. "Lack of Effect of Induced Menses on Symptoms in Women with Premenstrual Syndrome." *New England Journal of Medicine* 324:1174–1179.

Severino, S. K., and M. L. Moline. 1995. "Premenstrual Syndrome. Identification and Management." *Drugs. Practical Therapeutics* 49 (1):71–82.

Severino, S. K., and K. A. Yonkers. 1994. "A Literature Review of Psychotic Symptoms Associated with the Premenstruum." *Psychosomatics* 34:299–306.

Smith, R. N., J. W. Studd, D. Zamblera, and E. F. Holland. 1995. "A Randomized Comparison over 8 Months of 100 Micrograms and 200 Micrograms Twice Weekly Doses of Transdermal Oestradiol in the Treatment of Severe Premenstrual Syndrome." *British Journal of Obstetrics and Gynaecology* 6:475–484.

Smith, S., and I. Schiff. 1993. *Modern Management of Premenstrual Syndrome.* New York. Norton.

Smith, S., I. Schiff, and D. E. Stewart. 1989. "Positive Changes in the Premenstrual Period. *Acta Psychiatrica Scandinavica* 79:400–05.

Steinberg, S. 1991. "Mini Review: The Treatment of Late Luteal Phase Dysphoric Disorder." *Life Sciences* 49:767–802.

Steiner, M., S. Steinberg, D. Stewart, D. Carter, C. Berger, R. Reid, D. Grover, and D. Streiner. 1995. "Fluoxetine in the Treatment of Premenstrual Dysphoria." *New England Journal of Medicine* 332:1529–34.

Stone A. B., T. B. Pearlstein, and W. A. Brown. 1990. "Fluoxetine in the Treatment of Premenstrual Syndrome. *Psychopharmacology Bulletin* 26:331–335.

Thy-Jacobs, S., S. Ceccarelli, and A. Bierman. 1989. "Calcium Supplementation in Premenstrual Syndrome: A Randomized Cross Over Trial." *Journal of General Internal Medicine* 4:183.

Walther, M. 1981. ["Contribution to Local Topical Therapy of Mastodynia."] *Schweizrische Rundshau fur Medizin Praxis* 70:973–74.

Watts, J. F., W. R. Butt, and R. L. Edwards. 1987. "A Clinical Trial Using Danazol for the Treatment of Premenstrual Tension." *British Journal of Obstetrics and Gynaecology* 94:30-34.

Wilson, C. A., C. W. Turner, W. R. Keye, Jr. 1991. "Firstborn Adolescent Daughters and Mothers with and without Premenstrual Syndrome: A Comparison." *Journal of Adolescent Health* 12:130–137.

Wood, C., and D. Jakubowicz. 1980. "The Treatment of Premenstrual Syndrome with Mefenamic Acid. *British Journal of Obstetrics and Gynaecology* 87:627–630.

Yonkers, K. A., and S. J. Chantilis. 1995. "Recognition of Depression in Obstetric/Gynecology Practices." *American Journal of Obstetrics and Gynecology* 173:632–638.

Chapter 5: Serious Changes: Cardiovascular Disease and Osteoporosis

Bass, K. M., C. J. Newschaffer, M. J. Klag, and T. L. Bush. 1993. "Plasma Lipoprotein Levels as Predictors of Cardiovascular Deaths in Women." *Circulation* 153:2209.

Eastman, Peggy. 1997. "Osteoporosis: New Treatment." AARP Bulletin 38 (3).

Gurwitz, J. H., F. Nananda, and J. Avorn. 1992. "The Exclusion of the Elderly and Women from Clinical Trials in Acute Myocardial Infarction." *Journal of the American Medical Association* 268:1417.

Klibanski, A., B. M. Biller, D. A. Shoenfeld, D. B. Herzog, and V. C. Saxe. 1995. "Effects of Estrogen Administration on Trabecular Bone Loss in Young Women with Anorexia Nervosa." *Journal of Clinical Endocrinology and Metabolism* 80:898–904.

Lloyd, T., M. B. Andus, N. Rawlings, J. K. Martel, J. R. Landis, L. M. Demers, D. F. Eggli, K. Kiesehorst, and H. E. Kulin. 1993. "Calcium Supplementation and Bone Mineral Density in Adolescent Girls." *Journal of the American Medical Association* 270:841-844.

Michelson, D. 1996. "Bone Mineral Density in Women with Depression." *New England Journal of Medicine* 335:1176–1181.

Murphy, S. "Milk Consumption and Bone Density." 1994. *British Medical Journal* 308:939–41.

Nachtigall, Lila E., and Joan Rattner Heilman. 1995. *Estrogen: The Facts Can Change Your Life*. New York: Harper Collins.

Prince, R. L., M. Smith, I. M. Dick, R. I. Price, P. G. Webb, and N. K. Henderson. 1991. "Prevention of Postmenopausal Osteoporosis: A Comparative Study of Exercise, Calcium Supplementation, and Hormone Replacement Therapy." *New England Journal of Medicine* 325:1189–95.

Raisz, L. G. 1996. "Bone Formation and Resorption in Menopausal Women Using Estrogen and Androgen." *Journal of Endocrinology and Metabolism* 81:37–43.

Speroff, Leon. 1994. "Estrogen and Cardiovascular Disease." *Ob/Gyn Clinical Alert* 10:86–88.

Speroff, Leon. 1995. "Bisphosphonates Will Prevent Osteoporotic Fractures." *Ob/Gyn Clinical Alert* 12:20–21.

Theistz., G. 1992. "Bone Mass Accumulation in Adolescent and Young Adult Women." *Journal of Clinical Endocrinology and Metabolism* 75:1060–65.

Wenger, N. K., L. Speroff, and B. Packard. 1993. "Cardiovascular Health and Disease in Women." *New England Journal of Medicine* 329:72–75.

Chapter 6: The Great Imitator: Thyroid Change Can Fool You

Danese, M. 1996. "Screening for Mild Thyroid Failure at the Periodic Health Exam." *Journal of the American Medical Association.* 276:285-92.

Eskin, B. A., and L. S. Dumas. 1995. *Midlife Can Wait*. New York: Ballantine Books.

Hayslip, C. C. 1988. "The Value of Serum Antimicrosomal Antibody Testing in Screening for Symptomatic Postpartum Thyroid Dysfunction." *American Journal of Obstetrics and Gynecology* 159:203–9.

Chapter 7: Frightening Changes—Cancer

American College of Obstetricians and Gynecologists. 1993. "Routine Cancer Screening." *ACOG Committee Opinion No. 128*. Washington, D.C.: ACOG.

American College of Obstetricians and Gynecologists. 1995. "Health Maintenance for Perimenopausal Women. Technical Bulletin 210, Washington, D.C.: ACOG.

American College of Obstetricians and Gynecologists. 1997. "ACOG Maintains Mammography Screening Guidelines for Women Ages 40–49." *ACOG Newsletter* 41 (3):8.

American College of Obstetricians and Gynecologists. 1996. "Breast-Ovarian Cancer Screening." ACOG Committee Opinion No. 176. Washington, D.C.: ACOG.

American Cancer Society. April 1994. "Cancer Facts and Figures." Atlanta: American Cancer Society.

Anthonisen, N. R., J. E. Conneett, J. P. Kiley, M. D. Altose, W. C. Bailey, and A. S. Buist. 1994. "Effects of Smoking Intervention and the Use of an Inhaled Anticholinergic Brochodilator on the Rate of Decline of FEV. The Lung Health Study." *Journal of the American Medical Association* 272:1497–1505.

Bennicke, K., C. Conrad, S. Sobroe, and H. C. Sorensen. 1995. "Cigarette Smoking and Breast Cancer." *British Medical Journal* 310:1431–33.

Braly, P. S. May 1997. "The NIH Consensus Conference on Cervical Cancer: Implications for Practice." Presentation at 45th Annual Clinical Meeting of the American College of Obstetricians and Gynecologists.

Bosch, F. X., M. M. Manos, N. Munoz, M. Sherman, A. M. Jansen, and J. Petro. 1995. "Prevalence of Human Papillomavirus in Cervical Cancer: A Worldwide Perspective." International Biological Study on Cervical Cancer (IBSCC) Study Group. *Journal of the National Cancer Institute* 87:796–802.

Calle, E. E., and M. J. Thun. 1997. "The Epidemiology of the Effects of Estrogen and Aspirin on Colorectal Cancer." *Menopausal Medicine* 5(1):9–12.

Celentano, D. D., and G. deLissovoy. 1989–90. "Assessment of Cancer Screening and Follow-Up Programs." *Public Health Review* 17:173–240.

Colditz, G. A., W. C. Willet, D. J. Hunter, M. J. Stampfer, J. E. Manson, C. H. Hennekens, B. A. Rosner. 1993. "Family History, Age and the Risk of Breast Cancer. Prospective Data from the Nurses' Health Study." *Journal of the American Medical Association* 270:338–43.

Gambrell, R. D. 1983. "Decreased Incidence of Breast Cancer in Postmenopausal Estrogen-Progestogen Users. *Obstetrics and Gynecology* 62:435–43.

Gemmell, J., D. M. Holmes, and I. D. Duncan. 1990. "How Frequently Need Vaginal Smears Be Taken After Hysterectomy for Cervical Intraepithelial Neoplasia?" *British Journal of Obstetrics and Gynaecology* 91:67–72.

Gershenson, D. 1996. "Genetic Testing for Cancer Susceptibility." *Ob/Gyn Clinical Alert* 13 (4):31–32.

Gershenson, D. 1997. "ERT in Patients with a History of Endometrial Cancer." *Ob/Gyn Clinical Alert* 13 (10):79–80.

Grady, D., T. Gebretsadik, and K. Kerlikowske. 1995. "Hormone Replacement and Endometrial Cancer Risk: A Meta-Analysis." *Obstetrics and Gynecology* 85:304.

Grodstein, F., M. J. Stampfer, G. A. Colditz, W. C. Willet, J. E. Manson, M. Joffe, B. Rosner, C. Fuchs, S. .E Hankinson, D. J. Hunter, C. H. Hennekens, F. E. Speizer. 1997. "Postmenopausal Hormone Therapy and Mortality." *New England Journal of Medicine* 336:1769–75.

Hankinson, S. E., G. A. Colditz, and D. J. Hunter. 1992. "A Quantitative Assessment of Oral Contraceptive Use and Risk of Ovarian Cancer." *Obstetrics and Gynecology* 80:708–14.

Hankinson, S. E., D. J. Hunter, G. A. Colditz, W. C. Willet, M. J. Stampfer, B. Rosner, C. H. Henneken, and F. I. Speizer. 1993. "Tubal Ligation, Hysterectomy and Risk of Ovarian Cancer." *Journal of the American Medical Association* 270:2813–18.

Hoskins, K. F., J. E. Stopfer, K. A. Calzone, S. D. Merajuver, F. R. Rebbeck, and J. E. Garber. 1995. "Assessment and Counseling for Women with a Family History of Breast Cancer: A Guide for Clinicians." *Journal of the American Medical Association* 273:577–85.

Kinney, W. March 1997. Gynecologic Oncologist, Kaiser Permanente of Northern California. Personal communication.

Koutsky, L. A., K. K. Holmes, C. W. Critchlow, C. E. Stevens, J. Paavonen , and A. M. Beckman. 1992. "A Cohort Study of the Risk of Cervical Intraepithelial Neoplasia Grade 2 or 3 in Relation to Papillomavirus Infection." *New England Journal of Medicine* 327:1272–78.

Melbye, M., J. Wolfahrt, J. H. Olson, M. Frisch, T. Westergard, K. Helweg-Larson, and P. K. Anderson. 1997. "Induced Abortion and the Risk of Breast Cancer." *New England Journal of Medicine* 336:81–85.

Michels, K. B. 1996. "Birth Weight As a Risk Factor for Breast Cancer." *Lancet* 348:1542–46.

Nawa, A., Y. Nishiyama, T. Kobayashi, Y. Wakahara, T. Okamoto, F. Kikkawa. 1995. "Association of Human Leukocyte Antigen-B1*03 with Cervical Cancer in Japanese Women Aged 35 Years and Younger." *Cancer* 75:518–21.

Newcomb, P. A., B. E. Stoner, M. P. Longnecker, R. Mittendorf, E. R. Greenberg, and W. C. Willet . 1996. "Pregnancy Termination in Relation to Risk of Breast Cancer." *Journal of the American Medical Association* 275:283–87.

Newcomb, P. A., R. Klein, B. E. Klein, S. Hoffner, J. Mares-Perlman, P. M. Cruickshank, Marcus. 1995. "Association of Dietary and Lifestyle Factors with Sex Hormones in Postmenopausal Women." *American Journal of Epidemiology* 142:788–95.

Noller, K. L. 1997. "Computerization of Pap Smear Screening." *Ob/Gyn Clinical Alert* 13 (11):87–88.

Notelovitz, M., and D. Tennessen. 1993. *Menopause and Midlife Health.* New York: St. Martin's Press.

Reichman, J. 1996. *I'm Too Young To Get Old: Health Care for Women After Forty.* New York: Times Books.

Risch, H. A. 1994. "Dietary Fat Intake and the Risk of Epithelial Ovarian Cancer." *Journal of the National Cancer Institute*86:1409–15.

Schildkraut, J. M., and W. D. Thompson. 1988. "Familial Ovarian Cancer: A Population-Based Case-Controlled Study." *American Journal of Epidemiology* 128:456–66.

Seltzer, V. L. 1996. Presentation on breast cancer at ACOG 44th Annual Clinical Meeting.

Shattuck-Eidens, D., M. McClure, J. Simard, T. Labrie, S. Narod, F. Cerich, K. Hoskins, B. Weber, L. Castilla, and M. Erdos. 1995. "A Collaborative Survey of 80 Mutations in BRCA1 Breast and Ovarian Cancer Susceptibility Gene." *Journal of the American Medical Association* 273:535–41.

Speroff, L. 1996. "Pregnancy Termination in Relation to Risk of Breast Cancer." *Ob/Gyn Clinical Alert* 12 (11):82.

Tarone, R. July 1996. "Breast Cancer Death Rate Continues to Decline." *News from the National Cancer Institute.*

The Cancer and Steroid Hormone Study of The Centers for Disease Control and The National Institute of Child Health and Human Development., 1987. "The Reduction in Risk of Ovarian Cancer Associated with Oral Contraceptive Use." *New England Journal of Medicine* 316:650–55.

Thun, I., T. Brenn, E. Lund, M. Gaard. 1997. "Physical Activity and the Risk of Breast Cancer." *New England Journal of Medicine* 336:1269–75.

Whittemore, A. S., R. Harris, J. Intyre. and The Collaborative Ovarian Cancer Group. 1992. "Characteristics Relating to Ovarian Cancer Risk." *American Journal of Epidemiology* 136:1184–1203.

Willet, W. C., D. J. Hunter, M. J. Stampfer, G. A. Colditz, J. E. Manson, D. Spiegelman, B. Rosner, C. H. Hennekens, and F. E. Speizer. 1992. "Dietary Fat and Fiber in Relation to Risk of Breast Cancer: An 8-Year Follow-Up. *Journal of the American Medical Association* 268:2037–44.

Willet, Walter, 1994. "Diet and Health: What Should We Eat?" *Science* 264:532–37.

Chapter 8: You Can Change Your Hormones: The Case for Hormone Replacement Therapy

American College of Obstetricians and Gynecologists. 1994. "Estrogen Replacement Therapy in Women with Previously Treated Breast Cancer." *ACOG Committee Opinion No. 135.* Washington, D.C.: ACOG.

Adami, H. O. 1992. "Long-term Consequences of Estrogen and Estrogen-Progestin Replacement." *Cancer Causes and Control* 3 (1):83–90.

Areneo, B. A., T. Dowell, M. Woods, R. Daynes, M. Judd, and T. Evans. 1995. "DHEAS as an Effective adjuvant in Elderly Humans: Proof-of-Principle Studies." *Annals of the New York Academy of Science* 774:232–48.

Ayton, R., G. Darling, A. Murkies, E. Farrell, E. Weisberg, I. Selinus, and I. Fraser. 1996. "A Comparative Study of Safety and Efficacy of Continuous Low Dose Oestradiol Released from a Vaginal Ring Compared with Conjugated Oestrogen Vaginal Cream in the Treatment of Menopausal Urogenital Atrophy. *British Journal of Obstetrics and Gynecology;* 103:291–92.

Bates, G. W., R. Egerman, J. Buster, and P. Casson. 1995. "Dehydroepiandrosterone Attenuates Study-Induced Declines in Insulin Sensitivity in Postmenopausal Women." *Annals of the New York Academy of Science* 774:291–93.

Baulieu, E. 1995. "Dehydroepiandrosterone (DHEA) Is a Neuroactive Neurosteroid." *Annals of the New York Academy of Science* 774:82–110.

Beresford, S. A., N. S. Weiss, L. F. Voigt, and B. McKnight. 1997. "Risk of Endometrial Cancer in Relation to Use of Oestrogen Combined with Cyclic Progestagen Therapy in Postmenopausal Women." *Lancet* 349:458–61.

Bergkvist, L., H. Adami, I. Persson, R. Hoover, and C. Schairer. 1989. "The Risk of Breast Cancer after Estrogen and Estrogen-Progestin Replacement." *New England Journal of Medicine* 321:293–97.

Berman, J. S., et al. 1996. "Compliance with Postmenopausal Hormone Therapy." *Journal of Women's Health* 5:213–20.

Birge S. 1996. "Is There a Role for Estrogen Replacement Therapy in the Prevention and Treatment of Dementia?" *Journal of the American Geriatrics Society* 44:865–70.

Brody, J. March 4, 1997. "Drug Researchers Working to Design Customized Estrogen." *New York Times.*

Colditz, G. A., S. E. Hankinson, D. J. Hunter, W. C. Willet, J. E. Manson, M. J. Stampfer, C. Hennekens, B. Rosner, and F. E. Speizer. 1995. "The Use of Estrogens and Progestins and the Risk of Breast Cancer." *New England Journal of Medicine* 332:1589–93.

Cauley, J. A., D. G. Seeley, K. Ensrud, B. E. Hinger, and D. Black. 1995. "Prevention of Fractures Requires Long-Term Estrogen Treatment." *Annals of Internal Medicine* 122:9–16.

Cutler, W., 1990. *Hysterectomy:Before and After.* New York: Harper Row.

Cutler, W., and C. R. Garcia. 1992. *Menopasuse: A Guide for Women and the Men Who Love Them.* New York: W.W. Norton.

Cummings, S. R., D. M. Black, and S. M. Rubin. 1989. "Lifetime Risk of Hip, Colles', or Vertebral Fracture and Coronary Heart Disease among White Postmenopausal Women." *Archives of Internal Medicine* 149:458–61.

Dupont, W. D., and D. L. Page. 1991. "Menopausal ERT and Breast Cancer: A Meta-Analysis." *Archives of Internal Medicine* 151:67–72.

Ettinger, B. 1996. "Continuation Rates with Postmenopausal Hormone Therapy." *Menopause* 3:185–89.

Fantl, J. A., L. Cardozo, and D. R. McLish. 1994. "Estrogen Therapy for Urinary Incontinence in Postmenopausal Women." *Obstetrics and Gynecology* 83:12–18.

Felson, D. T., Y. Zhong, D. T. Hannan, D. P. Kiel, P. W. Wilson, and J. J. Anderson,. 1993. "Hormone Replacement Therapy Compliance." *New England Journal of Medicine* 329:1141–46.

Folsom, A. R., P. J. Mink, T. A. Sellers, C. P. Hong, W. Zheng, and J. D. Potter. 1995. "Hormone Replacement Therapy and Morbidity and Mortality in a Prospective Study of Postmenopausal Women." *American Journal of Public Health* 85:1128–32.

Gambrell, R. D., R. C. Maier, and B. I. Sanders. 1983. "Decreased Incidence of Breast Cancer in Postmenopausal Women." *Obstetrics and Gynecology* 62:435–43.

Gershenson, D. 1996. "Genetic Testing for Cancer Susceptibility." *Ob/Gyn Clinical Alert* 13 (4):31–32.

Grady, D., T. Gebretsadik, and K. Kerlikowske. 1995. "Hormone Replacement and Endometrial Cancer Risk: A Meta-Analysis." *Obstetrics and Gynecology* 85:304.

Greenblatt, R. B, 1987. "The Use of Androgens in the Menopause and Other Gynecologic Disorders." *Obstetric and Gynecologic Clinics of North America* 14 (1):251–68.

Grodstein, F., M. J. Stampfer, G. A. Colditz, W. C. Willet, J. E. Manson, M. Joffe, B. Rosner, C. Fuchs, S. E. Hankinson, D. J. Hunter, C. H. Hennekens, and F. E. Speizer. 1997. "Postmenopausal Hormone Therapy and Mortality." *New England Journal of Medicine* 336:1769–75.

Henderson, V. W. 1995. "Alzheimer's Disease in Women: Is There a Role for Estrogen Replacement Therapy?" *Menopausal Management* 4 (6): 10–13.

Judd, H. J. 1996. "The Impact of Ovarian Hormone Replacement on Selected Risk Factors of Coronary Heart Disease." *Menopausal Medicine* 4 (1):9–11.

Landau, C., M. G. Cyr, and A. W. Moulton. 1994. *The Complete Book of Menopause: Every Woman's Guide to Good Health*. New York: G. P. Putnam's Sons.

Leventhal, J. 1997. April 1, 1997. "Libido and Menopause." Lecture given to the Women's Health Department, Kaiser, Walnut Creek, CA..

Nestler, J. E. 1995. "Regulation of Human Dehydroepiandrosterone Metabolism by Insulin." *Annals of The New York Academy of Science* 774:ix–xi.

Notelovitz, M., and D. Tonnessen. 1993. *Menopause and Midlife Health*. New York: St. Martin's Press.

Parsons, A. 1993. "Sonography: A New Method to Evaluate the Endometrium. *Menopausal Medicine* 1:9-11.

Reichman, J. 1996. *I'm Too Young to Get Old: Health Care for Women After Forty*. New York: Times Books.

Rosenberg, S., D. Bosson, A. Peretz, A. Caufriez, and C. Robyn. 1988. "Serum Levels of Gonadotropins and Steroid Hormones in Post-Menopause and Later Life." *Maturitas* 10:215–24.

Schwartz, A. and L. L.Pashko. 1995. "Mechanism of Cancer Preventive Action of DHEA: Role of Glucose-6-Phosphate Dehydrogenase." *Annals of the New York Academy of Science* 774:121–27.

Sherwin, B., and M. Gelfand. 1985. "Sex Steroids and Affect in the Surgical Menopause: A Double Blind, Cross-Over Study." *Psychoneouroendocrinology* 3:325–35.

Skolnick, A.1996. "Scientific Verdict Still Out on DHEA." *Journal of the American Medical Association* 276:1365–67.

Speroff, L., 1995. "Postmenopausal Hormone Therapy and Breast Cancer Risk." *Ob/Gyn Clinical Alert* 12 (4):25–26.

Speroff, L. 1994. "Estrogen and Cardiovascular Disease." *Ob/Gyn Clinical Alert* 10 (11):86–88.

Speroff, L. 1994. "Managing Therapy-Related Postmenopausal Bleeding." *Ob/Gyn Clinical Alert* 11 (8):62–64.

Stanford, J., N. S. Weiss, L. F. Voight, J. R. Daling, L. A. Habel, and M. Rossing. 1995. "Combined Estrogen and Progesterone Replacement Therapy in Relation to Risk of Breast Cancer in Middle-Aged Women." *Journal of the American Medical Association* 274:137–42.

Schwartz, A. 1995. "Dehydroapeandrosterone (DHEA) and Aging." *Annals of the New York Academy of Science* 774:121–27.

Wild, R. A. 1996. "Estrogen Effects on the Cardiovascular Tree." *Obstetrics and Gynecology* 87:275–355.

Wolkowitz, O. M., V. Reus, E. Roberts, F. Manfredi, T. Chan, S. Ormiston, R. Johnson, J. Canick, L. Brizendine, and H. Weingartner. 1995. "Antidepressant and Cognition-Enhancing Effects of DHEA in Major Depression." Presentation to The New York Academy of Science. *Annals of The New York Academy of Science*; 774:337-39.

Woodruff, J. D., and J. H. Pickar. 1994. "Incidence of Endometrial Hyperplasia in Postmenopausal Women Taking Conjugated Estrogen (Premarin) with Medroxyprogesterone Acetate or Conjugated Estrogens Alone." *American Journal of Obstetrics and Gynecology* 170:1213.

Writing Group for the PEPI Trials, 1995, "Effects of Estrogen or Estrogen/Progestin on Heart Disease Risk Factors on Postmenopausal Women." *Journal of the American Medical Association*. 273:199-08.

Zhang, Y., D. P. Kiel, B. E. Kreger, L. A. Cupples, R. C. Ellison, J. F. Dorgan, A. Schatzkin, D. Levy, D. Felson. 1997. "Bone Density and Risk of Breast Cancer in Postmenopausal Women." *New England Journal of Medicine* 336:611–17.

Chapter 9: Alternative Medical Disciplines: Are They a Good Choice for You?

Aldercreutz, H., H. Honjo, and A. Higashi. 1991. "Urinary Excretion of Lignans and Isoflavenoids: Phytoestrogens in Japanese Men and Women Consuming a Traditional Diet." *American Journal of Clinical Nutrition* 54:1093–1100.

Bienfield, H., and E. Korngold. 1991. *Between Heaven and Earth: A Guide to Chinese Medicine*. New York: Ballantine Books.

Chopra, D. 1990. *Quantum Healing: Exploring the Frontiers of Mind/Body Medicine*. New York: Bantam.

Bettinger, B. 1997. Personal communication.

Khoo, S. K., C. Munro, and D. Battistutta. 1990. "Evening Primrose Oil and Treatment of PMS." *Medical Journal of Australia* 153:189–92.

Kleijmen, J. 1994. "Evening Primrose Oil Currently Used in Many Conditions with Little Justification." *British Medical Journal* 309:824–25. (Also see comment of the editor 309:1437).

Ojeda, L. 1995. *Menopause without Medicine*. Alameda, CA.: Hunter House.

Reichman, J. 1996. *I'm Too Young To Get Old: Health Care for Women After Forty*. New York: Times Books.

Tyler, V. E. 1997. "The Bright Side of Black Cohosh." *Prevention* 4:76–79.

Ullman, D. 1991. *Discovering Homeopathic Medicine for the 21st Century*. Berkeley: North Atlantic Books.

Wolfe, H. L. 1990. *Second Spring: A Guide to Healthy Menopause through Traditional Chinese Medicine*. Boulder: Blue Poppy Press.

Chapter 10: Wellness for a Change: Good Nutrition, a Healthful Diet, and Exercise

Ainsworth, B. E., W. L. Haskell, A. S. Leon, D. R. Jacobs, H. J. Montoye, J. F. Sellis, and R. S. Paffenbarger, Jr. 1992. "Compendium of Physical Activities: Classification of Energy Costs of Human Physical Activitied." *Medical Science in Sports and Exercise*; 24 (1):71–80.

American College of Obstetricians and Gynecologists, 1992. *Planning for Pregnancy, Birth and Beyond*; New York: Dutton

Bellerson, K. 1993. *The Complete Fat Book.* Garden City Park, N.Y: Avery Publishing.

Benson, H. and E. Stuart. 1993. *The Wellness Book: A Comprehensive Guide to Maintaining Health and Treating Stress-Related Illness.* New York: Fireside.

Blair, S. N., H. Kohl, R. Paffenbarger, D. Clark, K. Cooper, L. Gibbons. 1989. "Physical Fitness and All-Cause Mortality: A Prospective Study of Healthy Men and Women." *Journal of the American Medical Association* 262:2395–2401.

Block, G. 1991. "Dietary Guidelines: The Results of Food Consumption Surveys. *American Journal of Clinical Nutrition* 53:356(S)-357(S.)

Brink, S. 1995. "Health Guide, 1995." Interview with R. Rikli, Co-Director, Lifespan Wellness Clinic at California State University, Fullerton, CA. *U.S News and World Report* May 15, 1995:76–84.

Colvin, R. M., and S. R. Pinell. 1996. "Topical Vitamin C in Aging." *Clinics in Dermatology, Skin Aging, and Photoaging* 14:227–34.

Davis, R. 1996. "Yoga and You." *Weight Watchers* 29 (11):55–61.

Dreon, D. M., K. M. Vranizan, R. Krauss, M. A. Austin, and P. Wood. 1990. "The Effects of Polyunsaturated Fat vs. Monounsaturated Fat on Plasma Lipoproteins." *Journal of the American Medical Association* 263:2461–66.

Frisch, R. E., G. Wyshak, N. L. Albright, T. E. Albright, and I. Schiff. 1987 "Lower Prevalence of Reproductive System Cancers among Former College Athletes." *Medical Science in Sports and Exercise* 21:83–90.

Garrick, J. G., R K. Requa. 1988. "Aerobic Dance: A Review." *Sports Medicine* 6:169–79.

Hallfrisch, J., V. Singh, and D. Muller. 1994. "High Plasma Vitamin C Associated with High Plasma HDL and LDL-2 Cholesterol." *American Journal of Clinical Nutrition* 60:100–105.

Hunter, D., J. Manson, and G. Colditz. 1993. "A Prospective Study of the Intake of Vitamins C, E, and A and the Risk of Breast Cancer." *New England Journal of Medicine*: 329:234–40.

Jandak, J., and S. Richardson. 1989. "Alpha-tocopherol and Effective Inhibition of Platelet Adhesion." *American Journal of Clinical Nutrition* 60:100–05.

Kardinaal, A., F. Kok, and J. Ringstad. 1994. "Antioxidants in Adipose Tissue and Risk of Myocardial Infarction: The EURAMIC Study. *Lancet* 342:1379–84.

Krasinski, A., R. Russell, C. Otradovec, J. Sadowski, S. Hartz, R. Jacobs, and R. McGandy. 1989. "Relationship of Vitamin A and Vitamin E Intake to Fasting Plasma Retinol, Retinol-Binding Protein, Retinyl Esters, Carotene, Tocopherol, and Cholesterol among Elderly People and Young Adults: Increased Plasma Retinyl Esters Among Vitamin A Users." *American Journal of Clinical Nutrition* 49:112–20.

Kromhaut, D., E. Bosschieter, and C. Coulander. 1985. "The Inverse Relation Between Fish Consumption and 20 Year Mortality from Coronary Heart Disease." *New England Journal of Medicine* 312:1205–09.

Landau, C., M. Cyre, and A. Moulton. 1994. *The Complete Book of Menopause: Every Woman's Guide to Good Health.* New York: G. P. Putnam's Sons.

Lapidus, L. 1986. "Ischemic Heart Disease, Stroke, and Mortality in Women: Results from a Prospective Population Study in Gothenburg, Sweden." *Acta Medicus Scandinavia (Supplement)* 219:1–42.

Levine, M. 1987. "Vitamin C Utilization with Stress." *Annals of the New York Academy of Science* 498:424–44.

Lohman, W. 1987. "Ascorbic Acid and Cancer." Third Conference on Vitamin C. *Annals of the New York Academy of Science* 498:402–17.

McDowell, M. A., R. R. Briefel, K. Alaimo, A. M. Bischof, C. R. Caughman, and M. D. Caroll. 1994. "Third National Health and Nutrition Examination Survey with Data from National Center for Health Statistics." Washington, D. C: Government Printing Office.

Medical Research Council Vitamin Study Research Group. 1991. "Prevention of Neural Tube Defects: Results of the Medical Research Council Vitamin Study." *Lancet* 338:131–37.

Notelovitz, M. and D. Tonnessen. 1993. *Menopause and Midlife Health.* New York: St Martin's Press.

Ojeda, L. 1995. *Menopause without Medicine.* Alameda, CA. Hunter House.

Pauling, L. 1986. *How to Live Long and Feel Better.* New York: Freeman.

Pollack, M. L. and J. H. Wilmore. 1990. *Exercise in Health and Disease.* Philadelphia: W. B. Saunders.

Pollack, M.,and V. Froelicher. 1990. "Position Stand of the American College of Sports Medicine: The Recommended Quantity and Quality of Exercise for Development and Maintaining Cardiorespiratory and Muscular Fitness in Healthy Adults." *Journal of Cardiopulmonary Rehabilitation* 10:235–45.

Reichman, J. 1996. *I'm Too Young To Get Old: Health Care for Women After Forty.* New York: Times Books.

Rexrode, K. M. and J. E. Manson. 1996. "Antioxidants in Cardiovascular Disease Prevention: Fact or Fiction?" *Menopausal Medicine* 4 (3):8–12.

Stampfer, M., C. Hennekens, and J. Manson. 1993. "Vitamin E Consumption and the Risk of Coronary Disease in Women." *New England Journal of Medicine* 328:1444–49.

Stampfer. M., and W. Willet. 1993. "Homocysteine and Marginal Vitamin D Deficiency: The Importance of Adequate Vitamin Intake." *Journal of the American Medical Association* 270:2726–27.

"Nutrition and Your Health: Dietary Guidelines for Americans." 1995. *Home and Garden Bulletin No. 232.* Washington, D. C: U. S. Department of Agriculture and U. S. Department of Health and Human Services.

"Dietary Goals for the United States." 1990. Washington, D. C.: U. S. Senate Select Committee on Nutrition and Human Needs.

Wallace, J. P,. et al. 1982. "Changes in Menstrual Function, Climacteric Syndrome, and Serum Concentrations of Sex Hormone in Pre- and Postmenopausal Women Following a Moderate Intensity Training Program." *Modern Science in Sports and Exercise* 14:154.

Willet, W. 1994. "Diet and Health: What Should We Eat?" *Science* 264:532–37.

Willet, W., M. Stampfer, and J. Manson. 1993. "Intake of Trans Fatty Acids and Risks of Coronary Heart Disease Among Women." *Lancet* 341:581–85.

Von Schacky, C. 1987. "Prophylaxis of Atherosclerosis with Marine Omega-3 Fatty Acids." *Annals of Internal Medicine* 107:890–99.

Zannoni, T. 1987. "Ascorbic Acid, Alcohol, and Environmental Chemicals." Third Conference on Vitamin C. *Annals of the New York Academy of Science* 498:364–88.

Chapter 11: Wellness from Lifestyle Changes: Weight Control, and Detoxifying Your Body and Mind

Abenhaim, J., Y. Moride, F. Brenot, S. Rich, J. Benichou, X. Kurz, T. Higgenbottam, C. Oakley, E. Wonters, M. Aubier, G. Simmoneau, and B. Begard. 1996. "Appetite Suppressant Drugs and the Risk of Pulmonary Hypertension." *New England Journal of Medicine* 335:609–15.

American College of of Obstetrics and Gynecology. 1994. "Substance Abuse. *ACOG Technical Bulletin 19.* Washington, D.C.: ACOG.

American Diabetes Association. 1994. "Nutrition Recommendations and Principles For People with Diabetes Mellitus." *Diabetes Care* 17:519–22.

Autti-Ramo, I., E. Gaily, and M. L. Granstrom. 1992. "Dysmorphic Features in Offspring of Alcoholic Mothers." *Archives of Diseases in Children* 67:712–16.

Baron, R. B. 1977. "Treating Obesity: Diet, Exercise, and Phen-Fen." *Audio-Digest Obstetrics and Gynecology* 44 (5).

Brody, J. June 27, 1991. "Research Suggests Pulling the Strings on Yo Yo Dieting." *New York Times.*.

Butts, N. K., and S. Price. 1994. "Effects of a 12-Week Weight Training Program on the Body Composition of Women over 30 Years of Age." *Journal of Strength Conditioning Research* 8:265–69.

Fontham, E. T. H. 1994. "Environmental Tobacco Smoke and Lung Cancer in Nonsmoking Women." *Journal of the American Medical Association* 271:1752–59.

Frezza, M. 1990. "The Role of Gastric Alcohol Dehydrogenase Activity and First Pass Metabolism." *New England Journal of Medicine* 322:967–76.

Gold, M. 1991. *The Good News about Drugs and Alcohol.* New York: Random House.

Horm, J., and K. Anderson. 1993. "Who in America is Trying to Lose Weight?" *Annals of Internal Medicine* 119:672–76.

Institute of Medicine. 1995. *Weighing the Options: Criteria for Evaluating Weight-Management Programs*. Washington, DC: National Academy Press.

Insull, W., M. Henderson, and D. Thompson, 1990. "Results of a Randomized Feasibility Study of a Low-Fat Diet." *Archives of Internal Medicine* 150:421–27.

Johannessen, S., and H. Liu. 1986. "High-Frequency, Moderate-Intensity Training in Sedentary Middle-Aged Women. *Physician Sportsmedicine* 14:99–102.

Kayman, S., W. Bruvold, and J. Stern. 1990. "Maintenance and Relapse after Weight Loss in Women: Behavioral Aspects." *American Journal of Clinical Nutrition* 52:800–07.

Kuczmarski, R.J., K. M. Flegal, S. M. Campbell, and C. L. Johnson. 1994. "Increasing Prevalence of Overweight among U.S. Adults." *Journal of the American Medical Association* 272:205–11.

Landau, C., M. Cyr, and A. Moulton. 1994. *The Complete Book of Menopause: Every Woman's Guide to Good Health*. New York: G.P. Putnam's Sons.

Langreth, R. September 16, 1997. "Alternatives to Redux Still Are Years Away." *Wall Street Journal*.

Larson, Joan. 1993. *Seven Weeks to Sobriety: The Proven Program to Fight Alcoholism Through Nutrition*. New York: Columbine Fawcett.

Longnecker, M. P. 1988. "A Meta-Analysis of Alcohol Consumption in Relation to Risk of Breast Cancer." *Journal of the American Medical Association* 260:652–56.

Notelovitz, M., and D. Tonnessen. 1993. *Menopause and Midlife Health*. New York: St. Martin's Press.

Ojeda, L. 1995. *Menopause without Medicine*. Alameda, CA.: Hunter House.

Prochaska, J. P., J. C. Norcross, and C. DiClemente. 1992. "In Search of How People Change: Applications to Addictive Behavior." *American Psychologist* 47: 1102–14.

Physicians' Desk Reference (PDR). 1997. Montvale, NJ: Medical Economics Company.

Rigotti, N. 1992. "Smoking Cessation Strategies for Women." Paper presented on "Primary Care of Women" to Harvard Medical School.

Roubenoff, R., G. E. Dallal, and P. W. F. Wilson. 1995. "Predicting Body Fatness: The Body Mass Index vs. Estimation by Bioelectrical Impedance." *American Journal of Public Health* 85:726–28.

Stampfer, M. J., and W. Willet, 1988. "A Prospective Study of Moderate Alcohol Consumption and the Risk of Coronary Disease and Stroke in Women." *New England Journal of Medicine* 318:267–73.

van Veer, P., F. J. Kok, R. J. Hermus, and F. Sturmans. 1989. "Alcohol Dose, Frequency, and Age at First Exposure in Relation to the Risk of Breast Cancer." *International Journal of Epidemiology* 18:511–17.

Warner, K. E. 1991. "Health and Economic Implications of a Tobacco Free Society." *Journal of American Medical Association* 258:2080–88.

Willet, W. 1994. "Diet and Health: What Should We Eat?" *Science* 264:532–37.

Young, T. B. 1989. "A Case-Control Study of Breast Cancer and Alcohol Consumption Habits." *Cancer* 64(2):552-58.

Goldring, L. A. C. R. Myers, and W. E. Sinning, eds. 1989. *Y's Ways to Physical Fitness*, 3rd ed. Chicago: Human Kinetics.

Chapter 12: Relax for a Change

American College of Obstetricians and Gynecologists. 1993. "Depression in Women." *Technical Bulletin No. 182*. Washington, D.C.: ACOG.

Benson, H., and E. Stuart. 1993. *The Wellness Book: The Comprehensive Guide to Maintaining and Treating Stress-Related Illness*. New York: Fireside.

Brown, G. W., et al. 1986. "Life Stress, Chronic Subclinical Symptoms, and Vulnerability to Clinical Depression." *Journal of Affective Disorders* 11:1–9.

Depression Guideline Panel. 1993. *Depression in Primary Care: Detection, Diagnosis, and Treatment*. AHCPR Publication No. 93-0552. Rockville, MD: U.S. Department of Health and Human Services, Public Health Service, Agency for Health Care Policy and Research.

Diagnostic and Statistical Manual of Mental Disorders, 3rd ed. 1987. Washington, D.C.: American Psychiatric Association.

Gise, L. H. 1996. "What You Can Do about Depression at Menopause." *Menopausal Medicine* 4 (1):1–5.

Hauri, P., and S. Linde. 1990. *No More Sleepless Nights*. New York: John Wiley and Sons.

Kaplan, A. G. 1986. "The 'Self in Relation:' Implications for Depression in Women." *Psychotherapy: Theory, Research, and Practice* 23:235–42.

Kiecolt-Glaser, J., and R. Glaser. 1991. "Stress and Immune Function in Humans." In *Psychoneuroimmunology*, 2nd ed.(R Ader, D. L. Felten, and N. Cohen, eds.) San Diego: Academic Press.

Kiecolt-Glaser, J. 1996. "The Negative Influence of Stress on the Immune System." Presentation at the annual meeting of The International Society of Neuroimmunomodulation.

Kiecolt-Glaser, J., L. Fisher, P. Ogrocki, J. Stout, C. Speicher, and R. Glaser. 1987. "Marital Quality, Marital Disruption, and Immune function." *Psychosomatic Medicine* 49:13-34.

Kobasa, S., S. Maddi, and S. Kahn. 1982. "Hardiness and Health: A Prospective Study." *Journal of Personality and Social Psychology* 42:168–77.

Landau, C., M. Cyre, and A. Moutlon. 1994. *The Complete Book of Menopause: Every Woman's Guide to Good Health*. New York: G. P. Putnam's Sons.

McGrath, E., G. P. Ketia, B. R. Strickland, and N. F. Russo. 1990. *Women and Depression: Risk Factors and Treatment Issues*. Washington, D.C.: American Psychological Association.

McKinlay, J., S. McKinlay, and D. Brambilla. 1987. "The Relative Contributions of Endocrine Changes and Social Circumstances to Depression in Mid-Aged Women." *Journal of Health and Social Behavior* 28:345–63.

Moyers, B. 1993. *Healing and the Mind*. New York: Bantam Doubleday Dell.

Nolen-Hoeksema, S. 1987. "Sex Differences in Unipolar Depression: Evidence and Theory." *Psychological Bulletin* 101:259–82.

Notelovitz, M., and D. Tonnessen. 1993. *Menopause and Midlife Health*. New York: St. Martin's Press.

O'Hara, M. W. 1991. "Postpartum Mental Disorders." In *Gynecology and Obstetrics*, vol. 6 (J. J. Sciarra, ed.). Philadelphia: J. B. Lippincott.

Ojeda, L. 1995. *Menopause without Medicine*. Alameda, CA: Hunter House.

Reichman, J. 1996. *I'm Too Young to Get Old: Health Care For Women after Forty*. New York: Times Books.

Sherwin, B. 1993. "Menopausal Depression: Myth or Reality?" Chair of symposium at Fourth Annual Meeting of the North American Menopausal Society, San Diego, CA.

Somer, E. 1993. *Nutrition for Women*. N.Y.: Henry Holt

Wilde, L. April 22, 1997. "Humor: Rx for Healing, Health, and Happiness." Presentation at Rogue Valley Medical Center, Medford, Oregon.

Weissman, M. M., R. Bland, G. Canino, C. Faravelli, S. Greenwald, H. Hwu, P. Joyce, E. Karam, C. Lee, J. Lellouch, J. Lepine, S. Newman, M. Rubio-Stepic, E. Wells, P. Wickramatne, H. Wittchen, E. Yeh. 1996. "Cross-National Epidemiology of Major Depression and Bipolar Disorder." *Journal of the American Medical Association* 276:293–99.

Yerkes, R. M., and J. D. Dodson. 1989. "The Relation of Strength of Stimulus to Rapidity of Habit Formation." *Journal of Comparative Neurology* 18:459–82.

Chapter 13: Good Sex Doesn't Need to Change

Bachman, G. A., and S. R. Leiblum. 1991. "Sexuality in Sexagenarian Women." *Maturitas* 13:43-50.

Bolen, J. D. 1993. "The Impact of Sexual Abuse on Women's Health." *Psychiatric Annals* 23:446-53.

Cohen, P. 1994. "The Role of Androgens in Menopausal HRT." From J. Lorran (ed.), *Comprehensive Management of Menopause*. London: Sonnger Verag.

Cone, F. K. 1993. *Making Sense of Menopause*. New York: Simon and Schuster.

Edelman, D. 1992. *Sex in the Golden Years*. New York: Donald I. Fine.

Helstrom, L. 1994. "Sexuality after Hysterectomy: A Model Based on Quantitative and Qualitative Analysis of 104 Women Before and After Subtotal Hysterectomy. *Journal of Psychosomatic Obstetrics and Gynecology*.4:219–29.

Kegel, A. M. 1951. "Physiologic Therapy for Urinary Stress Incontinence." *Journal of the American Medical Association* 146:915–17.

Keverne, E., N. D. Martensz, and B. Tuite. 1989. "Beta-Endorphin Concentration in Cerebrospinal Fluid of Monkeys Are Influenced by Grooming Relationships." *Psychoneuroendocrinology* 14(1-2):155–61.

Landau, C., M. Cyre, and A. Moutlon. 1994. *The Complete Book of Menopause: Every Woman's Guide to Good Health*. New York: G.P. Putnam's Sons.

Lechner, M. E., M. E. Bogel, L. M. Garcia-Shelton, J. L. Leichter, and K. R. Steibel. 1993. "Self-Reported Medical Problems of Adult Female Survivors of Childhood Sexual Abuse." *Journal of Family Practice* 36 (6):633–37.

Leventhal, J. 1997. "Libido and Menopause." Lecture given to the Women's Health Department, Kaiser, Walnut Creek, CA.

Masters, W., and V. Johnson, 1966. *Human Sexual Response.* Boston: Little Brown.

Masters, W., and V. Johnson. 1970. *Human Sexual Inadequacy.* Boston: Little Brown.

"Drugs That Cause Sexual Dysfunction: An Update." 1992. *Medical Letter: Drug Therapy;* 34:74-77.

Nachtigall, L., and J. R. Heilman, 1995. *Estrogen: The Facts Can Change Your Life.* New York: Harper Perennial.

Notelovitz, M. and D. Tonnessen, 1993. *Menopause and Midlife Health.* New York: St. Martin's Press

Reichman, J. 1996. *I'm Too Young to Get Old: Health Care for Women after Forty.* New York: Times Books.

Russell, D. 1986. *The Secret Trauma.* New York: Basic Books.

Sarrel, P. M. 1990. "Sexuality and Menopause." *Obstetrics and Gynecology* 75 (4):26S–30S.

Sachs, J. 1991. *What Women Should Know About Menopause.* New York: Bantam Doubleday Dell.

Sheehy, G. 1977. *Passages: The Predictable Crises of Adult Life.* New York: Bantam Books.

Sherwin, B., and M. Gelfand. 1985. "Sex Steroids and Affect in the Surgical Menopause: A Double Blind, Cross-Over Study." *Psychoneouroendocrinology* 3:325–35.

Chapter 14: Looking Good While Changing: Skin Care, Hair Care, and Cosmetic Surgery

Alster, T. S., and S. Garg. 1996. "Treatment of Facial Rhytides with a High-Energy Pulsed Carbon Dioxide Laser." *Plastic and Reconstructive Surgery* 98(5):791-94.

Chemical Peeling. 1994. Brochure No. 003. Schaumberg, Ill.: American Society for Dermatologic Surgery

Eyelid Surgery: Blepharoplasty. 1993. Brochure No. 1252. Arlington Heights, Ill.: American Society of Plastic and Reconstructive Surgeons.

Facelift: Rhitidectomy, 3rd ed. 1994. Brochure. Arlington Heights, Ill.: American Society of Plastic and Reconstructive Surgeons.

Surgery of the Abdomen: Abdominoplasty. 1993. Brochure No. 1259. Arlington Heights, Ill.: American Society of Plastic and Reconstructive Surgeons.

Breast Augmentation: Mammoplasty. 1993. Brochure No. 1255. Arlington Heights, Ill.: American Society of Plastic and Reconstructive Surgeons.

Breast Lift: Mastopexy. 1993. Brochure No. 1262. Arlington Heights, IL: American Society of Plastic and Reconstructive Surgeons.

Brumberg, E. 1977. Ageless: What Every Woman Needs to Know to Look Good and Feel Good. New York: Harper Collins.

Cone, F. K. 1993. *Making Sense of Menopause.* New York: Simon and Schuster.

Darr, D., S. Dunstan, H. Faust, and S. R. Pinnell. 1996. "Effectiveness of Antioxidants (Vitamins C and E) with and without Sunscreens As Topical Photoprotectants." *Acta Dermato-Venereologica* 76:264–68.

Dover, J. S. 1996. "CO2 Laser Resurfacing: Why All the Fuss?" Editorial. *Plastic And Reconstructive Surgery* 98:506–09.

Epps, R. P. and S. C. Stuart. 1995. *Women's Complete Health Book*. New York: Delacorte.

Eskin, B. A., and L. S. Dumas. 1995. *Midlife Can Wait: How to Stay Young and Healthy After 35*. New York: Ballantine.

Fisher, A. A. 1995. *Contact Dermatitis*, 3rd ed. Philadelphia: Lea and Febiger.

Fulton, J. E., G. Pluwig, and A. M. Kilgman. 1996. "Effect of Chocolate on Acne Vulgaris." *Journal of the American Medical Association* 210:2071–74.

Glick, D., Y. Dlugosz, and F. Yuspa. 1994. "Regulating Normal Function by Polypeptide Growth Factors." *Cosmetics and Toiletries* 109:55–60.

Hayman, G. 1996. *How Do I Look?*. New York: Random House.

Idson, B. 1992. "Dry Skin, Moisturizing, and Emolliency." *Cosmetics and Toiletries* 107:69–78.

Idson, B. 1993. "Vitamins and the Skin." *Cosmetics and Toiletries* 108:79–94.

Leverette, K. 1991."The Glycololic Bandwagon: Fact and Fiction." *Dermascope* 4:50–51.

Lewis, A. B. and E. C. Genderl. 1996. "Resurfacing with Topical Agents: A Review Article. *Seminars in Cutaneous Medicine and Surgery* 15(33):139–44.

Love, S. 1995. *Dr. Susan Love's Breast Book*. Reading, Mass: Addison-Wesley.

Mackenzie, R., and L. Sauder. 1990. "Cytokines and Growth Factors: Functions in Skin Immunity and Homeostasis. *Dermatologic Clinics*, 8:649–61.

McCallion, R., and A. Li Wan Po. 1993. Dry and Photo-Aged Skin: Manifestations and Management." *Journal of Clinical Pharmaceutical Therapeutics* 18:15–32.

Moy, L. S. 1995. "Glycolocic Acid: A Safe Alternative for Chemical Peel." Presentation at Orlando, Fla., meeting on Cosmetic Dermatology. sponsored by Northwestern University School of Medicine.

Nakamura, T., S. R. Pinnell, and J. W. Streilein. 1995. "Ántioxidants Can Reverse the Deleterious Effects of Ultraviolet (UVB) Radiation on Cutaneous Immunity." *Journal of Investigative Dermatology* 104:600–05.

Notelovitz, M. and D. Tonnessen. 1993. *Menopause and Midlife Health*. New York: St. Martin's Press.

Ojeda, L., 1995. *Menopause Without Medicine*. Alameda, CA.: Hunter House.

Olson, K. R. 1994. *Poisoning and Drug Overdose*, 2nd ed. Norwalk, Conn.: Appleton and Lange.

Podolsky, D, and B. Streisand. 1996. "The Price of Vanity." *U.S. News and World Report* October 14:72–80.

Radd, B. 1997. "Antiwrinkle Ingredients." *Skin, Inc* 9(1):88–99.

Reichman, J. 1996. *I'm Too Young to Get Old: Health Care for Women after Forty*. New York: Times Books.

Roenigk, H. H. 1995. "Treatment of the Aging Face." *Dermatologic Clinics* 13:245–61.

Sies, H., W. Stahl, and A. Sundquist. 1992. "Antioxidant Functions of Vitamins." *Annals of the New York Academy of Science* 669:7–20.

Slovak, R. March 1997. Personal communication.

Sporn, M. B., and A. B. Roberts. 1991. *Peptide Growth Factors and their Receptors*, New York: Springer-Verlag.

Stiller, M., J. Bartoloni, S. Stein, S. Smith, R. Kollis, R. Gillies, and L. A. Drake 1996. "Topical 8% Glycolic Acid and 8% L-lactic Acid Creams in the Treatment of Photo-Damaged Skin." *Archives of Dermatology.* 132:631–36.

Tajima, S., and S. R. Pinnell. 1996. "Ascorbic Acid Preferentially Enhances Type I and III Collagen Gene Transcription in Human Fibroblasts." *Journal of Dermatological Science* 11:250–53.

Wilson, J. 1992. *Guide to Cosmetic Surgery*. New York: Simon and Schuster.

Chapter 15: Gynecologic Surgery and Medical Treatment: If Something Has Changed

Alexander, D. A., A. A, Naji, S. B. Pinion, J. Mollison, H. C. Kitchener, D. E. Parkin, D. R. Abramovich, and I. T. Russell. 1996. "Randomized Trial Comparing Hysterectomy with Endometrial Ablation for Dysfunctional Uterine Bleeding: Psychiatric and Psychosocial Aspect." *British Medical Journal* 312(7026): 280–284.

Appell, R. A. 1997. "Medications for Urge Incontinence." *Audio Digest Obstetrics and Gynecology* 44(4).

Ayton, R. A., G. M. Darling, A. L. Murkies, E. A. Farrell, E. Weisberg, I. Selinus, and I. S. Fraser. 1996. "A Comparative Study of Safety and Efficacy of Continuous Low Dose Oestradiol Released from a Vaginal Ring Compared with Conjugated Equine Oestrogen Vaginal Cream in the Treatment of Postmenopausal Urogenital Atrophy." *British Journal of Obstetrics and Gynaecology* 103:351–358.

Baggish, M., M. Paraiso, E. M. Breznock, D.V.M., and S. Griffey, D.V.M. 1995. A Computer-Controlled, Continuously Circulating, Hot Irrigating System for Endometrial Ablation." *American Journal of Obstetrics and Gynecology* 173(6):1842–1848.

Baggish, M. S, E. H. M. Sze. 1996. "Endometrial Ablation: A Series of 568 Patients Treated over an 11-Year Period." *American Journal Obstetrics and Gynecology* 174(3):908–13.

Bergman, A. and G. Elia. 1995. "Three Surgical Procedures for Genuine Stress Incontinence: Five-Year Follow-Up of a Prospective Randomized Study." *American Journal of Obstetrics and Gynecology* 173:66–71.

Brill, A. I. 1995. "What Is the Role of Hysteroscopy in the Management of Abnormal Uterine Bleeding?" *Clinical Obstetrics and Gynecology* 38:319–45.

Brown, J. 1996. "Episiotomy and Pelvic Floor Exercise for Incontinence." *Audio Digest: Obstetrics and Gynecology* 43 (21):Side A.

Burch, J. C. 1961. "Urethrovaginal Fixation to Cooper's Ligament for Correction of Stress Incontinence, Cystocele, and Prolapse." *American Journal of Obstetrics and Gynecology* 81:281–86.

Cadeddu, J. A., and L. R. Kavoussi. 1996. "Correction of Stress Urinary Incontinence: Transperitoneal Approach." *Journal of Endourology* 10:241–45.

Cameron, I. T., R. Haining, M. A. Lumsden, V. R. Thomas, and S. K. Smith. 1990. "The Effects of Mefenamic Acid and Norethisterone on Measured Menstrual Blood Loss." *Obstetrics and Gynecology* 76:85–8.

Carlson K. J. 1993. "Indications for Hysterectomy." *New England Journal of Medicine* 328:856–60.

Casper, R. F. , and M. T. Hearn. 1990. "The Effect of Hysterectomy and Bilateral Oophorectomy in Women with Severe Premenstrual Syndrome." *American Journal of Obstetrics and Gynecology* 162:105–09.

Cosiski-Marana, H.R., J. Moreira de Andrade, M. Matheus de Sala, R. Duarte, and R. R. Fonzar-Marana. 1996. "Evaluation of Long-Term Results of Surgical Correction of Stress Urinary Incontinence." *Gynecologic and Obstetric Investigation* 41:214–19.

Cramer, D. W. 1994. "Chapter 5: Epidemiology and Biostatistics." *Practical Gynecologic Oncology*, 2nd ed. Baltimore: Williams and Wilkins.

Creasman, W. T. 1997. "Ovarian Cancer Screening." *ACOG Clinical Review* 2 (2):1–2,14-15.

DeLancey, J. O. L. 1993. "Childbirth, Continence, and the Pelvic Floor." *New England Journal of Medicine* 329:1956–57.

Derman, S. G., J. Rehnstrom, and R. S. Neuwirth. 1991. "The Long-Term Effectiveness of Hysteroscopic Treatment of Menorrhagia and Leiomyomas." *Obstetrics and Gynecology* 77:591–94.

Dicker, R. C., J. R. Greenspan, and L.T. Strauss. 1982. "Complications of Abdominal and Vaginal Hysterectomies among Women of Reproductive Age in the United States." *American Journal of Obstetrics and Gynecology* 144:841–48.

Dwyer N., J. Hutton, and G. M. Stirrat. 1993. "Randomized Controlled Trial Comparing Endometrial Resection with Abdominal Hysterectomy for the Treatment of Menorrhagia." *British Journal of Obstetrics and Gynaecology* 100:237–243.

Elia, G., and A. Bergman. 1993. "Pelvic Muscle Exercises: When Do They Work? *Obstetrics and Gynecology* 81:283–86.

Fairbanks, V. F., and E. Bentler. 1995. "Chapter 46: Iron Deficiency." p492 *William's Hematology*, E. Bentler, M. A. Lichtman, B. S. Coller, and T. J. Kipps, eds, 5th ed. New York: McGraw-Hill.

Falconer, C., and B. Larsson. 1995. "Correction of Urinary Stress Incontinence in Women." *Neurorological Urodynamics* 14:365–70.

Fantl, J. A., L. Cardoza, and D. R. McLish. 1994. "Estrogen Therapy for Urinary Incontinence in Post Menopausal Women." *Journal of Obstetrics and Gynecology* 83:12–18

Ferry, J., and L. Rankin. 1994. "Low Cost, Patient Acceptable, Local Analgesia Approach to Gynaecological Outpatient Surgery: A Review of 817 Consecutive Procedures." *Australian and New Zealand Journal of Obstetrics and Gynaecology* 34:453–456.

Fraser, I. S., S. Angsuwathana, F. Mahmoud, and S. Yezerski. 1993. "Short and Medium Term Outcomes after Rollerball Endometrial Ablation for Menorrhagia." *Medical Journal of Australia* 158:454–57.

Gainey, H. L. 1955. "Postpartum Observation of Pelvic Tissue Damage: Further Studies." *American Journal of Obstetrics and Gynecology* 70.800–07.

Gambone, J., R. Reiter, and J. Lench. 1992. "Short term Outcome of Incidental Hysterectomy at the Time of Adnexectomy for Benign Disease." *Journal of Women's Health* 1:197–200.

Garnet, J. 1964. " Uterine Rupture during Pregnancy." *Obstetrics and Gynecology* 23:898–905.

Goldfarb, H. A. 1995. "Laparoscopic Coagulation of Myoma (Myolysis)." *Obstetrics and Gynecology Clinics of North America* 22:807–19.

Goldfarb, H. A. 1990. "A Review of 35 Endometrial Ablations Using the Nd:Yag Laser for Recurrent Menometrorrhagia." *Obstetrics and Gynecology* 76:833–35.

Goldrath, M. H., T. A. Fuller, and S. Segal. 1981. "Laser Photovaporization of Endometrium for the Treatment of Menorrhagia." *American Journal of Obstetrics and Gynecology* 40 (1):14–19.

Goldrath, M. H. 1990. "Use of Danazol in Hysteroscopic Surgery for Menorrhagia." *Journal of Reproductive Medicine.* 35 (Supplement 1 of Issue 1):91–96

Gomel, V. 1995. "For Tubal Pregnancy, Surgical Treatment Is Usually Best." *Clinical Obstetrics and Gynecology* 38:353–61.

Grimes, D. 1997. "Sense and Sensuality: Contraceptives." *Audio-Digest, Obstetrics and Gynecology* 44 (2).

Grimes, D. A. 1982. "Diagnostic Dilation and Curettage: A Reappraisal." *American Journal of Obstetrics and Gynecology* 142:1–6.

Hahn, I., I. Milsom, M. Fall, and P. Ekelund. 1993. "Long-Term Results of Pelvic Floor Training in Female Stress Urinary Incontinence." *British Journal of Urology* 72:421–27.

Handa, V. L., T. A. Harris, and D. R. Ostergard. 1996. "Protecting the Pelvic Floor: Obstetric Management to Prevent Incontinence and Pelvic Organ Prolapse." *Obstetrics and Gynecology* 88:470–78.

Harris, W. J. 1992. "Uterine Dehiscence Following Laparoscopic Myomectomy." *Obstetrics and Gynecology* 80:545–46.

Helstrom, L. 1994. "Sexuality after Hysterectomy: A Model Based on Quantitative and Qualitative Analysis of 104 Women before and after Subtotal Hysterectomy." *Journal of Psychosomatic Obstetrics and Gynecology.*15:219–29.

Helstrom, L., D. Sorbom; and T. Bäckström.1995. "Influence of Partner Relationship on Sexuality after Subtotal Hysterectomy." *Acta Obstetricia et Gynecologica Scandinavica* 74:142–46.

Hendricks-Matthews, M. K. 1991. "The Importance of Assessing a Woman's History of Sexual Abuse Before Hysterectomy." *Journal of Family Practice* 32:631–32.

Henriksson, L., M. Stjernquist, L. Boquist, I. Cedergren, and I. Selinus. 1996. "A One-Year Multicenter Study of Efficacy and Safety of a Continuous, Low-Dose, Estradiol-Releasing Vaginal Ring (Estring) in Postmenopausal Women with Symptoms and Signs of Urogenital Aging." *American Journal of Obstetrics and Gynecology* 174:85–92.

Herrmann, Jr., U. J, G. Locher, and A. Goldhirsch. 1987. "Sonographic Patterns of Ovarian Tumors: Prediction of Malignancy" *Obstetrics and Gynecology* 69:777–81.

Hufnagel, V. G. 1988. "Opinion: The conspiracy Against the Uterus." *Journal of Psychosomatic Obstetrics and Gynecology* 9(1):51–58.

Jaffe, S. B., and R. Jewelewicz. 1991 "The Basic Infertility Investigation" *Fertility and Sterility* 56:599–613.

Kelly, H. A. 1913. "Incontinence of Urine in Women." *Urologic and Cutaneous Review* 17:291–99.

Kjolhede, P., and G. Ryden. 1994. "Prognostic Factors and Long-Term Results of the Burch Colposuspension: A Retrospective Study." *Acta Obstetrics Gynecology Scandinavia* 73:642–47.

Klutke, J. J., and A. Bergman. 1996. "Chapter 37: Nonsurgical Management of Stress Urinary Incontinence." In D. R. Ostergard, A. E. Bent, eds, *Urogynecology and Urodymanmics: Theory and Practice,*4th ed. Baltimore: Williams and Wilkins.

Langer, R., A. Raziel, R. Ron-El, A. Golan, I. Bukovsky, and E. Caspi. 1990. "Reproductive Outcome after Conservative Surgery for Unruptured Tubal Pregnancies—A 15-Year Experience." *Fertility and Sterility* 53:227–31.

Lefler, H. T., G. H. Sullivan, and J. F. Hylka. 1991. "Modified Endometrial Ablation: Electrocoagulation with Vasopressin and Suction Curettage Preparation." *Obstetrics and Gynecology.* 77:949–56.

Leventhal, J. October 1996. "Premenstrual Dysphoric Disorder." Lecture given to the Women's Health Department, Kaiser, Walnut Creek, CA.

Liapis, A., E. Pyrgiotis, A. Kontoravdis, C. Louridas, and P. A. Zourlas. 1996. "Genuine Stress Incontinence: Prospective Randomized Comparizon of Two Operative Methods." *European Journal of Obstetric and Gynecological Reproductive Biology* 64 (1):69–72.

Loffer, F. D. 1987. "Hysteroscopic Endometrial Ablation with the Nd:YAG Laser Using a Nontouch Technique." *Obstetrics and Gynecology* 69 (4):679-682

Loft, N. L. 1993. "Ovarian Function after Premenopausal Hysterectomy." *Ugeskrift for Laeger* 155:3818–22.

Lund, J. J. 1955. "Early Ectopic Pregnancy." *Journal of Obstetrics and Gynaecology of the British Empire.* 62:70–76.

Lyons, T. L. 1995. "Minimally Invasive Treatment of Urinary Stress Incontinence and Laparoscopically Directed Repair of Pelvic Floor Defects." *Clinical Obstetrics and Gynecology*38:380–91.

Lyons, T. L., and W. Parker. 1996. "Highlights from the International Congress of Gynecologic Endoscopy." *Audio-Digest, Obstetrics and Gynecology* 43 (17).

McGuire, E. J., and R. D. Cespedes. 1996. "Proper Diagnosis: A Must Before Surgery for Stress Incontinence." *Journal of Endourology* 10:201–205.

McLucas, B., and S. Goodwin. 1996. "Embolic Therapy for Myomata." *Minimally Invasive Therapy and Allied Technology.* 5:1-3.

Magos, A. L., R. Baumann, G. M. Lockwood, and A.C. Turnbull. 1991. "Experience with the First 250 Endometrial Resections for Menorrhagia." *Lancet* 337:1074-78.

Maiman, M., V. Seltzer, and J. Boyce. 1991. "Laparoscopic Excision of Ovarian Neoplasms Subsequently Found to Be Malignant." *Obstetrics and Gynecology* 77:563–65.

Maiman, M. 1995. "Laparoscopic Removal of the Adnexal Mass: The Case for Caution." *Clinical Obstetrics and Gynecology* 38:370–379.

Malone, L. 1969. "Myomectomy: Recurrence after Removal of Solitary and Multiple Myomas." *Obstetrics and Gynecology* 34:200–03.

Mancuso, A., R. D'Anna, C. Dugo, and R Leonardi. 1991. "The Residual Ovary after Hysterectomy." *Clinical Experimental Obstetrics and Gynecology* 18 (2) :117–19.

Marshall, V. E., A. A. Marchetti, and K. E. Krantz. 1949. "The Correction of Stress Incontinence by Simple Vesicourethral Suspension Surgery." *Obstetrics and Gynecology* 88:509–14.

Marrs, R. 1991. "The Use of Potassium-Titanyl-Phosphate Laser for Laparoscopic Removal of Ovarian Endometriomas." *American Journal of Obstetrics and Gynecology* 164: 1622–28.

Maymon, R., A. Shulman, B. B.Maymon, F. Bar-Levy, M. Lotan, and C. Bahary. 1992. "Ectopic Pregnancy, the New Gynecological Epidemic Disease: Review of the Modern Work-Up and the Nonsurgical Treatment Option." *International Journal of Fertility* 37 (3):146–64.

Mecke, H., E. Lehmann-Willenbrock, M. Ibrahim, and K. Semm. 1992. "Pelviscopic Treatment of Ovarian Cysts in Premenopausal Women." *Gynecologic and Obstetric Investigations* 34 (1):36–42.

The Medical Letter 1995. "Antimicrobial Prophylaxis in Surgery." *The Medical Letter* 37(957):79–82.

Montz, F. J., and J. B. Schlaerth. 1995. "Laparoscopic Surgery: Does It Have a Role in the Management of Gynecologic Malignancies?" *Clinical Obstetrics and Gynecology*38:426–433.

Mouritsen, L., C. Frimodt-Moller, and M. Moller. 1991 "Long-Term Effect of Pelvic Floor Exercises on Female Urinary Incontinence." *British Journal of Urology* 68 (1):32–37.

Munro, M. G., and J. Neprest. 1995. "Laparoscopic Hysterectomy: Does It Work? A Bicontinental Review of the Literature and Clinical Commentary." *Clinical Obstetrics and Gynecology* 38:401–25.

Nachitgall, L. E., J. R. Heilman. 1994. *Estrogen: The Facts Can Change Your Life.* New York: Harper Perennial.

National Center for Health Statistics. 1987. Pokras, R., V. G. Hufnagal. *Hysterectomies in the United States, 1965–1984.* Vital and health statistics. Series 13 no. 92. Washington, DC: Government Printing Office. DHOWS publication no. (PAS)88–1753.

Notelovitz, M., and D. Tonnessen. 1993. *Menopause and Midlife Health: America's leading authority on menopause and midlife health reveals what every woman must know about Menopause.* New York: St. Martin's Press.

Ostergard, D. R. 1997. "Biofeedback and Other Treatments for Incontinence." *Audio Digest Obstetrics/Gynecology* 44 (4).

Parker, W. H. 1995. "The Case For Laparoscopic Management Of Adenexal Mass." *Clinical Obstetrics and Gynecology* 38:362–369.

Parker, W. H. 1995. "Myomectomy: Laparoscopy or Laparotomy?" *Clinical Obstetrics and Gynecology* 38:392–400.

Ranney, B. 1990. "Decreasing Numbers of Patients for Vaginal Hysterectomy and Plasty." *South Dakota. Journal of Medicine* 43 (1):7–12.

Ravina, J. H., D. Herbreteau, N. Ciraru-Vigneron, J. J. Bouret, E. Houdart, A. Aymard, and J. J. Merland. 1995. "Arterial Embolisation to Treat Uterine Myomata." *Lancet* 346(8976):671–672.

Reggiori, A., M. Ravera, E. Cocozza, M. Andreata, and F. Mukasa. 1996. "Randomized Study of Antibiotic Prophylaxis for General and Gynaecological Surgery from a Single Centre in Rural Africa." *British Journal of Surgery* 83:356–59.

Reich, H., J. DeCaprio, and F. McGlynn. 1989. "Laproscopic Hysterectomy." *Journal of Gynecologic Surgery* 5 (2):213–216.

Schildkraut, J., E. Bastos, and A. Berchuck. 1997. "Relationship between Lifetime Ovulatory Cycles and Overexpression of Mutant N Epithelial Ovarian Cancer." *Journal of the National Cancer Institute.* 89(13)932–938

Seifer, D. B., J. N. Gutmann, W. D. Grant, C. A. Kamps, and A. H. DeCherney. 1993. "Comparison of Persistent Ectopic Pregnancy after Laparoscopic Salpingostomy versus Salpingostomy at Laparotomy for Ectopic Pregnancy." *Obstetrics and Gynecology* 81:378–82.

Silva, P. D., A. M. Schaper, and B. Rooney. 1993. " Reproductive Outcomes after 143 Laparoscopic Procedures for Ectopic Pregnancy." *Obstetrics and Gynecology* 81:710–15.

Snooks, S. J., M. Swash, M. M. Henry, and M. Setchell. 1986. "Risk factors in Childbirth Causing Damage to the Pelvic Floor." *International Journal of Colorectal Diseases* 1 (1) :20–24.

Stovall, T. G. 1995. "Medical Management Should Be Routinely Used As Primary Therapy for Ectopic Pregnancy." *Clinical Obstetrics and Gynecology* 38:346–52.

Stovall, T. G., F. W. Ling, L. A. Gray, S. A. Carson, and J. E. Buster. 1991. "Methotrexate Treatment of Unruptured Ectopic Pregnancy: A Report of 100 Cases." *Obstetrics and Gynecology* 77:749–53.

Tanos, V., and N. Rojansky. 1994. " Prophylactic Antibiotics in Abdominal Hysterectomy." *Journal of the American College of Surgeons* 179:593-600.

Thorp, Jr., J. M., and V. L. Katz. 1991. "Submucous Myomas Treated with Gonadotropin Releasing Hormone Agonist and Resulting in Vaginal Hemorrhage: A Case Report." *Journal of Reproductive Medicine* 36:625-626.

Townsend, D. E., R. M. Richart, R. A. Paskowitz, and R. E. Woolfork. "'Rollerball' Coagulation of the Endometrium." *Obstetrics and Gynecology* 76:310–13.

Trockman, B. A., and G. E. Leach. 1996. "Needle Suspension Procedures: Past, Present, and Future." *Journal of Endourology* 10:217–220.

Tulandi, T., C. Murray, and M.Guralnick. 1993. "Adhesion Formation and Reproductive Outcome after Myomectomy and Second-Look Laparoscopy." *Obstetrics and Gynecology* 82:213–15.

Valle, R. F. 1993. "Endometrial Ablation for Dysfunctional Uterine Bleeding: Role of GnRH Agonists." *International Journal of Gynecology and Obstetrics* 41 (1):3–15.

Van Den Eeden, S. K., M. Glasser, S. D. Mathias, H. H. Colwell, D. J. Pasta, and K. Kunz. 1997. "Quality of Life: Health Care Utilization and Costs among Women Undergoing Hysterectomy in a Managed Care Setting." Submitted for publication.

Voss, E., M. R. Steel, and J. Erian. 1993. "Laparoscopic Hysterectomy: A Valid Alternative to Conventional Surgery." *British Journal of Hospital Medicine* 50:537–39.

West, S., and P. Dranov. 1994. *The Hysterectomy Hoax: A Leading Surgeon Explains Why 90% of All Hysterectomies Are Unnecessary and Describes All the Treatment Options Available to Every Women, No Matter What Age.* New York: Doubleday.

Whittemore, A. S., and V. McGuire. 1997. "Ovulations, p53 Mutations, and Ovarian Cancer—A Causal Link. *Journal of the National Cancer Institute* 89:906-07.

Index

anovulation, and entrometrial cancer
risk, 119
ANS. *see* autonomic nervous system
(ANS)
antioxidants, 58, 192–195
antithyroid medication, 102
antitubercular and anticonvulsive
drugs, effect of birth control pills
on, 47
appearance changes, during
perimenopause, 275–301
aromitization, 119
arthritis and orthopedic problems,
effect on sex life, 266
artificial insemination, 42–44
asperin, role in preventing colorectal
cancer, 126
assisted hatching, 42
assisted reproductive technologies
(ARTs), 42–44
atherosclerosis, 77
atrophy, of skin and mucous
membrane, 7
atypical squamous cells of
undetermined significance
(ASCUS), 131
autonomic nervous system (ANS), 22

B

baby boomers, changes brought about
by, 5
barrier methods of contraception, 44–45
behavioral modification
for mild PMS, 60
principles of, 178–179
for weight loss, 225–226
beta-carotenes, role in preventing
colorectal cancer, 126
biofeedback
for stress reduction, 249
treating urinary incontinence
with, 334
bioflavinoids, 173
biological markers, in perimenopause,
6–8
birth control pills
diabetes management while
taking, 46–47
during perimenopause, 46–49

effect of antitubercular and
anticonvulsive drugs on, 47
effect on fibroid tumors, 47
effect on migraine headaches, 47
effect of stopping, 37
hypertension risks, 47
risk if you smoke, 46
use of low-dose for controlling
hot flashes, 23
black cohosh, 148, 172
blepharoplasty (eyelid lift), 297
body-mass index (BMI), 212–213
bone mass, loss of, 7. *see also*
osteoporosis
brain cell changes, in perimenopause,
7, 24–29
BRCA1 and BRCA2 genes, cancer risks
from, 108–109
breast cancer
and combined HRT, 153
effect of alcohol consumption on,
109–110, 229
effect of estrogen on, 109, 141–144
effect of exercise on, 111
effect of obesity and high fat diet
on, 109
familial, 106–107
new developments in screening
for, 115–116
odds of developing, 108
prior abortion and, 111
risk of, 107–111
screening for, 111–116
effect of smoking on, 109
treatment of, 116–118
ultrasound screening for, 115
breast examination, physician, 112
breast implants, effectiveness of
mammography with, 114
breast self-examination (BSE), 111–112
breast tenderness, treating with
androgen, 158
B vitamins, 195–196

C

calcitonin, 84, 90
calcium, 197
preventing osteoporosis with,
83–84

T

TAH & BSO (total abdominal hysterectomy and bilateral salpingo-oophorectomy), 314, 315
t'ai chi, 248
Tamoxifen, in breast cancer treatment, 117
teeth, care of during perimenopause, 293
telomerase, 106
testosterone (T), 155–156
    role in treating osteoporosis, 83
    treating menstrual migraine headaches with, 71–72
T4 (thyroxine), 96
thyroid disease, 8
    diagnosis of, 99–101
    and infertility, 41, 99
    laboratory tests for, 101
    and loss of sexual desire, 99
    and menstrual irregularity, 98
    physical symptoms of, 100
    and postpartum blues, 99
    symptoms of, 93–95, 96
    treatment for, 101–103
thyroid gland, 95–98
thyroiditis, 99
thyroid stimulating hormone. see TSH (thyroid stimulating hormone)
thyroid stimulating immunoglobulin. see TSI (thyroid stimulating immunoglobulin)
thyroxine. see T4 (thyroxine)
tobacco
    effect of during pregnancy, 38
    role played in aging of skin, 28
    effects of use in perimenopause, 15
tranquilizers, and PMS, 64
transition, 3–4
tricyclic antidepressants, 336
triglycerides (TG), 191
triiodothyronine. see T3 (triiodothyronine)
triple marker tests, for abnormal pregnancies, 36
trisomy 21 (Down syndrome), 33–34

TSH (thyroid stimulating hormone), 96–97
TSI (thyroid stimulating immunoglobulin), 96, 97–98
T3 (triiodothyronine), 96–97
tubal disease, as cause of infertility, 41
tubal ligation, 50–51
tubal pregnancy. see ectopic pregnancy
tumor, 37, 47

U

ultrasound
    for diagnosing osteoporosis, 90
    for measuring endometrial thickness, 120
ultraviolet light, effect on aging of skin, 27, 276
unopposed estrogen, 163
urethra, 331
urge incontinence. see urinary incontinence
urinary incontinence, 28–29, 331–338
    effect of estrogen on, 139–140, 338
    genito-urinary system, 331–332
    nonsurgical treatments for, 333–336
    siphon (Type III), 336
    stress (Type I), 333–334
    surgical options for, 337–338
    types of, 332–336
    urge (Type II), 334–336
uterine bleeding
    abnormal, 13, 304–308
    causes of, 304–305
    diagnosis, 305
    summary of treatment for abnormal, 325–326
UV (ultraviolet), 21, 27, 278–280

V

vagina, changes in, 7
vaginal cones, treating urinary incontinence with, 334
vaginal dryness and thinning (atrophy), preventing with estrogen, 139

vaginal ultrasound, for endometrial
thickness, 120
vaginismus, 261
varicose veins, 291–292
vasoconstrictors, for treating menstrual
migraine headaches, 71
vasomotor instability, 20–23
viral infections, abnormal pregnancies
from, 34, 38
visualization, 246
vitamin B6, in treatment of PMS, 58
vitamin D, 196–197
vitamine E, in treatment of PMS, 58
vitamins and minerals, 191–198
antioxidants, 192–195
B vitamins, 195–196
in treatment of PMS, 57–59

W

warts (human papilloma virus), 39
weight control, 212–226
body-mass index, 212–213
causes of overweight, 215–216
fat distribution, 214–215
role of exercise in, 222–225
weight loss
diet pills, 221–222
diets, 217–219
low-calorie liquid diets for,
220–221
plans, 219–220
wellness. *see also* exercise; nutrition
for a change, 177–210
from lifestyle changes, 211–236
women's health care advisor, selecting,
12
wrinkles
causes of, 27–28
effect of estrogen replacement
therapy on, 140

XYZ

yin and yang, 168–169
yoga, for stress reduction, 248
Yuzpe method, 49

Some Other New Harbinger Self-Help Titles

Dr. Carl Robinson's Basic Baby Care, $10.95
Better Boundries: Owning and Treasuring Your Life, $13.95
Goodbye Good Girl, $12.95
Being, Belonging, Doing, $10.95
Thoughts & Feelings, Second Edition, $18.95
Depression: How It Happens, How It's Healed, $14.95
Trust After Trauma, $13.95
The Chemotherapy & Radiation Survival Guide, Second Edition, $13.95
Heart Therapy, $13.95
Surviving Childhood Cancer, $12.95
The Headache & Neck Pain Workbook, $14.95
Perimenopause, $13.95
The Self-Forgiveness Handbook, $12.95
A Woman's Guide to Overcoming Sexual Fear and Pain, $14.95
Mind Over Malignancy, $12.95
Treating Panic Disorder and Agoraphobia, $44.95
Scarred Soul, $13.95
The Angry Heart, $13.95
Don't Take It Personally, $12.95
Becoming a Wise Parent For Your Grown Child, $12.95
Clear Your Past, Change Your Future, $12.95
Preparing for Surgery, $17.95
Coming Out Everyday, $13.95
Ten Things Every Parent Needs to Know, $12.95
The Power of Two, $12.95
It's Not OK Anymore, $13.95
The Daily Relaxer, $12.95
The Body Image Workbook, $17.95
Living with ADD, $17.95
Taking the Anxiety Out of Taking Tests, $12.95
The Taking Charge of Menopause Workbook, $17.95
Living with Angina, $12.95
Five Weeks to Healing Stress: The Wellness Option, $17.95
Choosing to Live: How to Defeat Suicide Through Cognitive Therapy, $12.95
Why Children Misbehave and What to Do About It, $14.95
When Anger Hurts Your Kids, $12.95
The Addiction Workbook, $17.95
The Mother's Survival Guide to Recovery, $12.95
The Chronic Pain Control Workbook, Second Edition, $17.95
Fibromyalgia & Chronic Myofascial Pain Syndrome, $19.95
Flying Without Fear, $12.95
Kid Cooperation: How to Stop Yelling, Nagging & Pleading and Get Kids to Cooperate, $12.95
The Stop Smoking Workbook: Your Guide to Healthy Quitting, $17.95
Conquering Carpal Tunnel Syndrome and Other Repetitive Strain Injuries, $17.95
Wellness at Work: Building Resilience for Job Stress, $17.95
An End to Panic: Breakthrough Techniques for Overcoming Panic Disorder, Second Edition, $17.95
Living Without Procrastination: How to Stop Postponing Your Life, $12.95
Goodbye Mother, Hello Woman: Reweaving the Daughter Mother Relationship, $14.95
Letting Go of Anger: The 10 Most Common Anger Styles and What to Do About Them, $12.95
Messages: The Communication Skills Workbook, Second Edition, $13.95
Coping With Chronic Fatigue Syndrome: Nine Things You Can Do, $12.95
The Anxiety & Phobia Workbook, Second Edition, $17.95
The Relaxation & Stress Reduction Workbook, Fourth Edition, $17.95
Living Without Depression & Manic Depression: A Workbook for Maintaining Mood Stability, $17.95
Coping With Schizophrenia: A Guide For Families, $13.95
Visualization for Change, Second Edition, $13.95
Postpartum Survival Guide, $13.95
Angry All the Time: An Emergency Guide to Anger Control, $12.95
Couple Skills: Making Your Relationship Work, $13.95
Self-Esteem, Second Edition, $13.95
I Can't Get Over It, A Handbook for Trauma Survivors, Second Edition, $15.95
Dying of Embarrassment: Help for Social Anxiety and Social Phobia, $12.95
The Depression Workbook: Living With Depression and Manic Depression, $17.95
Men & Grief: A Guide for Men Surviving the Death of a Loved One, $13.95
When the Bough Breaks: A Helping Guide for Parents of Sexually Abused Children, $11.95
When Once Is Not Enough: Help for Obsessive Compulsives, $13.95
The Three Minute Meditator, Third Edition, $12.95
Beyond Grief: A Guide for Recovering from the Death of a Loved One, $13.95
Hypnosis for Change: A Manual of Proven Techniques, Third Edition, $13.95
When Anger Hurts, $13.95

Call **toll free, 1-800-748-6273,** to order. Have your Visa or Mastercard number ready. Or send a check for the titles you want to New Harbinger Publications, Inc., 5674 Shattuck Ave., Oakland, CA 94609. Include $3.80 for the first book and 75¢ for each additional book, to cover shipping and handling. (California residents please include appropriate sales tax.) Allow two to five weeks for delivery.

Prices subject to change without notice.